Longitudinal Studies in Child Psychology and Psychiatry

WILEY SERIES ON
STUDIES IN CHILD PSYCHIATRY

Series Editor
Michael Rutter
Institute of Psychiatry
London

The First Year of Life
Psychology and Medical Implication of Early Experience
Edited by
David Shaffer and Judy Dunn

Out of School
Modern Perspectives in Truancy and School Refusal
Edited by
Lionel Hersov and Ian Berg

The Clinical Psychiatry of Adolescence
by Derek Steinberg

Longitudinal Studies in Child Psychology and Psychiatry
Practical lessons from research experience
Edited by
A. R. Nicol

Further titles in preparation

Longitudinal Studies in Child Psychology and Psychiatry

Practical Lessons from Research Experience

Edited by
A. R. Nicol
Nuffield Psychology and Psychiatry Unit
University of Newcastle upon Tyne

JOHN WILEY & SONS
Chichester · New York · Brisbane · Toronto · Singapore

Library of Congress Cataloging in Publication Data:
Main entry under title:

Longitudinal studies in child psychology and psychiatry.

  (Wiley series on studies in child psychiatry)
  Includes index.
  1. Child psychology—Longitudinal studies. 2. Problem
children—Longitudinal studies. 3. Problem families—
Longitudinal studies. 4. Child psychiatry—Longitudinal
studies. I. Nicol, A. R. (Arthur Rory) II. Series.
BF721.L5785   1985   155.4   84-11802
ISBN 0 471 10441 8

British Library Cataloguing in Publication Data:
Longitudinal studies in child psychology
  and psychiatry—(Wiley series on studies
  in child psychiatry)
  1. Child psychiatry—Longitudinal studies
  I. Nicol, A. R.
  618.92′89′00722   RJ499

  ISBN 0 471 10441 8

Phototypeset by Dobbie Typesetting Service, Plymouth, Devon
Printed by Page Bros., (Norwich) Ltd.

Series Preface

During recent years there has been a tremendous growth of research in both child development and child psychiatry. Research findings are beginning to modify clinical practice but to a considerable extent the fields of child development and of child psychiatry have remained surprisingly separate, with regrettably little cross-fertilization. Much developmental research has not concerned itself with clinical issues, and studies of clinical syndromes have all too often been made within the narrow confines of a pathological condition approach with scant regard to developmental matters. The situation is rapidly changing but the results of clinical-developmental studies are often reported only by means of scattered papers in scientific journals. This series aims to bridge the gap between child development and clinical psychiatry by presenting reports of new findings, new ideas, and new approaches in a book form which may be available to a wider readership.

The series includes reviews of specific topics, multi-authored volumes on a common theme, and accounts of specific pieces of research. However, in all cases the aim is to provide a clear, readable, and interesting account of scientific findings in a way which makes explicit their relevance to clinical practice or social policy. It is hoped that the series will be of interest to both clinicians and researchers in the fields of child psychiatry, child psychology, psychiatric social work, social paediatrics, and education — in short all concerned with the growing child and his problems.

This fourth volume in the series provides a very direct bringing together of developmental and clinical issues in terms of its consideration of the practical lessons to be learned from longitudinal studies. The research questions posed in the investigations described in this volume vary greatly. Some focus on highly specific issues such as the changes in the family as the result of the birth of a second child or the development of children with Down's syndrome; others tackle broader topics, such as the determination of continuities and discontinuities in psychosocial 'deprivation' across the generations; yet others aim to evaluate the effects of different forms of treatment. What the investigations have in common is the use of measurement of changes over time to gain an understanding of the processes and mechanisms involved in both

v

normal development and in problem behaviour. The findings are important in their emphasis on the variety of factors that serve to influence children's development, on the need to take account of both continuities and discontinuities, and on the protective function of good experiences as well as the damaging effects of bad ones. The results of the research reported in this volume have wide-ranging implications for policy and practice in the fields of child care and clinical services.

Preface

This book explores a method, the longitudinal study, and the rich harvest it has yielded for the practising professional and for students in the social and medical sciences. The exploration consists of thirteen studies, each described by the active research workers who pioneered them. They range in origin from Sweden, Britain and the United States and they constitute considerable variety both in character and in the lessons that can be drawn from them.

Over the last two decades there has been a healthy development of interest in research findings among practising professionals in the child care field. This is reflected in massive and discriminating attendance at professional meetings and heavy sales of books which summarize and review research. There is a wide recognition that knowledge derived from field experience, *a priori* theorizing or clinical intuition is unsatisfactory. Rigorously conducted research has become an essential framework for guiding practice. This volume is aimed at exploding another myth: that research 'facts' can, as it were, be written on tablets of stone. What is really needed is a *critical interpretation* of research findings and this cannot be made unless the methodology and design of the research is understood. For the busy practitioner this is extremely difficult if the research is scattered in journal articles or presented in long, complex reports.

The book presents brief, but comprehensive research reports of longitudinal studies. Here the methods used tend to be complex yet clear understanding is particularly important if the results are to realize their full value. For this reason the methodology of the different studies is presented simply and clearly. The book will be of particular value to students of educational and clinical psychology, psychiatry and the social sciences who want to develop their understanding of the uses of longitudinal research. The findings will help practising professionals in making everyday decisions about such things as sibling rivalry, the management of toddler problems, the effects of childhood deprivation on parenting capacities, adolescents who are disruptive in school and the effects of smoking. The therapeutic enthusiast should get help in deciding how to bend his efforts to best account and what positive factors in any given situation can be encouraged and promoted.

Most important, the information is presented in such a way that practitioners can make up their own minds about the relevance of research to their particular practical problems.

Contributors

M. Bohman	*Barn och Ungdomspskiatriska Kliniken, Umea Universitet, 901 85 Umea, Sweden*
J. Dunn	*MRC Unit on the Development and Integration of Behaviour, Madingley, Cambridge, CB3 8AA*
H. Fells	*Human Development Unit, 1 Tankerville Terrace, Newcastle upon Tyne, NE2 3AH*
K. Fogelman	*National Children's Bureau, 8 Wakley Street, London EC1V 7QE*
R. F. Garside	*(Deceased)*
A. Gath	*The Drummond Clinic, Mill Road, Bury St Edmunds, Suffolk IP33 3PP*
P. J. Graham	*Academic Department of Child Psychiatry, Hospital for Sick Children, Great Ormond Street, London WC1N 3JH*
K. A. Hibbert	*Child and Family Guidance Service, Arthur's Hill Clinic, Douglas Terrace, Newcastle upon Tyne, NE4 5QX*
C. Hulbert	*Earl's House Hospital, Lancaster Road, Durham City*
S. Kruk	*Family Research Unit, 16 Walden Street, London, E1*
I. Kolvin	*Human Development Unit, 1 Tankerville Terrace, Newcastle upon Tyne, NE2 3AH*
I. M. Leitch	*London School of Hygiene and Tropical Medicine, Kepple Street, London WC1*

ix

A. MacMillan — Department of Psychological Services and Research, Johnson House, Crichton Royal Hospital, Bankend Road, Dumfries DG1 4TG

F. J. W. Miller — Department of Child Health, Social Pediatrics, Medical School, Newcastle upon Tyne, NE1 7RU

A. R. Nicol — Human Development Unit 1 Tankerville Terrace, Newcastle upon Tyne, NE2 3AH

D. Quinton — Institute of Psychiatry, De Crespigny Park, London, SE5 8AF

N. Richman — Academic Department of Child Psychiatry, Hospital for Sick Children, Great Ormond Street, London, WC1N 3JH

M. L. Rutter — Institute of Psychiatry, De Crespigny Park, London, SE5 8AF

S. Sgvardsson — Barn och Ungdomspskiatriska Kliniken, Umea Universitet, 901 85 Umea, Sweden

J. Stevenson — Department of Human Biology, University of Surrey, Guildford

E. E. Werner — University of California, Davis, California 95616, USA

C. B. Willcox — Human Development Unit, 1 Tankerville Terrace, Newcastle upon Tyne, NE2 3AH

S. N. Wolkind — Family Research Unit, 16 Walden Street, London, E1

F. Wolstenholme — School Psychological and Child Guidance, Moss Side Child Guidance and Support Centre, Westwood Street, Manchester M14 4SW

R. M. Wrate — The Young People's Unit, Tipperlin House, Tipperlin Road, Edinburgh EH10 5HF

Contents

Series Preface v
Preface vii
Contributors ix

1 Introduction 1
   A. R. Nicol

Section I   Short-term studies which ask a specific question

2 The arrival of a sibling 15
   J. Dunn
3 What sort of children are suspended from school and what can we
   do for them? 33
   A. R. Nicol, C. Willcox and K. Hibbert

Section II   Short-term studies which ask broader questions

4 From child to parent: early separation and the adaptation to
   motherhood 53
   S. Wolkind and S. Kruk
5 Sex difference in outcome of pre-school behaviour problems . 75
   N. Richman, J. Stevenson and P. J. Graham
6 Family pathology and child psychiatric disorder: a four-year
   prospective study 91
   D. Quinton and M. Rutter

Section III   Long-term studies which ask a specific question

7 A prospective longitudinal study of adoption 137
   M. Bohman and S. Sigvardsson
8 Parenting behaviour of mothers raised 'in care' 157
   D. Quinton and M. Rutter
9 Down's Syndrome in the first nine years 203
   A. Gath

Section IV   Long-term studies which ask broader questions

10 Becoming deprived: a cross-generation study based on the Newcastle
   upon Tyne 1000-Family Study   223
   F. J. W. Miller, I. Kolvin and H. Fells
11 Exploiting longitudinal data: examples from the National Child
   Development Study   241
   K. Fogelman

Section V   Treatment and prevention

12 Helping seriously disturbed children   265
   R. M. Wrate, I. Kolvin, R. F. Garside, F. Wolstenholme,
   C. M. Hulbert, and I. M. Leitch
13 What sort of therapy should be given for what sort of problem?   319
   A. R. Nicol, A. Macmillan, I. Kolvin and F. Wolstenholme
14 Stress and protective factors in children's lives   335
   E. E. Werner
15 Family and school influences: meanings, mechanisms
   and implications   357
   M. Rutter

Index   405

Chapter 1

Introduction

A. R. Nicol

In his *Introductory Lectures on Psychoanalysis* (1973), Freud warned his audience: 'If, however, there should actually turn out to be one of you who did not feel satisfied by a fleeting aquaintance with psychoanalysis but was inclined to enter into a permanent relationship with it, I should not merely dissuade him from doing so, I should actually warn him against it.'

For different, but to some extent overlapping, reasons the same advice might be given to the enthusiastic young scientist bent on undertaking a longitudinal study or to the far-sighted clinician or administrator who wishes to interpret the results. The promise of satisfying one's curiosity over what happens to such and such a group of patients, the seductive promise of being able to predict the future and to uncover the secrets of causation may drive him on. What he must be sure of is that the years of labour and the scanty reinforcement with results during the course of the investigation are not in vain. Properly planned, longitudinal studies can be intensely exciting and yield knowledge that cannot be obtained in any other way. They can address questions of great practical importance as we shall see here. They are not for the timid, but need to be approached with open eyes and a clear head. It is our hope that this book will help that process as well as communicating research findings.

The material here constitutes a bringing together of different styles of longitudinal study. Some of these have not been reported elsewhere and in some the data is freshly examined or added to in the light of new developments. For this reason, it will be of interest to the mature investigator as well as the neophyte. This introduction, however, is aimed to provide an integration of some of the features of the longitudinal method to guide the reader through the various chapters. Reports of thirteen separate studies follow. These have been selected for their different approaches to longitudinal methodology as much as for the different practical lessons that can be drawn from them. Underlying the differences are important general themes and it is as well to highlight these now as an introduction. The variety in the approaches is more likely to speak for itself in the separate chapters.

BUILDING THEORETICAL PERSPECTIVES

The fact that the title of this book could be taken to suggest that practical questions can be answered by the simple application of longitudinal techniques makes it especially important to emphasize the place of theoretical perspectives. Theory and experiment interact with each other with, in some cases experiment confirming or refuting theory and in others research results leading, in a more inductive way, to the development of theoretical ideas and hypotheses. The treatment study in Chapter 13 can be taken as an example. The original hypotheses were that the treatments, parent–teacher counselling, group therapy and behaviour modification, would be more effective than no treatment, that they would differ in effectiveness from each other and that some would be more suitable for some types of disorders and for boys rather than girls or vice versa. As described in Chapter 13, group therapy and behaviour modification in particular were effective but the outcomes were remarkably similar. This leads on to an inductive approach: we ask further questions and see how they fit the data. This in turn may lead to further fieldwork to test the ideas that have arisen. Those whose main aim is to extract practical lessons from research find this process frustrating since the scientist will always seem tentative and questioning—unwilling to commit himself. This has a lot to do with the process of theory building since one of the traps a scientist can fall into is to become so emotionally committed to a pet theory that he finds it difficult to relinquish if it ceases to be useful.

Over the last twenty years there has been a great change in the types of theories that developmental psychologists and psychiatrists have employed. It is important that this change in theorizing is communicated to practitioners as well as the evidence in support of the various theories that have been put forward. Traditionally, there was a rather sharp distinction between what Hartup (1978) has called 'social-mold' theories on the one hand and those of maturational development on the other. The former type of theory, typically derived from learning theory, tended to emphasize the child's response to environmental stimuli and to pay less attention to individual differences or developmental stages. Perhaps the most extreme of these theories are those of Skinner's operant conditioning. In contrast stands the work of authors such as Gesell (1948) on maturation: here there is little reference to the caretaker or the environment but a concentration on age-related maturational stages.

These very distinct concerns have in themselves led to a vast body of research of the utmost practical importance. From the 'social-mold' perspective has come the theoretical and experimental basis of behaviour modification and the concepts of identification and social learning (Ross, 1981; Bandura, 1977). From the maturational school has come the basis of developmental paediatrics. As explanatory frameworks, however, both positions have been eroded and extended almost beyond recognition.

The first of these changes in perspective has been towards taking account of the *specificity of behaviour* to particular situations or between particular people. While this trend is hampered by our, as yet, poor understanding of human relationships in general (Hinde, 1979) and has long been recognized in relation to attachment theory, it is now recognized as important in all descriptions of behaviour. In Chapter 8, for example, mothering difficulties were not restricted to the 'in care' group but were present also in the control group. Attention to the specifics of these difficulties, however, revealed important differences. In the case of the 'in care' mothers, the parenting problems were part of a wider disturbance, quite different from the control mothers whose difficulty tended to be confined to the parenting role alone. A second example comes from the study of children suspended from school (Chapter 3). Here the misbehaviour of the suspended group is not only more aggressive than that of the comparison group of difficult youngsters but also more indiscriminate in that it is manifest both in formal classroom situations as well as in informal settings and in the playground.

This brings us to a second shift of perspective from the 'social-mold' theories. If the individuals are more than a sort of social plasticine, they will relate to a seemingly similar environment in an individual way so that in a sense the environment is rather different for each person in it. Thus, in Chapter 3, the school environment as experienced by the suspended children seems to have been manifestly more hostile than that of the control children or even of the other 'difficult' children: they were isolated and rejected by the other children, failing educationally and seldom at school anyway.

The individual will also influence the environment they are in as well as the other way round. This is elegantly shown in Chapter 2 on the effects of the birth of a sibling on the interaction between the mother and the firstborn. Observations of the child revealed more attention demanding and negative behaviour on the part of the child as well as some positive behaviour changes. The picture became more comprehensible when the mother's behaviour was also taken into account. Here the children received less attention from their mothers, were put in the situation of having to initiate more of the interactions and what attention they did get was more likely to be a prohibition than before the birth. The resulting changes (and sometimes difficulties) can be understood as a two-way process much more adequately than by trying to understand the child in isolation.

Such multiple and two-way causation is part of the bedrock of modern theories of development. Further, these influences may operate in different ways. First, there may be a direct effect—mother lessening their interactions to the older child after the birth of the sibling in the above example. Second, the causative influences may interact with each other so that the resultant influence is more powerful than the sum of the individual components—an interactional effect. A good example is the study of the progress of different groups of maladjusted children in different educational and hospital settings (Chapter 12). The authors report that the maladjusted children in the ESN schools show the worst outcome. This finding persisted even after allowing for the many adversities that fell most heavily on this group. One explanation could be that consideration of the separate individual adversities was not enough: there is an added effect due to the overall weight of adversity. This is called an *interaction* effect. The third way in which causative influences can act is by operating indirectly in a situation to alter the probabilities of a particular outcome—the so-called *transactional* effect. The Waltham Forest Study of pre-school children (Chapter 5) provides an illustration. At the original three-year survey, it was clear that boys were more likely to show restlessness. At eight-years follow-up, we see that, in addition to this, restlessness, when present in boys, is more likely to persist than it is in girls. Thus the high level of restlessness in 8 year olds was arrived at by two mechanisms: a transactional effect being common in boys in the first place *and* the interactional effect that the restlessness in boys was more persistent.

The longitudinal method is probably necessary for the investigation of the perspectives discussed so far. It becomes essential, however, when we consider that different causal relationships may not only operate in two or more directions nor even directly or indirectly at one given point in time but they may operate also at different points in development. In Chapter 11, data is used from the National Child Development Study to show the relative transience of such potentially adverse social factors as being a member of a one-parent family or of living in substandard accommodation. This leads on to the idea of *chains of influence* that can operate at different stages of maturation during development. To take an example, the mothers raised in care (Chapter 8) for the most part spent their early years in the sort of disrupted and discordant environments that are normally associated with poorly developed attachments. The traditional 'social-mold' hypothesis might be that, as children, their capacity to relate is so damaged in these early encounters that it adversely effects their own parenting capacity a generation later. The evidence cited in Chapter 8 raises the possibility of a much more elaborate and optimistic picture. First, one-third of the mothers demonstrated perfectly good parenting capacity despite their disadvantages. Further, the authors were able to unravel a chain of events and circumstances: whether the mother had demonstrated a psychiatric disturbance in childhood, the circumstances of her rehabilitation home, the age and circumstances of her first pregnancy and her choice of spouse, each of which had a bearing on outcome. The most important current factor was the quality of the marriage. There seems to be a characteristic string of events each of which operated directively, interactively or transactively to effect outcome. It seems probable that these chains of factors operating at different stages of development are common. In Chapter 13 for example, the groups of children who benefited from the various treatments seemed to go on improving even after the active treatment had been discontinued—possibly chains of helpful experiences in the school had been set in motion as a result of the initial improvement which continued to operate after specific treatment had finished.

The idea that early experience does not necessarily predict outcome, but frequently does so because the social situations of families tend to persist is the basis of the Swedish Adoption Study (Chapter 7). Here considerable leverage is gained on the possibilities of change by comparing children brought up in utterly different environments through the adoption and fostering process. The very different results of these different arrangements brings up the question of *protective factors* in children's development. This in turn is the subject of Chapter 14 which draws on data from the Kauai Longitudinal Study. A whole series of factors are identified which mark the child who, despite severe disadvantages, develop well through childhood and adolescence. It is equally illuminating to examine those families that get into difficulties during the upbringing of the children against a general background of improving social conditions in society at large, since this may reveal particular risk factors that may be amenable to early intervention. This subject is addressed using data from the 1000-Family Study (Chapter 10).

In all these three studies; mothers brought up in care, the children of Kauai and those of Newcastle upon Tyne, a common theme that emerges is the pervasive influence of supportive family and social networks as a protective factor against adversity—one might also quote the supportive commitments of adoptive parents in the Swedish study (Chapter 7) and the parenting study from the London Hospital group (Chapter 4) among others. Are there other pervasive influences such as this? It seems highly likely that there are and two come to mind. The first of these is the role of the individual as a predicting and appraising modifier of events one likely to be influenced to great effectiveness by a belief in his or her own worth and ability to influence events. Chapters 3 and 14 report studies where attempts are made to measure such attributes although as Wylie (1974) has shown, there are great difficulties methodologically. In a more indirect (but not necessarily less effective) way, measures of capacity to plan for the future were found to be associated with favourable outcome in the 'in care' mothers in Chapter 8.

The second group of factors which has been little investigated is genetic factors. Certainly, there are important indicators of the potential importance of such factors, the study reported in Chapter 7 being a distinguished example (see also Chapter 15). In Chapter 8 also, an attempt is made to assess genetic factors. At the same time when we consider the potential of genetic mechanisms to turn on and off at different stages on the individual's life, it may be that chains of events as complex as the social factors described above are in operation. The big difference is that such effects are so far largely hidden from view.

NATURAL EXPERIMENTS

An important point of similarity of the thirteen studies in this book is in their epidemiological nature. This means that they are studies of disorders in their natural environment. It is not necessary for longitudinal studies to have this epidemiological basis, since a longitudinal study is simply one where the measurements are taken at two or more points in time. However, the term seems usually to be applied to those that do, and this is so in this book. The accent on epidemiology leads us to the idea of the natural experiment, which also merits some discussion as an underlying theme.

An experiment is a demonstration of the truth (or more accurately potential falsehood) of a question rather than the posing of the question in the first place. We have already explored the importance of theory and indeed mental health workers have shown themselves gifted at developing ideas and speculations, which, with appropriate humility, can be re-couched as questions. It is left to the scientist to do so and to design and carry out the necessary experimental demonstration. In doing this, the epidemiologist has great advantages over the laboratory scientist but also added difficulties. It is convenient to mention some of the difficulties first.

The main characteristic of epidemiological experiments is that they are opportunistic. The experimenter cannot arrange conditions in his laboratory but has to make use of natural situations that come to hand. This is well demonstrated in many of the studies in this book. For example, in the sibling study (Chapter 2), use was made of the natural birth of a second sibling to provide a comparison for the behaviour of the mother and the firstborn before and after the birth itself. Since the births in the sample were spaced differently from the birth of the firstborn, it was possible to exploit this natural variation to see whether the developmental stage of the firstborn made any difference to his or her reaction: it did not. The reader will find numerous examples of this sort of exploitation of natural variations of all sorts—not just time intervals—in the pages that follow.

The use of natural opportunities in this way, while often ingenious and elegant, carry grave disadvantages. The first of these has to do with the fact that opportunities are not always available, or if they were, would be almost impossible to exploit. For example, supposing that, using the methodology of repeated observations of a large population (as in Chapter 3), one wanted to chart the onset of a rare disorder such as disintegrative psychosis of childhood, one would need such an enormous base population as to make the whole enterprise quite unrealistic.

The second problem is perhaps even more important. Taking again the arrival of a sibling as an example, it seems likely that there are some systematic differences between those parents who have their families at close intervals and those who have them more widely spaced. In this case the difference may be trivial and largely irrelevant to the particular question under examination—however, the possibility exists and detracts to some extent from the conclusiveness of the results obtained. The one example in this book where this problem has been overcome is in the treatment study described in Chapter 13—yet there are few situations where random allocation as used in that study would be appropriate or could be employed. Various ways can be used to try to overcome this very grave difficulty of naturalistic experiments, in Chapter 6 for example, the investigators examine the possibility that the sex of the parent with psychiatric problems has some bearing on the sex of which child becomes disturbed. In order to simplify the situation, they examine only those families where there are two parents, thus avoiding the obvious possibility that the rules that hold for two-parent families do not hold for one-parent families, as regards sex identification. The problem with this method is that for every variable controlled in this way, the sample size is reduced, particularly if the attributes being examined are unusual ones. Very soon, the sample size becomes too small for meaningful statistical comparison. The other type of technique that is widely used is some sort of statistical correction. One such example is illustrated in Chapter 12 where a statistical method is used to attempt to allow for differences in the groups of children attending different types of school. The authors discuss the advantages and disadvantages of their techniques in some detail and I will not expand on it here. Another such technique is demonstrated in Chapter 11, where a number of variables are taken into account in looking at the association between, for example, smoking in pregnancy and the subsequent height and educational attainment of the child at various ages.

Perhaps the greatest strength of the natural experiment is that it approximates to real life. It is often possible to see an inverse relationship between the internal rigour of an experiment and the extent to which the findings can be generalized to real-life situations. Taking as an example the field of psychotherapy research, a body of research has been carried out on essentially normal young people with minor anxiety, but as college students they were cooperative and readily available to the experimenter. What is questionable is how much the results of this research is applicable to patient populations. In the same way, while the design of the random control evaluation reported in Chapter 13 is likely to lead to more rigorous results than the quasi-experimental evaluation of Chapter 12, it also is in more danger of raising expectations through its obtrusiveness and unusualness within the normal school curriculum than is the more low-key naturalistic approach of Chapter 12. In short, every approach carries its share of assumptions and disadvantages. The research worker must be aware of them and choose the best strategy for his purpose.

A further point merits attention before we leave the subject of the experiment. It will never be the case, except in very unusual circumstances (the clinical trial of penicillin for lobar pneumonia comes to mind), that one study will be conclusive. If associations of importance are found, their validity needs to be checked in different populations, at different times and from different centres. Nationwide studies such as that reported in Chapter 11 are important in giving a national overview but still cannot take the place of more detailed local studies. Findings also need to be critically examined by a convergence of different research techniques. For example, the finding concerning mothering capacity of girls raised in care (Chapter 8) represents an attempt to explore, in a longitudinal study, the common observation (see, for example, Chapter 4) that women who report adverse experiences in their own childhoods have difficulties in rearing children themselves. In Chapter 8, the authors use the converging strategies of interviewing the parents and of direct observation of the mothering itself with some interesting and illuminating discrepancies between the two techniques. Other confirmatory strategies could be added, for example, this is a situation which might be elucidated in the laboratory using animals with a relatively short intergenerational cycle—an elaboration of the classic experiments of Harlow and Suomi (1971) for example.

My opening paragraph suggested that longitudinal research is strictly for masochists. Some further modification of this impression is needed. Research with human populations carries many difficulties, one of which, for the developmental psychologist or psychiatrist is that the subjects mature and age at the same slow rate as themselves. Robins (1979) identified three strategies that should be considered in planning a study since there may be ways of short circuiting this long time span in some circumstances. The first study strategy is identified as the 'real time' study. This is the no-short-cuts technique of identifying a sample at the beginning of the study and following it through to the end. It carries the advantage that the investigator can plan the study in detail from the start and aim with precision at the question he hopes to answer. For short-term investigations (all the short-term studies here are of this type) this is the strategy of choice. With long-term studies the apparent advantages of the 'real-time' study begin to recede and the disadvantages increase. Research questions that seemed important fifteen to thirty years before may have dated and indeed the research team may have moved, retired, died or simply lost enthusiasm. Despite these hazards, some of the studies reported in this book have been carried out over long time spans on a prospective 'real-time' basis, and the reader can judge the rich prizes that can result from such persistence. Thus the study of Down's syndrome (Chapter 9) is still in progress while the National Child Development Study (Chapter 11) and the Kauai Study (Chapter 14) report findings here of sixteen and eighteen years respectively. It is notable that these studies are concerned with broad questions that are not likely to date, while Gath's study of Down's syndrome concerns a particular client group where the problems of long-term development have a special importance.

The remaining three long-term studies illustrate an alternative technique: the 'catch-up' study. This is dependent on finding past documentation of a population sample that can serve as a base line, the sample then being contacted and re-examined as a follow up. Examples here are in Chapter 8 and 9 where previous research records were used to mount follow up studies to explore research questions which have become more clearly emphasized since the original study was done. Chapter 7 shows a mixed strategy since the original population consisted of adoption records yet the study also incorporates a real-time follow-up. Although the early data in this design is collected for a different purpose, many researchers have been able to turn such data to good purpose and some of the most important developmental studies have employed such designs. The third type of design is not represented in this book but has been called the 'follow-back' study. The distinction is that the study group is identified at follow-up rather than at baseline as in the 'catch-up' study. Previous records are then identified to provide the baseline measures. The type of questions that can be tackled by this method are rather different from those tackled by the 'catch-up' study. For example it will not give an accurate estimate of how often an antecedent condition (say discordant parents' marriage) leads to a subsequent problem (say childhood disturbance) as any marriage problems not followed by disturbance will be missed. The follow-back strategy is particularly useful for very rare disorders, as any other strategy would involve massive numbers at the baseline. The long-term component of Chapter 4 might qualify as a follow-back study had records of the parents childhood been sought. As it stands the distinction between the different backgrounds of the mothers is made on the basis of their memory which makes the study a retrospective one.

DEFINITIONS AND INSTRUMENTATION

While not peculiar to longitudinal research, it is necessary in this integrative introduction to give some attention to these basic building blocks of psychosocial research. Careful definition of populations studied and behaviour measured is of course particularly important in expensive long-term research projects and sufficient time should be given to it. To take examples from this book, there are two studies, reported in Chapters 4 and 8 which examine the parenting of mothers who have themselves been in care. One might think that this would offer a useful opportunity for replication of findings. However, closer examination reveals that the 'in-care' groups are in fact different. In Chapter 8 the children were in care primarily because of the breakdown of parenting whereas in Chapter 4 a wider group was used—some of whom were in care as a result of behaviour difficulties. While psychiatric problems was a feature of the girls in both studies, this difference in these ostensibly comparable groups seems particularly likely to effect outcome. On the other hand, the two studies do complement each other in interesting ways, for example both show the same association of parental marital discord with early pregnancy.

Regarding instrumentation, this has purposely not been a main focus in this book about practical lessons. However, the importance of using reliable and valid measuring instruments cannot be over-emphasized.

THE USE OF LONGITUDINAL STUDIES

Since uses is the main message of the next fourteen chapters, it will not be dwelt on here but a few general points need to be made. The most obvious use of longitudinal studies is the search for causation. However, it would be quite wrong to see this as their sole usefulness. First, longitudinal studies have an indispensable role in the *description* of development. Examples of this use abound in the chapters that follow but they have a particularly important application for long standing handicapping conditions such as Down's syndrome (see Chapter 9). Cross-sectional studies may be of some use if groups of different ages are compared; however, a currently adult subject is likely to have had very different early experiences from those of a currently young child. To chart the course of the disorder under current conditions adequately, longitudinal studies are needed. Comparison with previous comparable studies may show the effects of changes in attitude and management of the disorder. Other examples to be found here concern asthma and wheezy bronchitis (Chapter 11). Secondly, longitudinal studies may be needed to estimate the *prevalence* of disorder. This is particularly true where persistent disorders have to be differentiated from transient adaption reactions (see Chapter 6) or where an estimate is needed of the period prevalence of remitting and relapsing disorders. Longitudinal studies are important also in the *delineation of syndromes*. In the absence, for the most part of a single necessary and sufficient causative factor for psychological disorders (Down's syndrome is an exception) there is a need to chart the progress of disorders to check the stability of their features. *Continuities and discontinuities* in social circumstances may also be investigated in longitudinal studies as may features of children's educational progress. These matters are also very clearly reported in Chapter 11. Another important use is in the *evaluation of services* of various types. This is the central theme of Chapters 12 and 13.

Concerning the search for causes, there is a common misconception that simple application of longitudinal method will reveal causation. It should already have become apparent that, helpful as longitudinal studies are, causative mechanisms are only likely to be uncovered by careful sifting of evidence derived from converging approaches to a problem and consideration of the many possible mechanisms involved. This search is the theme of Chapter 15.

REFERENCES

Bandura, A. (1977). *Social Learning Theory*, Prentice Hall, Englewood Cliffs, New York.

Freud, S. (1973). *Introductory Lectures on Psychoanalysis*, Penguin, Harmondsworth Middlesex.

Gesell, A. (1948). *Studies in Child Development*, Harper Row, New York.

Harlow, H. F. and Suomi, S. J. (1971). Social recovery by isolation reared monkeys. *Proc. Nat. Acad. Sci.*, **68**, 1534–1538.

Hartup, W. W. (1978). Perspectives on child and family interaction: Past, present and future, in (Eds R. M. Lerner and G. B. Spanier) *Child Influences on Marital and Family Interaction*, Academic Press, New York.

Hinde, R. A. (1979). *Towards Understanding Relationships*, Academic Press, London.

Robins, L. N. (1979). Longitudinal methods in the study of normal and pathological development, in (Eds K. P. Kisker, J.-E. Meyer, C. Müller and E. Stromgren) *Psychiatrie der Gegenwart Band 1. 'Grundlagen und Methoden der Psychiatrie', 2 Auflage.* Springer-Verlag, Heidelberg.

Ross, A. O. (1981). *Child Behaviour Therapy*, Wiley, New York.

Wylie, R. (1974). *The Self Concept*, Vol. 1, University of Nebraska Press, Nebraska.

Section I

Short-term Studies which ask a Specific Question

Longitudinal Studies in Child Psychology and Psychiatry
Edited by A. R. Nicol
© 1985 John Wiley and Sons Ltd.

Chapter 2

The Arrival of a Sibling

J. Dunn

The idea that the arrival of a sibling can lead to disturbed behaviour, and to long-term changes in a child's personality is one that has been widely held (Adler, 1928, 1959; Winnicott, 1977; Petty, 1953; Black and Sturge, 1979). Yet there has been relatively little careful study of the ways in which family relationship change with the birth of another child, and very little direct study of children before and after such a change. Parents' manuals frequently refer to jealousy and rivalry between siblings, but because of the lack of systematic evidence on the subject, the advice they offer is often confusing and contradictory. Spock (1969) holds that jealousy is inevitable—Close (1980) that it is not, but arises from parental fears and expectations. The results of interview studies certainly suggest that disturbance following the birth of a sibling is common (Henchie, 1963; Legg *et al.*, 1974; Trause *et al.*, 1981). But without direct study of the children and their parents, crucial questions on the nature of the children's response and its long-term significance cannot be answered. How common are the reactions of disturbance? How long do they persist? How do different patterns of parental behaviour relate to the children's behaviour after the birth? Which children are most vulnerable to the stressful changes accompanying the birth of a sibling?

These questions are of direct practical importance to parents and to clinicians. They also have more general clinical implications. We know very little about the origins of individual differences in children's responses to stressful changes in their environment. Yet in every study of children experiencing such changes— periods in hospital, or in institutions, divorce or separation of parents, periods of separation from the mother, or in group care—it is noted that children differ very much in their apparent vulnerability to the change. That many such changes are extremely common experiences for children under 5 years old lends urgency to our understanding more clearly what might account for the differences between children in their responses. Only careful systematic research which follows children over time can provide the basis from which we can begin to understand which children are most vulnerable, and which parental strategies can best aid them.

To address some of these questions, a sample of forty firstborn children and their families were followed over the period when a second child was born, and through the infancy of the second child (Dunn and Kendrick, 1982) and at follow-up visits when the firstborn were 6 years old (Stillwell-Barnes, 1982). The families lived in Cambridge, or in housing estates in surrounding villages; in terms of the occupation of the fathers, the families were largely lower middle class or non-manual working class. The children were aged between 18 and 43 months at the time of the sibling's birth (mean age 23 months), and there were twenty-one boys and nineteen girls.

In the study a variety of methods were employed: direct, unstructured observations of the children, interviews, rating scales, and assessment of temperamental characteristics. All observations and interviews were carried out in the homes. A full account of the study, with reliability of methods, details of analyses and results is given in Dunn and Kendrick 1982 (see also Dunn and Kendrick, 1980a,b, 1981a,b). In this chapter some of the main findings with practical implications for parents and for clinicians will be briefly outlined, and the lesson to be drawn from the findings discussed. The families were visited at four time points: before the birth of the second baby, during the first three weeks after the birth, when the baby was 8 months old, and when he or she was 14 months old. At each time point, observations were carried out and the mothers were interviewed (see Table 2.1). We attempted to minimize the intrusive effect of an observer by visiting the families before we began to observe, by

Table 2.1   Outline of study

Mother pregnant with second child	Two pre-sib-birth observations with mother (with and without father) Interview Rating of temperamental characteristics
Birth of second child	
2 weeks post-birth	Post-sib-birth observation child with mother and sibling
3 weeks post-birth	Observation (including feed) Interview (with and without father)
Second child 8 months old	Two observations: siblings with mother (with and without father) Interviews Rating of temperamental characteristics
Second child 14 months old	Two observations: siblings with mother (with and without father) Interviews
	Follow-up for sub-sample when first child 6 years old.

becoming a familiar visitor to the house, and by putting a premium on establishing rapport with the family. Both mothers and children talked freely to us in the course of the observations.

The observations consisted of a pencil and paper record of a series of pre-coded categories of behaviour, noted in 10-second intervals in a lined notebook (based on the method of Clarke-Stewart, 1973). This method also allowed us to make narrative notes on other aspects of the family interaction, on the details of the child's play, and so on. A portable stereotape recorder was used during the observations to record the conversation, and this was transcribed by the observer immediately after the observation.

THE CHILDREN'S REACTION TO THE BIRTH

Clear changes were evident in the behaviour of the firstborn children in the 2–3 weeks following the birth of the sibling—documented in our direct observations and in the reports by the mothers (Dunn *et al.*, 1981; Table 2.2).

Table 2.2   Numbers of children reported to show changes in behaviour after sibling birth ($n = 40$)

(a) Increases in behaviour	Rare/ absent	Occasional	Frequent	Constant
Tearful	16	11	10	3
Clinging	17	12	9	2
Withdrawn	29	9	2	-
Demanding	3	13	22	2
Negative behaviour towards mother	9	8	22	1

(b) Increase in incidence of problems (4-point scale)	No change	1-point increase	2-point increase	Extreme breakdown
(1) Sleep problems	29	7	3	1
(2) Feed problems	37	3	—	—
(3) Toilet-training problems ($n = 26$)	14	4	5	3

However, the nature of these changes varied considerably between the children. Most children showed an increase in demands for attention and in negative behaviour directed towards the mother. Incidents of deliberate naughtiness were observed to increase markedly after the birth. However, while some children became withdrawn others became much more clinging or aggressive. Several children showed disturbance in bodily functions: sleeping problems increased, and of the children who were toilet trained at the time of the birth, several suffered setbacks or regressed completely to an untrained state.

In addition to these increased problems, about half the sample also showed more positive changes—increased independence over feeding or dressing, an insistence on going to the toilet alone, a new preparedness to play independently; and friendly behaviour towards the baby—concern over his/her distress, a wish to entertain and cuddle him or her, and to 'help' the mother in caregiving was very common (Table 2.3). Signs of hostility to the baby were also shown: many children irritated the baby by pinching him, taking away the dummy, shaking or banging the pram or cot (Table 2.4). It was notable that many of the children who showed clear signs of disturbed behaviour or hostility to the baby *also* showed a friendly interest in and affection towards him. Ambivalence was evident both in the children's behaviour, and in their comments about the baby.

Table 2.3   Numbers of children showing positive interest in the baby sibling ($n = 40$)

	Absent or rare	Occasional	Frequent	Constant
Verbal references and comments	8	20	12	
Concern shown when baby cries	16	14	9	1
Attempts to help mother in care of baby	2	16	21	1
Entertains baby	18	11	11	
Affectionate physical interest	10	21	8	1

Table 2.4   Behaviour towards the new baby: Numbers of children showing irritating or negative behaviour, or imitating the baby ($n = 40$)

Behaviour towards the new baby	Absent/rare	Occasional	Frequent
Irritates baby	19	13	8
Negative behaviour to baby	31	6	3
Imitates baby	10	15	5

The differences in the children's behaviour towards the new baby, and the changes in their behaviour following the birth were documented both in the maternal interviews and in the observations, and an encouraging level of agreement was found between the two sources of data. Since the interviews were carried out after the observations at each time point there may have been a 'halo' affect contributing to this agreement. The interviewer could have been biased in her rating of the mothers' replies. But it is important to note that the interview questions were focused upon detailed descriptions of the child's behaviour, rather than requests to the mother for general comments on the child's behaviour, and were thus less open to 'halo' effects than global ratings would have been. The comparison of the interview and observations indicated that under the circumstances in which the mothers talked to us they gave accurate descriptions of their children; this agreement between observation and interview information on the children was found, indeed, at every point in the study.

In attempting to understand *why* the children reacted in these ways to the arrival of the sibling, it is important to note that the observations of the families before and after the birth showed that there were major changes in the interaction between mother and first child following the birth (Dunn and Kendrick, 1980a). First, the children received much less attention from their mothers. In particular, mothers and children spent less time playing together, or doing things together. There was also increased conflict between them. Second, analysis of their conversations showed that the mothers made fewer friendly comments and suggestions, and were less likely to start a new conversation by suggesting a new activity or by starting a verbal game or fantasy. In contrast they were much more likely to start a conversation by prohibiting the first child. Thirdly, there was a change in the balance of responsibility for initiating interaction. After the sibling birth, the mothers were less likely to start an exchange, and the children took a greater part in the responsibility for starting an interaction.

How far were these changes the consequences of the mothers' involvement with her new baby? We compared the interaction between mother and firstborn during the times when she was involved in feeding, bathing or holding the new baby, and the times when the baby was out of sight. The results showed that there was indeed more confrontation between mother and first child, more demands and more naughtiness from the first child during the moments when the mother was bathing, holding or bottle feeding the new baby (Dunn and Kendrick, 1980a). Incidents of deliberate naughtiness, for instance, were three times more frequent when the mother was involved in caring for the baby in these ways. However, there was also more joint attention and play by mother and first child during the times when the new baby was being actively cared for. The overall decrease in maternal attention and play which followed the sibling birth was not, therefore, a result of the mother's involvement with caring for the baby, but reflected a decrease in attention to the firstborn at those periods when the new baby was not in evidence. Interestingly, the escalation of conflict which was evident in bottle feeds did not in fact take place during breast feeds. It appeared that this was partly due to the more elaborate preparations made by mothers who were about to breast feed — books, crayons, potty, drink — all were collected in readiness for the increased demands which the first children made when feeding began.

For the firstborn children, then, the arrival of the new baby involved not only a symbolic displacement, but a sharp decrease in sensitive maternal attention, and an escalation of conflict and punishment. These changes were of course closely associated with the increase in demands and in naughtiness by the children: we are not in a position to make causal inferences about the direction of change. However, the findings do suggest that one practical lesson of importance is that mothers should attempt to minimize the drop in the level of attention and play that they are able to devote to their firstborn which accompanies the sibling birth.

The findings also suggest that the advice of many parent manuals—that breastfeeding is particularly traumatic for the first child to witness, (see Spock, 1969)—is misplaced. Mothers should not be made to feel that by choosing to breast feed they are placing their firstborn under particular extra stress. But they should be aware that demands and naughtiness are likely to increase at those times when the new baby is being cared for. The advantages of being ready, with distractions, to cope with the increased demands, are obvious.

INDIVIDUAL DIFFERENCES IN THE CHILDREN'S REACTIONS

Signs of disturbance and difficult behaviour were, then, very common among the firstborn children in the first month after the sibling's birth. For mothers it is encouraging to know just how common the increase in demands and naughtiness were. But individual differences in the form of the reaction were very marked. Some children showed marked withdrawal, others became very difficult and aggressive. The pattern of these changes contrasted very much with the consistency of the mother's behaviour: although as we have seen there were overall decreases in maternal attention and increases in maternal prohibitions and restraint, the relative playfulness and punitiveness of the mothers remained very stable from before to after the birth. But the children changed dramatically in their behaviour relative to one another. Some remained cheerful and assertive, concentrating on play, and endlessly starting conversations with their mothers. Others, who had been bright and assertive before the birth became tearful, quiet and miserable, or withdrawn. What accounted for these differences? Were they attributable to the age of the firstborn, to their sex, to personality differences or to differences in the relations with the parents? What practical lessons could be learnt from studying these differences?

AGE GAP AND SEX

Within the relatively narrow age range of the children in the study, we found that age differences were relatively unimportant in accounting for differences in reaction to the birth, either in the disturbance or in friendly interest in the baby, though the younger children did tend to become particularly clinging. Sex differences were also relatively unimportant, but there were marked differences between the children in families where the siblings were of the same sex and those where they were of different sex. Firstborn with a sibling of the same sex showed much more friendly interest in the baby than those with a sibling of a different sex, and these differences continued to be important throughout the next year.

HOME AND HOSPITAL DELIVERY

Many mothers who were to deliver their second child in hospital were concerned about the effects of the separation on the first child, and such separations have of course been shown to have marked effects on children (Robertson and Robertson, 1971; Bowlby, 1973). However, in our study there were few differences in the reactions of children whose mothers went to hospital, compared with those who stayed at home. Two points should be noted on the issue of separation. The first is that while most of the children whose mothers went to hospital were not accustomed to being away from their mothers, they were almost all very familiar with and attached to the grandparent or father who cared for them while the mother was in hospital. In these families the separation was probably far less traumatic than the separation experienced by many children who do not have close relationships with relatives living close by. A second point is that we must recognize that even when the mother stayed at home to have the baby, there were major changes in the daily life and routine of the firstborn children. These changes were considered by the mothers to be very important in contributing to the unhappiness and restlessness shown by the firstborn. A practical lesson here, to which many mothers referred was that more could be done to ensure that the life and routine of the first child remained as normal as possible over the period of the birth. In the interviews we documented the changes experienced by the children, and they were many and varied. To many 2 and 3 year olds a familiar and regular routine to the day seems to be important, and this issue of individual differences in response to change, differences assessed as part of the *temperament* of the first child, was one which turned out to be of central importance.

TEMPERAMENT OF THE FIRSTBORN CHILD

Temperamental or personality differences between the firstborn children were clearly linked to the form of their reaction to the sibling birth. The assessment of the children's temperament was made before the sibling birth. Those who had been predominantly negative in mood, and intense in their emotional reactions were significantly more likely to react to the birth by becoming withdrawn, by increasing in sleep problems, or by becoming clinging than the rest of the sample. Those who had been assessed as withdrawn in temperament initially reacted to the new baby with much less friendly interest than the other children. The problem of how far such temperamental differences reflect differences in mothers' perception of their children, or differences in the mother–child relationship rather than differences in children's personalities is one which is considered elsewhere (Dunn and Kendrick, 1980b). The results of that analysis show that temperamental differences cannot be simply attributed to the biased perception of the mother, though they are (unsurprisingly) closely linked to differences in the relationship between child and mother.

MOTHER'S STATE

Many of the mothers became extremely tired, and some also became depressed, in the weeks following the birth of the second child. In these families the firstborn children were more likely to increase in withdrawal. It is clear that we cannot draw any conclusions about the direction of the cause of this association; however, its practical implications for the caring professions are clear.

RELATIONSHIP WITH FATHER

In families in which the first child had a close and intense relationship with the father, the escalation of conflict and difficulty between mother and child, and the drop in maternal attention, were less marked. It is not clear whether this link means that children with close relationships with their fathers were less upset by the baby's birth, or whether the father in these families provided more support for their wives, thus allowing them more time and energy for attending to the firstborn, or whether these fathers were caring for their firstborn more directly and more effectively after the sibling birth. But whatever the explanation for the link, the practical implications are obvious and important.

PREPARATION FOR THE NEW BABY

The question of how best to prepare a child for the arrival of the new baby is one which exercises many parents, and it is a topic on which books of advice for parents have much to say, though the advice varies widely (see, for instance, Spock, 1969; Ginott, 1969; Close, 1980; as compared with Homan, 1970). In our study we found that all the mothers had discussed the imminent birth with the firstborn; most had shown him or her pictures of babies, and many children had felt the baby kick in the mother's tummy. But we were not able to give any precise answer to the question of how differences in the extent of this preparation affected the children's reactions. The explanations offered, and the nature of the discussion inevitably had such different meanings for the children aged 18 months and the children aged 40 months that there was no adequate way of assessing the differences. But it is worth noting that in a study by Trause *et al.* (1981) there was no link found between the initial response to the birth, and the incidence of problems over the next few days and weeks. It seems likely that however well 'prepared' a child may be, and however well he appears to understand what is going to happen, he may well be overwhelmed by the real experience.

PERSISTENCE OF PROBLEMS

How long did the problems which had increased at the birth of the sibling persist?

When the answers to the interviews at each of the four time points were compared, the results showed that many of the problems which had increased at the sibling birth decreased markedly over the months that followed. By the 14-month visit, sleeping problems, demanding behaviour, and the incidence of *marked misery* (those children who were described as being frequently miserable most days, or unhappy for long periods on more than three days a week) all decreased sharply. It is encouraging for mothers to learn that though these problems commonly increase at the time of the sibling birth, they are unlikely to persist. It is also encouraging to know that the incidence of these problems did not relate to the development of a difficult relationship between the siblings. There was no association between the various indices of disturbed behaviour, and the quality of the relationship which developed between the children over the next year, with the exception of the reaction of increased withdrawal. In families where the first child withdrew at the sibling birth, both children were behaving in a relatively hostile way towards each other by the 14-month visit.

In marked contrast to these 'improvements', a number of aspects of anxious or unhappy behaviour shown by the first children increased over this period. The number of children who were described by their mothers as having marked specific fears, as having 'miserable or grumpy moods', or as showing frequent marked ritualistic behaviour all increased. Since the sample is small, we should clearly be cautious about generalizing from these findings. However, the grouping of these aspects of anxious behaviour does parallel the patterns of association found in the large scale study of Richman *et al.* (1982). Since in their study 'neurotic' behaviour, particularly fearful behaviour, in 3- and 4-year-old children was associated with persisting difficulties over the next five years, it is clearly important to investigate further *which* children showed this pattern in the year following the sibling birth. But first, the question of age changes must be considered. Were these increases in unhappy behaviour simply developmental changes, unrelated to the birth of a sibling? Without a control group of children who did not experience the birth of a sibling we cannot establish whether the increases were simply age effects. But we can examine which children showed the marked increase in or persistence of problems. Here the results showed that the age of the child was not important, but that temperamental differences between the children, and the pattern of the child's initial reaction to the birth *were* important. Children who had been described by their mothers as negative in mood and intense in emotional reaction, in the initial interview, were more likely to have increased in fears, worries and ritualistic behaviour. So by the time that the baby was 8 months old there were close links between the children's temperamental assessment before the sibling birth, and the incidence of a range of problems: worries, fears, miserable moods,

Table 2.5   Behaviour at 8-month interview and temperament: Significant differences between those children scoring above the median on particular temperament traits and the rest of the sample

Behaviour	Temperament trait	Extreme group greater or less than rest of sample	p level (Fisher exact probability)
Constant use of comfort object	Intensity	Greater	0.04
Marked fears	Intensity	Greater	0.001
Frequent worry	Intensity	Greater	0.04
Marked rituals	Intensity	Greater	0.001
Frequent miserable moods	Intensity	Greater	0.04
Feeding problems	Intensity and unmalleability	Greater	0.04
Sleeping problems	Negative mood	Greater	0.01
Tantrums	Withdrawal	Less	0.001
Marked affection for mother	Intensity	Greater	0.02
Marked affection for father	Intensity	Greater	0.02

rituals, sleep problems and feeding problems (Table 2.5). The incidence of these problems (with the exception of miserable moods) had *not* been associated with temperamental differences before the sibling birth.

Those children who had reacted to the sibling birth by increasing in withdrawal were more likely to have sleeping problems and to be 'worriers'. Ritualistic behaviour, marked fears, and increased use of comfort objects were more common among children who at the time of the birth had become more tearful. It seems likely then that the events surrounding the birth were influencing the increase in unhappiness over the year following the sibling birth. For the clinician, the importance of individual differences in temperament as an indicator of differences in vulnerability to potentially stressful events is again highlighted.

How far was the evidence that some children increased in fearful anxious and worried behaviour, obtained from the interviews with the mothers, confirmed by the observations? For several aspects of this anxious behaviour — such as fearful responses to particular TV programmes, or distress at the dark, we were not able to make systematic comparisons between interview and observations, since we visited the families during the daytime. But we were able to compare the 'anxious' children with the rest of the sample on behaviour such as the time they spent using comfort objects, wandering aimlessly, or sitting without playing. The results showed that those who had increased in marked fears and miserable moods, according to maternal interview, were spending more time during the observation in these ways. The observations showed too that while the dramatic increase in confrontation which occurred after the sibling birth decreased over the next few months, the level of joint play and maternal attention which dropped after the birth did not rise again. Indeed the level of 'child-centred' comments made by the mother decreased from the post-sibling birth observations to the 14-month observations. And at these visits the frequency of 'mutual looking' between mother and child was also significantly lower than before the sibling birth. Any attempt to understand the changes in the children's behaviour must, clearly, also take account of these changes in the relationship of mother and child in the year following the sibling birth— and *vice versa*.

THE RELATIONSHIP BETWEEN THE SIBLINGS

The observations of the children made when the second born were 8 and 14 months old revealed a dramatically wide range of individual differences in the quality of their relationship. In some families friendly approaches accounted for 90 per cent of the behaviour of the older child to the sibling, in others such friendly approaches were never seen. A similarly wide range of differences was apparent in the frequency and proportion of overtly aggressive or hostile actions. And by 14 months, the second-born children also varied very much in the friendliness or hostility of their behaviour to the older. Quarrels and fights were very frequent in some families, rare in others.

Now parent manuals frequently lay the responsibility for poor sibling relationships and frequent fighting upon the parents. 'When the baby is mobile this is when sibling quarrels usually get under way . . . how the parents handle all this determines whether or not this becomes a repetitive rivalrous situation.' (Calladine and Calladine, 1979). Clinicians writing for other clinicians also hold this view (Einstein and Moss, 1967); and Close (1980) argues that jealousy is not inevitable but arises through the indirect suggestion of others in the family.

How far did the results of our study support this view? The findings showed that the behaviour of the children towards one another was related to the behaviour of the mother towards each of the children, in a number of ways, but that it would have been deeply misleading to suggest that the parents were primarily responsible for the extent of jealousy and aggression shown by the siblings. Hostility and aggression were clearly related, for instance, to a number of other factors—the sex of the children, the temperament of the first child. The pattern of association between the family relationships was complex. First, the quality of the relationships between both father and mother and firstborn *before* the sibling birth was associated with differences in the quality of the relationship which developed between the siblings (Dunn and Kendrick, 1981a). In families where the mother had had a particularly close and intense relationship with her daughter, spending much time playing with her and attending to her, the elder girl behaved, over time, in a relatively hostile way towards her younger sibling. By 14 months, in these families, the younger child was relatively hostile to the older. But the mothers should surely not be *blamed* for the intensity of their relationships with their daughters.

A quite different aspect of the mothers' behaviour with their firstborn was also linked to the quality of the siblings' behaviour over the year following the birth. The mothers differed markedly in the first weeks after the birth, in the ways in which they discussed the new baby with their firstborn. Some drew attention to the baby's needs and feelings, discussed what his crying might mean, and consulted the firstborn about what should be done about caring for him, almost as if this was a matter of joint responsibility. The firstborn in these families were often treated almost as equals in discussing the interpretation of the baby's crying, and were consulted about possible courses of action. (Not surprisingly the advice they gave was often bizarre in the extreme.) In other families the mothers never discussed the baby as a person in this way with their firstborn, or drew attention to his feelings and needs. Over the next year the differences between the children's behaviour in these two groups of families were notable: friendly behaviour from each child to the other was more common in those families where the mothers had discussed the baby as a person and treated the first child more as an equal.

Now we certainly would not wish to infer that there was a simple causal link between this style of talking to the first child about the baby in the early weeks, and the children's behaviour towards one another one year later. Rather, the findings show that there were many differences in the conversational style between the mothers who talked in this way about the baby, and those who did not. Those who discussed the baby's needs and feelings were also more likely to enter the first child's pretend fantasies, they more frequently gave justification for controlling the child (though they were not less likely to attempt to control the child), they used language for more complex cognitive purposes, and they explored and discussed motives and intentions of both the child and of other people more frequently. These differences reflect, we would suggest, a different style of relating to the firstborn, a style perhaps similar to the one that Light (1979) describes in his study of the development of social sensitivity as reflecting a high degree of 'symmetry' in the relationship between mother and child. These mothers were not only prepared to treat the child more as an equal in discussing rules and control issues, but were more tuned into their child's world, in the sense that they entered and enjoyed the child's fantasies and games. Such evidence as we have then suggests that the link over time between the early discussion of the baby, and the later behaviour of the siblings was one between a particular *style* of mother–firstborn interaction, and the siblings' behaviour, rather than any one specific aspect of this style.

Books of advice to parents disagree very much on the issue of whether parents should talk to their first children about the baby. Some recommend that parents keep references to the baby to a minimum. But our findings support the other line of advice, given for example by Calladine and Calladine (1979): 'Talk with your children about each other's needs, if the sibling is a baby, talk with the old one about what babies are like.'

FOLLOW-UP: THE SIBLINGS THREE YEARS LATER

How far did the differences evident in the sibling relationship persist as the children grew up and entered the wider world of school and peers?

Twenty-five of the firstborn children were studied as 6 year olds, as part of a larger study of children's relationships with peers, siblings and parents (Stilwell-Barnes, 1983). Since the sample of children followed is so small the results must be regarded with caution; however, the patterns of continuity with the earlier findings are so striking that they deserve mention. Stilwell-Barnes interviewed the children and their mothers. She asked the children a number of questions about their siblings (e.g. Tell me about your brother/sister. What is it you really like about him/her? What is it you do not like about him/her?) The children's replies were scored in terms of the number of positive comments, the number of negative comments, and the relative proportion of positive to negative comments. From the maternal interview, measures of the aggression shown towards the sibling, and the quality of the relationship between the siblings were selected for comparison with earlier measures.

The results showed that the marked individual differences found among the 2–3 year olds in both observed behaviour and in comments during the 14-month observations about their siblings were correlated with differences in the children's comments, 3–4 years later, as 6 year olds about the sibling, and with differences in their mothers' accounts of the sibling relationship at the 6-year visit. There were, for instance, significant positive correlations between the 2–3-year-old children's hostile approaches at the 14-month visit, and aggression at 6 years, and significant negative correlations between friendly approaches at the 14-month visits and aggression at 6 years, and between hostile approaches at 14 months and the positive quality of the relationship at 6 years. There were also significant positive correlations between the frequency of friendly comments the children made as 2–3 year olds, and the friendly comments they made when interviewed as 6 year olds.

The evidence that the correlations over time were between measures of observed child behaviour at one time point and maternal interview measures at a different time point suggests that the continuity was in the *children's* behaviour itself, rather than simply in the maternal perception of the children. Although, as we have noted, it is very important to be cautious about extrapolating from such a small sample, one general point deserves comment. Research on aggressive behaviour in middle childhood has shown that sibling influence is of major importance in contributing to the manifestation of aggressive and antisocial behaviour (Patterson, 1975; Patterson and Cobb, 1971). The present study (which provides the only available information on the continuity of sibling behaviour between infancy, preschool and early childhood years) with its evidence for stability in aggression towards the sibling suggests that the processes shown by Patterson to be of real significance in middle childhood are already apparent in the infancy of the second child. The link between Patterson's work and our own suggests that the early years of the sibling relationship deserve attention from clinician and from developmental psychologist alike.

CONCLUSIONS

The practical implications for parents of the findings of the study centre on the importance of minimizing the changes in the child's life at the time of the sibling birth, especially the drop in maternal attention and play experienced by many children. The individual differences between children that are so important in accounting for their reaction to the second child are not features of the child's behaviour which parents could easily change, or for which parents should be held responsible. The findings suggest that it is important to talk with a first child—even one who is under 2 years—about the baby as a person with needs and feelings, to let him join in caring for the baby if he wishes, and to be well prepared with distractions for the demands that escalate.

What are the implications of the findings for research methodology? The first point that deserves comment concerns the good agreement found between observation and interview data. The encouraging findings suggest that if mothers are asked to give specific descriptions of their children's behaviour in particular situations the answers are likely to be accurate, in the sense that they agree well with an observer's record of the child. Does this mean that we do not need to embark on laborious and time-consuming observations, but can simply rely on mothers' reports? Hardly: first, many of the significant changes in the interaction between mother and child were not changes that the mothers could be expected to notice or report—changes in their own interaction with the child such as the decrease, after the sibling birth, in the likelihood that the child's *looks* to the mother would be responded to. Secondly, many of the differences between the families in the interaction which turned out to be importantly related to the differences in the developing relationship between the siblings, such as the differences in the way in which mother and firstborn discussed motives, intentions and feelings, would not have been revealed in an interview.

This point illustrates another general lesson from the study. It was clear that it was important to try to describe different aspects of the family interaction and the children's behaviour at different levels of detail. It was evident, for instance that neither a description of the child's behaviour in global terms of jealousy or affection, nor a description in terms of minute behavioural acts would have adequately captured the most interesting or complex features of the children's behaviour towards their siblings. And a further methodological point that the findings highlight is the importance of studying not simply the mother–dyad, but the different relationships within the family, and the pattern of mutual influence between these relationships both at one time point and over time.

The findings do have some general implications for those with responsibility for caring for families. The first is that mothers are very likely to need support in the first year after a second or third baby. They are often very tired (over half the mothers in the study were still getting less than 5 hours sleep a day one month after the second child's birth), they frequently have a very trying toddler to deal with, and the documentation of their daily lives which the study provided revealed that for many, a relentless and exhausting pattern continued during the year after the sibling birth. Comments from four mothers illustrate these problems:

I'm very tired. The baby wakes two or three times a night, and then they are both awake at 5.30. Some days I get very edgy. I have to watch myself.

It's the baby who drives me mad. She screams when she can't get her own way . . . and I get so tired with the broken nights, and my husband's away.

When she was about 6 months daily I felt over the top. I stayed in bed because I felt I might hit her.

I was so tired . . . Ronnie was waking five or six times a night. I was very miserable. I smacked Sue all the time. I was screaming and shouting at her. He's very easy in the day, very undemanding. Quite unlike her. If he'd been like her, I'd be in hospital.

The extreme tiredness and depression felt by several mothers in the first three weeks after the birth did not continue for very long: Only 28 per cent of the mothers who were very exhausted and depressed in the post-partum period were still so at eight months. But it is clear that the stresses facing some mothers with several small children are grave, that they desperately need support and help, and opportunities to escape, even if briefly, their domestic circumstances. We know from the work of Brown and Harris (1978) that the problems of mothers living with small children without support or escape must be taken very seriously. Given this bleak picture it is encouraging for both parents and those in the caring professions to know that many of the changes in the children's behaviour are short-lived, that the occurrence of disturbed behaviour following the birth of a sibling is very common, and that it is not something for which the parents should be blamed. For clinicians, the recurrent theme running through the study that temperamental differences are linked to later disturbance is one that should be noted. And finally the most encouraging findings were those showing that in families where the first child was interested and affectionate towards the new baby, a warm and loving relationship frequently developed which continued not just over the next months but over the next three or four years.

ACKNOWLEDGEMENTS

This study was supported by the Medical Research Council, and carried out in collaboration with Carol Kendrick. We are grateful to the families in the study for their generous help.

REFERENCES

Adler, A. (1928). Characteristics of the 1st, 2nd and 3rd child, *Children*, 3, 14 (Issue 5).
Adler, A. (1959). *Understanding Human Nature*, Premier Books, New York.
Black, D. and Sturge, C. (1979). The young child and his siblings, in *Perspectives in Infant Psychiatry*, (Ed. J. G. Howells), Oliver and Boyd, Edinburgh.
Bowlby, J. (1973). *Attachment and Loss*, vol. II, Separation, anxiety and anger, Hogarth Press, London.
Brown, G. W. and Harris, T. (1978). *Social Origins and Depression*, Tavistock, London.
Calladine, C. and Calladine, A. (1979). *Raising Siblings*, Delacorte Press, New York.
Clark-Stewart, K. A. (1973). Interactions between mothers and their children: Characteristics and consequences, *Monographs of the Society for Research in Child Development*, 38, 6–7 (Serial No. 153).
Close, S. (1980). *The Toddler and the New Baby*, Routledge and Kegan Paul, London.
Dunn, J. and Kendrick, C. (1980a). The arrival of a sibling: Changes in patterns of interaction between mother and first-born child, *Journal of Child Psychology and Psychiatry*, 21, 119–132.
Dunn, J. and Kendrick, C. (1980b). Studying temperament and parent–child interaction: A comparison of information from direct observation and from parental interview, *Developmental Medicine and Child Neurology*, 22, 484–496.
Dunn, J. and Kendrick, C. (1981a). Interaction between young siblings: associations with the interaction between mother and first born, *Developmental Psychology*, 17, 3, 336–343.
Dunn, J. and Kendrick, C. (1981b). Social behavior of young siblings in the family context: differences between same-sex and different-sex dyads, *Child Development*, 52, 1265–1273.
Dunn, J. and Kendrick, C. (1982). *Siblings: Love, Envy and Understanding*, Harvard University Press, Cambridge, Mass.
Dunn, J., Kendrick, C. and Macnamee, R. (1981). The reaction of first-born children to the birth of a sibling: Mothers reports, *Journal of Child Psychology and Psychiatry*, 22, 1–18.
Einstein, G. and Moss, M. S. (1967). Some thoughts on sibling relationships, *Social Case Work*, 48 (9), 549–555.
Ginott, H. G. (1969). *Between Parent and Child*, Avon Books, New York.
Henchie, V. (1963). Children's reactions to the birth of a new baby, Unpublished thesis, Institute of Education, London.
Homan, W. E. (1970). *Child Sense a Guide for Parents*, Thomas Nelson and Sons, London.

Legg, C., Sherick, I. and Wadland, W. (1974). Reaction of pre-school children to the birth of a sibling, *Child Psychiatry and Human Development*, **5**, 3–39.

Light, P. (1979). *The Development of Social Sensitivity*, Cambridge University Press, Cambridge.

Patterson, G. R. (1975). The aggressive child: Victim and architect of a coercive system, in *Behavior Modification and Families* (Eds L. A. Hamerlynck, E. J. Marsh and L. C. Handy), Brunner/Mazel, New York.

Patterson, G. R. and Cobb, J. A. (1971). A dyadic analysis of 'aggressive' behaviors, in *Minnesota Symposia on Child Psychology* (vol. 5) (Ed. J. P. Hill), University of Minnesota Press, Minneapolis.

Petty, T. A. (1953). The tragedy of Humpty Dumpty, *The Psychoanalytic Study of the Child*, **8**, 404–422.

Richman, N., Stevenson, J. and Graham, P. (1982). *Preschool to School: A Behavioral Study*, Academic Press, London.

Robertson, J. and Robertson, J. (1971). Young children in brief separation: A fresh look, *Psychoanalytic Study of the Child*, **26**, 264–315.

Spock, B. (1969). *Baby and Child Care*, Pocket Books, New York.

Stilwell-Barnes, R. (1983). Social relationships as seen by mothers, children and teachers, Unpublished PhD thesis, University of Cambridge.

Trause, M. A., Voos, D., Rudd, C., Klaus, M., Kennell, J. and Boslett, M. (1981). Separation for childbirth: The effect on the sibling, *Child Psychiatry and Human Development*, **12**, 32–39.

Winnicott, D. W. (1977). *The Piggle*, Hogarth Press and Institute of Psychoanalysis, London.

Longitudinal Studies in Child Psychology and Psychiatry
Edited by A. R. Nicol
© 1985 John Wiley and Sons Ltd.

Chapter 3

What Sort of Children are Suspended from School and what can we do for them?

A. R. Nicol, C. Willcox and K. Hibbert

Youngsters who are suspended from school for more than a temporary period present many practical problems. Given compulsory education, how does one educate them? What are they entitled to and what do they need in terms of scarce resources? Is there any way in which schools can be organized to cope with them better? More specifically, what sort of children are they and what does the suspension do to them?

The first point is of course the obvious one that the suspension itself is a reflection of the children's behaviour. An overview of suspensions in one education authority showed that 30 per cent of them had been precipitated by physical violence and 42 per cent by verbal abuse to staff or other children. It is also important to note, however, that suspension rates, even from inner city schools, can show an up to ten-fold difference from one school to another. This reflects different policy towards difficult behaviour in different schools and also the ability of the different schools as social organizations to meet the needs of the children and cope with misbehaviour (Rutter *et al.*, 1979; Reynolds and Sullivan, 1981). Galloway (1976) for example, found an excess of suspensions from previously selective schools. Nevertheless, although a somewhat elastic ruler, suspension from school can be an indication of serious behaviour problems in the child.

The second implication is that when children are finally suspended from school, they are put in a situation of great difficulty. No satisfactory way has been found to 'threat' such children, and once they have been finally suspended, it is the exception for them to be reintegrated into their own school (Galloway, 1982). Many spend long periods of time receiving home tuition or other forms of make-shift education which cannot offer them the full curriculum. For a group of youngsters who, in general, are likely to have restricted access to life's opportunities, this may be seen from their point of view as a further restriction on their limited horizons. Rutter (1979) has identified a number of such events in the adolescent period, including unemployment and early pregnancy and the implications are elaborated further in Chapter 15 of this volume.

In a study of children excluded from school in Edinburgh (York et al., 1972) only four of twenty-five excluded chidlren were living at home and attending ordinary school at one- and three-year follow-up.

On the other hand, it seems possible that these youngsters were making so little use of their educational opportunities anyway that their suspension from school was a relatively insignificant episode in a more generally antisocial career. Robins (1966) in her classic follow-up study of child guidance clinic attenders showed that 36 per cent of children suspended from school continued to show severe behavioural problems into adult life. However, the act of suspension itself did not contribute to the genesis of persistent antisocial behaviour. The Robins study was, of course, a long-term follow-up study and could not record short-term changes and trends, nor did it chart development in any other way than in terms of severe psychiatric disturbance.

In considering this problem, it seemed important to start an investigation of what happened *before* suspension. In the British school system, there is often a change of school at age 11 years, and this seemed an appropriate age at which to start looking at the difficulties of the children.

THE STUDY

In our study, we were interested in the following questions:

1 What sort of behaviour characterizes children who are suspended from school?
2 What about the behaviour of difficult children who could, nonetheless, be contained and integrated in the school? Does this give us any clues as to which behaviours are particularly unacceptable?

To examine these issues we set up a longitudinal study. We did this for several reasons. First, we recognized the need to gather information on the children who were destined to be suspended before the suspension itself. To suspend a child from school is a highly emotive and politically loaded act and retrospective reports are likely to be coloured by this fact. The second reason was that we wanted an ongoing log of the behaviour of the children in the weeks and months leading up to the suspension. It was necessary, therefore, to get frequent reports of behaviour, since infringements of discipline, except when very major, are not usually reported or remembered for any length of time. The third point was that we wanted equal and unbiased weighting in our reports of the suspended children and controls. Again, this was unlikely if the cases had already been suspended.

Three large, non-selective schools participated in the project. Three consecutive year cohorts of 11-year-old children, a total of 1827, formed the base population. All these children were given a battery of screen measures in their second term at school. The first of the year cohorts was followed up for three years (start of second to end of fourth years at the school). The second and third cohorts were followed up through their second and third years at the school. The key teachers who had responsibility for the welfare and discipline of the children in the school were the year tutors and the form tutors. These staff were systematically interviewed each month, using a standard interview. Two of the three schools served deprived inner-city areas, whereas the third served a more middle-class area of the town. During the course of the study, each of the schools had an internal small teaching unit for temporary management of behaviour problems within the school.

THE SCREEN

The screen had two aims. The main aim was to collect systematic and relevant information about the children's functioning at an early stage of their secondary school career and before there had been any move towards suspension. The second term of the first year was chosen as the time for screening in order to allow the children to settle (or not settle) into the school. With so many children the screening process was necessarily somewhat superficial. It had to be given to the children in class groups. It consisted of a self-concept scale developed especially for the project (details available from authors on request) sociometry, including isolation and rejection measures and 'guess who' measures (Macmillan *et al.*, 1976); the Widespan Reading Test (Brimer and Gross, 1972) and an attendance record compiled from the school register over the first two terms. Finally, the teachers were asked to complete a disruption questionnaire for each child (Kolvin *et al.*, in preparation). As can be seen from the measures, we were particularly interested in the child's social adjustment in school. We postulated that, despite the fact that group tests were used, a useful picture could be built up by tapping peer opinions, teacher reports, attendance and attainments.

Despite the great methodological difficulties in measurement (see Wylie, 1974) we hoped that the self-concept measure would also yield interesting insights. It included two independent scales which were judged to measure dimensions of goodness versus badness and toughness versus timidity in self concept. These scales were derived from a principal component analysis of the forty-five items of the self-concept questionnaire. The goodness versus badness component is of importance in this discussion. It contrasted the items: 'Good at school work'; 'Cheerful'; 'Happy'; 'Clever' and 'Well behaved' at the positive pole with: 'Forget what is learned'; 'Do bad things'; 'Slow in school work'; 'Unhappy' and 'Often in trouble' at the negative pole.

The second aim of the screen was to provide information for matching groups of children for the rest of the study, we will describe how this was done when we describe the design of the research below.

CONTINUOUS MEASURES

In order to answer the key questions posed above, we need to chart the behaviour of the children who would eventually be suspended and compare them with children who were not excluded. Since we did not possess a crystal ball, this meant we had to keep track of the behaviour of the entire sample—all 1827 of them. To do this we developed an interview schedule which could be used repeatedly with school staff. It consisted of a set of twenty-nine pre-coded behavioural items with information about the setting and social context of the behaviour as well as the response on the part of the school staff and the community. Details of parent behaviour and response was also recorded. Year tutors and form tutors were invited to go systematically down their class list and report any incident about any of the children in the class within the month. Care was taken not to record the same incident in two successive months. A high level of agreement was gained between two raters of the same interview for all the items in pilot studies involving twenty-seven children and five members of staff.

THE DESIGN

The answer the key question outlined above we had to wait until suspension occurred and the look back over the behaviour records of the suspended children: Had the suspension followed a long history of unacceptable behaviour or one major crisis? What types of behaviour had been particularly hard for the school to tolerate? To make valid judgements in answering these questions we needed to have comparisons with both a norm of behaviour for the school as a whole and also a comparison with other difficult children who had not actually been suspended from school. To cut a long story short, we attempted to deal with these questions as follows.

For each child who had a high score on the teachers questionnaire we selected a second child with a comparably high score. For this we developed a 4-point weighted score from the two teachers questionnaires such that agreement between teachers led to a higher score than a high by one teacher alone. Children were matched on this weighted score. The children who scored 0 on the teacher behaviour questionnaire were either matched with each other or were used as a second control group. The total population of 1827 children was thus formed into age and sex matched triplets, the teacher reported, (a) difficult children paired with, (b) an equally difficult child, and (c) with a 'non-difficult' child, and the remaining 'non-difficult' children also combined into groups of three. This process was carried out at the time of screening well before any suspensions occurred.

Thus, at the time of suspension, each child could be compared with a second 'difficult' child and with a 'non-difficult' child. There were four occasions when both of the 'difficult' children in a matched pair were suspended. In these cases a disruptive control child was reallocated in order to preserve the comparison group.

RESULTS

Thirty-five children were suspended during the course of the study. Six of these were suspended rather soon after the continuous observations began. These have been left out of the continuous observations analysis but included in the screen analysis. The continuous observations results are therefore based on twenty-nine suspended children, twenty-nine 'difficult' controls and twenty-nine 'non-difficult' controls. There were nine girls excluded and twenty boys. Table 3.1 shows the differences between the cases and controls as a comparison. Both the suspended and 'difficult' controls, not surprisingly, showed major differences from the 'non-difficult' children on all scales except the self-report 'tough–timid' component. We have no explanation as to why they did not show up on this particular scale. The major differences between the suspended children and the

Table 3.1   Screen results ($n = 35$ in each group)

Description of screen measure	Differences (χ^2 test)	
	Excluded children vs. 'difficult' children	Excluded child vs. 'non-difficult' child
Teacher behaviour rating scale	NS (the two groups were matched on this scale)	Excluded children score higher ($p < 0.1\%$)
Self report		
Component I (good vs. bad)	No difference	Excluded children lower self image ($p < 0.1\%$)
Component II (tough vs. timid)	No difference	No difference
Sociometry		Excluded more:
Isolation	No difference	Isolated ($p < 1\%$)
Rejection	Excluded more rejected ($p < 5\%$)	Rejected ($p < 0.1\%$)
'Guess who'		
Tough	Excluded rated tough ($p < 5\%$)	Tough ($p < 0.1\%$)
Touchy	No difference	Touchy ($p < 0.1\%$)
Fool around	Excluded rated more fooling around ($p < 5\%$)	Fool around ($p < 0.1\%$)
Widespan Reading Test	No difference	Excluded lower reading age ($p < 1\%$)
Attendance during first year of secondary education	Excluded have poor attendance ($p < 0.1\%$)	Excluded have poor attendance ($p < 0.1\%$)

'difficult' controls was in their attendance during the first year at the school. Here the 'difficult' controls showed an attendance pattern similar to the 'non-difficult' controls with 76 per cent of the children putting in over 80 per cent attendance. Of the suspended children, however, only 28 per cent put in over 80 per cent attendance. The extraordinary fact is that the children who were ultimately suspended from school were only putting in intermittent appearances from an early stage of their career at school anyway. On the Widespan Reading Test, over half of both the suspended children and the 'difficult' controls had a standard score reading quotient of less than 85.

On the sociometry the suspended children were shown to be particularly rejected by other children and were seen as being tough and fooling around.

A cautionary note needs to be made in interpreting the self-concept scale. As the suspended and 'difficult' groups were poor readers, it is possible that the results may be less reliable as a result of their difficulty with reading—this reducing the validity of the test (Wylie, 1974).

MONTHLY REPORTS

In the monthly reports our aim was to develop a picture of the pattern of events leading up to suspension. We therefore took the final report for each suspended child and the comparable controls. These reports were then summated and the percentage of positive reports was computed for the suspended group and each of the two controls. The same was then done for the penultimate reports and so on back to the sixth from last report. The result represents a six or more month lead-up to the suspension (the months were term-time months). Figures 3.1–3.3 show the results. The 'non-difficult' controls are not shown since there were very few reports of deviant behaviour.

Figure 3.1 shows the percentage of cases where there was a report of aggressive behaviour for the six months leading up to suspension. It can be seen that there are huge differences in the number of reports of aggressive behaviour in the suspended children when compared with the 'difficult' controls. Figure 3.2 shows the patterns of reported disruptive behaviour. Here there is a steep rise in reports of disruption in the months preceding suspension. The differences from the 'difficult' controls are far less clear cut. Figure 3.3 shows a continuation of the marked attendance problems in the excluded group which was detected at screen level.

In preparing Figures 3.1 to 3.3 the children were given a binary score; that is *any* deviant behaviour of the given type within a given month for each child scored 1 whereas *no* deviant behaviour during that month scored 0. The scores of all the children were then added. This meant that the total scores shown represent a spread of behaviour across the group rather than a possible very high score for a small number of individual children.

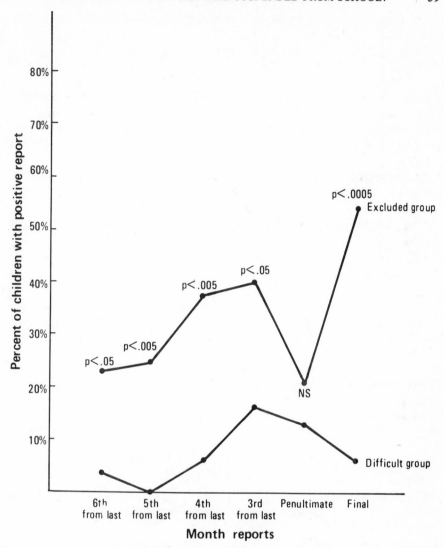

Fig. 3.1   Percentage of children reported as involved in episodes of aggressive behaviour in sequence of months leading up to exclusion

Aggression was itemized into eight categories: physical and verbal aggression to children and to adults, fun fights, bullying, tempers and other aggression. We then looked at the incidence of these types of behaviour in the suspended as compared with the 'difficult' controls. For this analysis we summed all the continuous measure reports. The most striking differences were in the area of physical aggression to adults. There were twenty-three instances of this in the

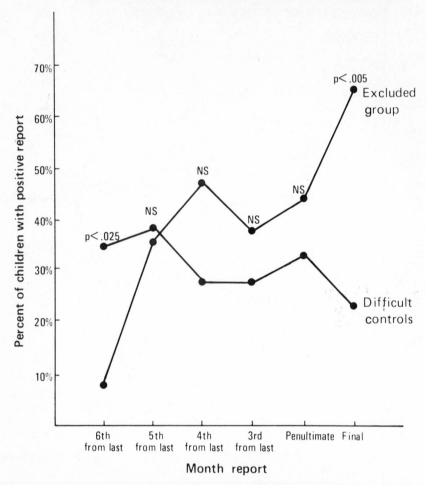

Fig. 3.2   Percentage of children reported as involved in episodes of disruptive behaviour
in sequence of months leading up to exclusion

suspension and only one in the 'difficult' control group. Similarly, verbal
aggression to adults was 12.75 times as common in the suspended group. It
should be remembered that these figures do not include the suspension incident
itself but are a sum of previous behaviour. The next biggest difference was
in bullying (defined as intimidating others who are younger or weaker).
This was four times as common in the suspended as compared to the
'difficult' group. The other categories also showed higher rates but it
does appear that it was in the above categories than the most outstanding
differences occurred.

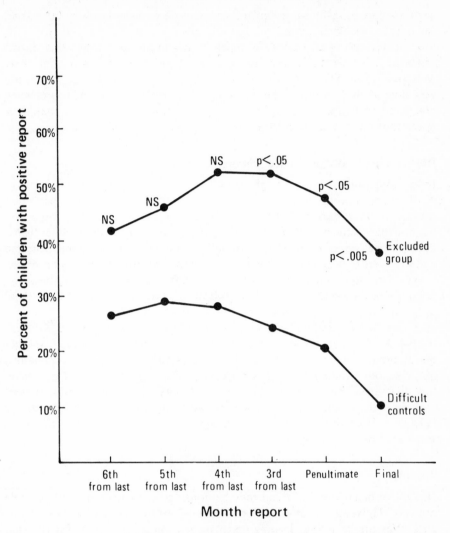

Fig. 3.3   Percentage of children reported as having attendance problems in sequence of months leading up to exclusion

The setting of misbehaviour

We believe, with Barker (1968), that a description of behaviour is not complete unless its environmental context is included. We were not in a position to carry out the detailed analysis and differentiation of settings that the Kansas workers did. However, we systematically reported the location of any behaviour that was reported to us. We were able to combine the various different settings so as to compare behaviour in school and in the playground and for non-attendance to compare the whereabouts of the child when not in class. In all cases, the level of deviance was, of course, much higher in absolute terms than in the 'difficult' controls. It was only in the case of aggression, however, that there were significant difference in the setting. In the suspended group, aggression was more likely to occur in the class context rather than the playground when compared with the control group ($\chi^2 = 6.03$, df $= 1$, $p < 0.02$). It should be noted that these data do *not* include the suspension incident itself.

Did we sample all 'suspended' children?

In any longitudinal study, the group who default from follow up are likely to be of special importance, particularly in behavioural research. In this particular project the children who left the schools are likely to be especially important because there is the possibility that among them are a proportion of either 'back-door' suspensions or of the restless, impulsive families who tend to move around and who were so well described by Robins (1966) as having widespread problems.

We identified eighty-nine children who left the schools from the study populations during the course of our follow up. We attempted to follow these up in their new schools but could only identify forty-two of them. We were able, however, to examine the screen data of all the eighty-nine leavers. Of these thirty-five (39 per cent) scored 4 or above on the combined teacher questionnaires. This contrasted with the total body of children who remained in the school. Among these 25.4 per cent of the children scored 4 or above, this difference being highly significant ($\chi^2 = 8.49$, df $= 1$, $p < 0.005$). It does look as if the children who left school had a higher incidence of disruptive behaviour than those who remained, and some of these might have been suspended had they stayed.

Sex differences

Disruptive behaviour in school may be considered as predominantly a male preserve. However, among the thirty-five suspended children there were nine girls. Was the behaviour leading up to suspension any different for the girls than the boys? We looked again at overall aggressive behaviour in boys and girls separately. In girls there was at least one episode of aggressive behaviour on 35 per cent of the possible occasions. In boys the comparable figure was 30 per cent. There seemed, therefore, no gross difference in the behaviour in the two sexes among the suspended children.

Teacher predictions

The teachers were asked the question of all the children at the time of screening: 'Do you think the child will present a management problem?' The answers clearly distinguished the excluded children and 'difficult controls' on the one hand from the 'non-difficult' group on the other where the teachers seldom predicted problems. There were no differences in prediction scores between the excluded and non-excluded but 'difficult' children.

Self reports and opinions

Following exclusion, both the excluded children and each of their two controls were interviewed. Among other information, they were asked about their aggressive behaviour. The interview used was developed by Nicol *et al.* (1972). The results (Table 3.2) show that youngsters own reports support the high aggressiveness of the excluded group. Further enquiry revealed that while their aggression was often directed towards the teacher, there was also more aggression directed towards family members and peers in the suspended group.

The suspended youngsters were asked for their opinion about the suspension. Forty per cent of them considered suspension a fair response by the school to their difficult behaviour.

Table 3.2   Self report of fights among cases and controls

	Cases	'Difficult' controls	'Normal' controls
Frequency of fights			
Less than one fight ever	10	15	32
Up to three fights in six months	7	12	3
More than three fights in six months	11	2	0
Target of violence (ever)			
Parents	4	2	1
Siblings	13	7	1
Peer individual	24	14	6
Peer group	15	6	6
Teacher	14	1	1
	$n = 28$	$n = 29$	$n = 35$

For frequency $\chi^2 = 20.68$ for less than 1 versus more than 1 df = 2 $p < 0.005$.

The parental viewpoint

Also following suspension, an extensive interview was undertaken with the parents of the suspended child and controls. Among other things, the parents were asked for their views about the suspension. Thirty per cent of the parents agreed that the suspension was justified, whereas 63 per cent thought that the suspension was either rather unreasonable or very unreasonable. Again, 29 per cent were prepared to hold the child responsible for the problem, whereas

63 per cent blamed some aspect of the school such as a particular teacher or lax discipline. It is interesting that the parents seemed, on the basis of these results, to be more likely to criticize the school than were the children themselves.

Follow-up

A brief follow-up enquiry was made one year after the completion of the study. At that time eleven of the twenty-nine children were at special day schools for maladjusted children or day units, three were in borstal, one was in detention centre, two had disappeared, four were in residential school, one in an adolescent unit and five had left school. Only two were receiving normal education but in schools different from those they had been excluded from. One of these two, a girl, seemed to have responded to a psychotherapeutic approach to her many problems of adjustment.

It should be emphasized that during the course of the research, a special unit was in operation with the aim of returning excluded children to their ordinary school. This was in addition to the Special Units within each of the three schools. The work done in this unit was of a high quality and many of the youngsters benefited by being there, unfortunately as we can see it did not result in the return of the children to their own school. This is consistent with the findings concerning off-site units in other areas (Galloway *et al.*, 1982).

DISCUSSION

Returning to the questions that were posed at the outset of this chapter, we can arrive at some clear answers. There do seem to be consistencies in the behaviour of the excluded youngsters. Suspension commonly follows a long record of aggressive behaviour. There is a tendency for this behaviour to be more commonly directed towards staff and to occur in classroom situations. It is often physical aggression. This is the sort of behaviour that teachers can tolerate least well and it would seem that children are largely suspended for extremes of behaviour rather than other, vaguer reasons such as 'reputation' or 'labelling' as has sometimes been suggested. Further, the behaviour does not occur as a sudden crisis but constitutes persistent difficulties over many months. The aggression reported by the teachers is supported by the youngster's own reports and, at screen level, by the responses of their peers.

The relationship difficulties of the suspended children were manifestly more widespread. They were more likely to indulge in bullying of other children and to be deeply unpopular and rejected by their peers. This pattern seemed to be established early in their school career. One might conclude that the suspended children had for long been an unwelcome sight in the school. The other remarkable feature of these children when compared with the control groups is their persistently high level of truancy from school. It could be that both these features constitute part of a global picture of severe and widespread deviance or it could be that the aggressiveness of these children leads in turn to their unpopularity and thence to their 'self' and 'official' exclusion. Certainly their aggressiveness is widely recognized. For example their peers, even at the time of the screen, identified them as significantly more 'tough' than the difficult controls. The subjects themselves were prepared to talk about their aggressiveness which was more frequent not only at school but also towards parents, siblings and peers.

Over the relatively short period of early adolescence, there does seem to be considerable consistency in the aggressive behaviour of these youngsters. Several authors, from the findings of their separate longitudinal studies, have commented on the apparent continuity of aggressive traits over time. Lefkowitz *et al.* (1977) studied a cohort of children at 8 years of age and again at 19 years in Columbia County, New York State. Forty-nine per cent of the original 875 children were traced and complete data obtained.

As in our study, a high proportion of the original sample who scored aggressive had moved away or were untraceable at follow-up. Aggressiveness was rated in several ways: at the 8-year-old level of peer ratings and parent reports and at 19 years by peer ratings again, self reports and questionnaire scores and arrest records. One of the notable findings was the consistency of aggression between these two ages. Peer nominations of the aggressive individuals showed marked consistency between the two ages. Also peer nominations at age 8 years predicted self rating of aggression ten years later. Lefkowitz and his colleagues used criminal records of violent crime as a check on the validity of their self-report questionnaire, but despite this, it is not possible to get a picture of the quality and severity of the aggressive behaviour of the subjects of Lefkowitz *et al.*'s (1977) study. Comparison with our own findings is therefore difficult. It seems likely that they were focusing on a wider spectrum of aggressive behaviour than that in our study. One point of similarity was that the aggressive children had poor school attainment.

The study of Olweus (1978, 1979) on the characteristics of aggressive and bullying adolescents also showed marked stability of aggressive behaviour at one- and three-year follow up. The main source of data was peer reports. In other respects, the aggressive boys in the study seem to have quite different characteristics from ours. Thus they were as popular, on average, as other members of the class and, in sharp contrast to our findings, seemed to have good self esteem and to be free from unhappiness as measured by self report. Also, the aggressives showed average IQ and attainment at school.

The study most comparable to our own in the type of population studied, is the Cambridge Study of Delinquent Development (summarized in West, 1982). All boys from a high-delinquency inner-city area were followed up from middle childhood until adult life. Again, there was a strong tendency for the same group of boys to be picked out on different measures of aggression taken from different sources and at different developmental stages over the course of the study. Aggressiveness at an early stage was characteristic of those boys who later became delinquent.

It would be wrong to equate a social problem such as exclusion from school with one type of behaviour problem such as the habitually aggressive youngster. Seven of the excluded youngsters in the twenty-nine suspended group of the present study had no record of aggressive behaviour in the six-month lead-up period to exclusion. Examination of the self reports of these seven revealed that four of them admitted to being involved in fights in which they used weapon or boots and one to have injured another youth to the extent that he had to be admitted to hospital in coma! It so happened that the behaviour that led to the exclusion was disruptive rather than aggressive, but the overall picture was of highly aggressive youths, even those without aggressive reports.

So far we have developed a picture of the quite marked differences between the excluded youngsters and the controls. We have also remarked that these children, at least partly as a result of their behaviour, inhabit, as it were, a more hostile environment than their peers within the school. This is true from an early stage of their school career. Social phenomena such as disruptive behaviour at school and the school's response to it are made up of subtle situational responses which cannot be understood in isolation from an analysis of the social situation, all the actors involved and the ethos of the school in general. As mentioned above, and as has been found in other studies (Galloway, 1976) the rates of exclusion in seemingly comparable schools can be sharply different. Some pioneering studies have focused on the school as the object of study and have been able to identify various characteristics of the school which are associated with low rates of behavioural deviance, delinquency and absenteeism and high rates of achievement. One of these studies (Rutter et al., 1979) is quite fully described in Chapter 15 of this volume. The authors identified two sorts of differences between the more and the less successful schools. First, in these mixed-ability schools, it was clear that an overall balanced intake of pupils with a fair proportion of the more able contributed to success. Second, there was a variety of characteristics of the psychological environment of the school which seemed important (see Chapter 15). In a similar study in Wales, Reynolds and his colleagues (Reynolds and Sullivan, 1981) have identified a range of somewhat similar variables as important. In particular, they were able to identify two styles of school, the more successful of which involved the children and their families in the school life and gave them responsibility. The Welsh study took place in schools where the intake was restricted to less-able children, but one overall possibility is that in both studies there were circumstances and social institutions that operated against the setting up of 'antisocial' subcultures among the children.

These studies adopt schools rather than pupils as the object of study. Whether or not their detailed findings are replicated, the message is clear, schools do make a difference. However, this assertion is likely to be closely followed by a question such as — what can the less successful schools do to more adequately meet the needs of these pupils? The answer to this is by no means obvious since so many of the features of the less successful school have the appearance of self-maintaining vicious circles. For example, it seems likely that a change from corporal punishment to positive reinforcement would be difficult if staff morale is low and the children either absent or very badly behaved. The school-based studies do not, by their design, give us any clue about careers of the most difficult and aggressive pupils. We might assume that their problems are less manifest in the more successful schools. However, this brings us to ask: What is the relative experience of the disadvantaged and conduct-disordered child in the different settings? Is it that he or she is actually involved in positive interactions in the 'good' schools, or merely deprived of the subcultural support that reinforces their deviances? Our findings suggest that the most disturbed youngsters only have a tenuous foothold in the school anyway, but a closer look at their grouping in the school would be of interest. In addition, from the parents' response to their exclusion, it does seem likely that the children get some tacit support for their problem behaviour from outside the school.

We conclude with a consideration of the practical implications of our findings. The climate of opinion concerning the best approach to intervention with disturbed children has undergone a radical change in recent years. Traditionally, children with all types of behaviour problem have been treated in isolation from the school in child guidance clinics and, where necessary, in special educational settings. This policy has applied to all types of problem from children with psychotic disorders to the problems of disruptiveness and aggressiveness that characterized the subjects of the present study. Many reviews (e.g. Robins, 1973) have concluded that this approach is of unproven effectiveness. One result has been a shift in emphasis in provision which has occurred on both sides of the Atlantic towards provision for the special needs of children in ordinary schools (Warnock Report, 1978; Strain and Kerr, 1981). Few could doubt that this shift in emphasis is likely to be of benefit to many children so long as it is adequately funded and accompanied by the setting up of the necessary programmes of evaluative research and the appropriate implementation of research findings. Our research, along with that of previous work suggests that it is with aggressive children that problems are likely to be most difficult to tackle. It seems unlikely that the persistent aggressive and antisocial behaviour of these children will respond to global attempts to modify the school 'social system' (Gillham, 1978) although in some schools this may be a necessary adjunct to other efforts. There is a danger that in rejecting the isolated individual approach of the past, we throw out the baby with the bathwater and reject all individual centred approaches. What is needed is an approach which starts with the individual child but which takes account of his or her *individual* environment in the school.

Our sociometry results suggest that this may be very different from that of the well-adjusted child and much less hospitable.

Also, as our parent and self reports suggest the behaviour is likely to be backed by hardened and alienated attitudes towards school. If an analysis of these factors preceded intervention it may be that interventions could tackle both the management of problems of aggression and of disruptiveness in the classroom, as in many successful behaviour modification programmes (Goldstein *et al.*, 1981; O'Leary and O'Leary, 1976) and also problems at home and with the peer group. Our work highlights the fact that there is usually plenty of warning of approaching difficulty so perhaps a thorough school-based assessment at an early stage could be helpful before problems get out of control and suspension becomes necessary.

REFERENCES

Barker, R. G. (1968). *Ecological Psychology: Concepts and Methods for Studying the Environment of Human Behaviour*, Stanford University Press, Stanford.

Brimer, A. and Gross, H. (1972). *Manual of the Widespan Reading Test*, Nelson, London.

Galloway, D. M. (1976). Size of school, socio-economic hardship, suspension rates and persistent unjustified absence from school, *Brit. J. Educ. Psychol.*, **46**, 40–47.

Galloway, D. M., Ball, T., Blomfield, D. and Boyd, R. (1982). *Schools and Disruptive Pupils*, Longman, London.

Gillham, B. (Ed.) (1978). *Reconstructing Educational Psychology*, Croom Helm, London.

Goldstein, A. P., Carr, E. G., Davidson, W. S. and Wehr, P. (1981). *In Response to Aggression: Methods of Control and Prosocial Alternatives*, Pergamon, New York.

Lefkowitz, M. M., Eron, L. D., Walder, L. P. and Rowell Heusimann, L. (1977). *Growing Up To Be Violent. A Longitudinal Study*, Pergamon, New York.

Macmillan, A., Walker, L., Garside, R. F., Kolvin, I., Leitch, L. M. and Nicol, A. R. (1978). The development and application of sociometric techniques for the identification of isolated and rejected children, *J. Assn. of Workers for Maladjusted Children*, **6**, 58–74.

Nicol, A. R., Gunn, J. C., Foggitt, R. H. and Gristwood, J. (1972). The quantitative assessment of violence in adult and young offenders. *Med. Sci. and the Law*, **12**, 275–282.

O'Leary and O'Leary, K. D. (1976). Behaviour modification in the school, in *Handbook of Behaviour Modification* (Ed. H. Leitenberg) Prentice Hall, Englewood Cliffs, New Jersey.

Olweus, D. (1978). *Aggression in the Schools, Bullies and Whipping Boys*, Hemisphere, Washington, DC.

Olweus, D. (1979). Stability of aggressive reaction patterns in males: a review, *Psych. Bull.*, **86**, 862–875.

Reynolds, D. and Sullivan, M. (1981). The effects of school: A radical faith re-stated, in *Problem Behaviour in the Secondary School* (Ed. Bill Gillam) Croom Helm, London.

Robins, L. N. (1966). *Deviant Children Grown Up*, Williams and Wilkins, Baltimore.

Robins, L. N. (1973). Evaluation of psychiatric services for children in the United States, in *Roots of Evaluation* (Eds J. K. Wing and H. Hafner) Oxford University Press (for the Nuffield Provincial Hospitals Trust), London.

Rutter, M. (1979). Protective factors in children's response to stress and disadvantage, *Primary Prevention of Psychopathology:* Vol. 3: *Social Competence in Children* (Eds M. W. Kent and J. E. Roff), University Press of New England, Hanover.

Rutter, M., Maughan, B., Mortimore, P. and Ouston, J. (1979). *Fifteen Thousand Hours*, Open Books, London.

Strain, P. S. and Kerr, M. M. (1981). *Mainstreaming of Children in Schools*, Academic Press, New York.

Warnock Report (1978). *Special Educational Needs*, Report of the Committee of Enquiry into the educational needs of children and young people. HMSO, London.

West, D. J. (1982). *Delinquency: Its Roots Careers and Prospects*, Heinemann, London.

Wylie, R. (1974). *The Self Concept*, vol. I, University of Nebraska Press, Nebraska.

York, R., Heron, J. M. and Wolff, S. (1972). Exclusion from school, *J. Child Psychol. Psychiat.*, **13**, 259–266.

Section II

Short-term Studies
which ask Broader Questions

Longitudinal Studies in Child Psychology and Psychiatry
Edited by A. R. Nicol
© 1985 John Wiley and Sons Ltd.

Chapter 4

From Child to Parent: Early Separation and the Adaptation to Motherhood

S. Wolkind and S. Kruk

The last fifteen years have seen a rapid growth of epidemiological research in child psychiatry. The development of measuring instruments has enabled data to be collected on the prevalence and patterns of psychiatric disorder amongst a wide variety of child populations (see, for example, Graham, 1978). One important result of this body of new knowledge has been to cause many clinicians to critically re-evaluate the type of service that they should be offering their communities. The rates of disorder that have been found are such that it is clear that conventional clinics will never see more than a small minority of those children who have disorders. We now know that these disorders are not trivial. Many children do not 'grow out' of them and in many cases they will persist through long periods of childhood (Graham and Rutter, 1973). In searching for a response to these worrying findings 'more of the same' does not really seem to be appropriate. The evidence for the efficacy of many current treatments is not very convincing, in particular, in the case of the commonest condition, namely conduct or antisocial disorder. There is, therefore, a growing tendency amongst clinicians and administrators to think instead, of developing programmes of early intervention and primary prevention.

This is a tempting possibility, but one which must be treated with some caution. Many questions must first be posed and answered. The controversy that still surrounds the US Head Start Project illustrates the backlash that can be generated by launching programmes before a sound theoretical model has been established (see, for example, Zigler and Valentine, 1979). Longitudinal studies may offer one of the best ways of providing the information we need. A first, if obvious, point, is that if we are hoping to start preventative work before problems become established, we need to determine the criteria by which we will identify those groups for whom intervention is justified. It does appear possible to do this without having to use longitudinal data. For example, it has been shown that children who are physically abused are more than four times as likely as controls to have been admitted to a special care unit after birth (Lynch *et al.*, 1976). From this important finding it would be tempting to suggest that intervention should be applied to all admitted children. This ignores the fact that, though abuse is commoner in this group, the vast majority will, of course, not be abused. In any given population we need to know what proportion of the originally identified 'risk' group actually develops the problem. A longitudinal study could reveal this and also far more about the characteristics of those that do not. It may also enable us to make an even more important step and find out how and why the original characteristic and the outcome are related. Merely finding an association will be of no help in deciding how to prevent the adverse outcome. If we do find a group where a poor outcome occurs, we may learn our greatest lessons from a longitudinal examination of those members of that group who, against our predictions, do well. Longitudinal studies are, by their nature, time consuming and to produce practical results it may be necessary to mount projects that combine the use of both retrospective and prospective data.

The clinical issues discussed above have exercised the Psychiatric Unit of The London Hospital Medical College for some years. The London Hospital serves one of the most deprived inner-city areas in the country. Various attempts have been made to provide community-based services, including early treatment for children usually considered too young to be referred to conventional child psychiatric clinics (Coleman *et al.*, 1977). In addition to the clinical innovations it was decided to mount a non-intervention longitudinal study following up a group of families in order to better understand why, in some families, child and parent problems become fixed and persistent. It was hoped that this could act as a prelude to preventative work.

In this paper we shall be comparing the outcome over four years for three groups of women and their firstborn children. Before describing the structure of our study and the detailed definitions which determined group membership, we shall first describe the rationale which led us to hypothesize that the women in two of these three groups could be considered to be 'at risk'. Our strategy has been to use retrospective data to select our samples who we have then followed prospectively.

The basic criterion determining sample membership concerned the family of origin of the mothers of the children we intended to study. There is a major assumption running through much psychiatric theory that it is in a woman's earliest socialization experiences that the foundations will be laid for her future rôle as a mother. This concept has been particularly emphasized in the psychoanalytic literature with special emphasis being laid on the woman's relationship with her own mother (Deutsch, 1947). Recent work based on empirical studies would seem to support this conclusion. Kezur (1978), for example, in a small study found that a woman's identification with her own mother was an important factor determining the quality of her attachment to her newborn baby. Hustoin-Stein and Higgins-Trenk (1978), in a review of life-span work on rôle identification in women, felt that the evidence suggested that amongst women the wish to remain childless was associated with negative experiences of their parents' marriage and of motherhood during their own childhood. The hypothesis we decided to examine was that women with experiences of that nature who *did* conceive would have particular problems with their own children. In 1973, when we selected our sample, the evidence suggesting this as a worthwhile hypothesis was relatively limited. There had been studies in relevant areas such as that of Melges (1968) which showed that the majority of women with post-partum psychosis had themselves had mothers who provided inadequate models for mothering, but the bulk of this work tended to lack controls. The research findings that appeared in time to help us make up our minds to examine this issue in some detail were those of Frommer and O'Shea (1973a,b). In a representative sample they demonstrated that amongst women going through an obstetric unit, those who had been separated from their own parents before the age of eleven, in a context suggesting family difficulties, were more likely than most to be depressed after the birth and to have difficulties in child rearing. In our study we used childhood separation as one of a number of easily determined factors which might suggest risk.

We shall describe how we selected the women for our three groups and then outline their progress through pregnancy to a point three-and-a-half years after the birth of the child. We shall look at their children and at their families. Though the women were selected with retrospective data the importance of the longitudinal approach will be demonstrated. Differences exist between the three samples but the way in which they differ from each other is not the same at all points of the study. We shall use this changing pattern to suggest how difficulties can become established and maintained. We shall discuss the contribution of our original selection criterion (i.e. childhood separation experiences) to the final picture and will consider whether our findings suggest any leads for early intervention.

THE STUDY

The study began in 1974; during that year we approached all British-born primiparous women aged 16 years and over who were, when they attended the antenatal booking clinics serving Tower Hamlets, living in that Inner London Borough. A research worker interviewed 534 women, representing over 95 per cent of those eligible. The majority of subjects were of working-class origin. They were given a short 'screening' interview which was used to obtain basic demographic information and also covered certain areas which we hypothesized might be related to the degree of risk for later family and child problems. The two major criteria used to detect increased risk were the childhood separation experiences which form the subject of this chapter and a history of a previous emotional or neurotic disorder. We shall not be discussing the women in this second risk group here but it is worth mentioning that they did indeed develop high rates of later problems. The screening interview was used in two ways to select samples for the study proper. First, the code number of each interview was used monthly to randomly select women who would be part of two samples. The first sample was a group who, at the time of booking, were married or in a stable cohabitation ($n = 105$). The second was a group who at the time of booking were unmarried and were not living with a man who would be regarded as the father of the child ($n = 81$).

Using a random selection process women from both of these samples have since been combined to form a true random sample ($n = 131$) with the correct proportion of each marital/cohabiting status as existed in the original total population. It is perhaps worth diverting briefly to consider the reasons for originally having groups selected according to marital status. It did seem reasonable to consider the single women, most of whom were teenagers, as being another example of a group at risk. Our findings on this point illustrate well the value of the longitudinal approach. During pregnancy and immediately after the birth much of our data did indeed suggest that children born to these mothers would be at considerable disadvantage. With marital status being such an easily identified criterion, early intervention would have appeared at this point to be both justified and necessary. As the study progressed over the three years following the birth a striking feature has been that the differences between the single and married groups rapidly diminished. Though the originally single women were at all stages more economically disadvantaged, three-and-a-half years after the birth they and their children were, on interview measures of family relationships and psychiatric state, doing as well as those in the married group. It is not difficult to imagine an intervention programme being started and claims being made for its effectiveness in producing beneficial change. We have described and discussed these findings in detail elsewhere (Kruk and Wolkind, 1982).

To return, however, to our screening interview. Its second purpose was, on the basis of certain replies, to select the risk group we have described previously. Clearly some women would of course be selected for both a random and a special-risk group. This was not, however, regarded as a problem, as the different samples would be used in different ways. The random sample would allow us to make estimates of the prevalence of various characteristics in the population. The risk group would give us a pool of subjects defined by a certain characteristic who could be compared with the subjects without that characteristic, drawn from the random sample. The risk group we are considering here comprised all women who had been separated from one or both parents for at least one month before the age of 5 years or for at least three months between the ages of 5 and 16 years *in a context suggesting continuing family disharmony or difficulties*. The criteria used for this comprised family break-up through divorce or separation, prolonged parental physical or psychological illness or the admission of the woman as a child to a boarding school for social or psychological reasons. We also included parental death as one of the categories as pilot work suggested that in this population it was followed by long-standing family problems.

For the purposes of this presentation this separation risk group has been divided into two and the three groups we will be comparing are:

1   All those women from the true random sample who had had no experience of childhood separation from their parents; the non-separated group ($n = 78$).
2   Women from the two original random samples *and* the special risk group who had had the type of separation described above but had remained with their family; the *disrupted* group ($n = 49$).
3   Women from the two original random samples and the special risk group who, in childhood, had been separated and in addition had been admitted to local authority or equivalent care; the *in care* group ($n = 33$).

It will be realized that certain women from the true random sample have been excluded from our analyses, i.e. those women ($n = 20$) who had been separated from their parents but not in a context suggesting family difficulties. Those women whose separations were due either to their own illness or to factors such as a parent temporarily leaving because of work differed only slightly from those in the non-separated group (Wolkind *et al.*, 1976).

METHODS OF INVESTIGATION

A feature of our study has been to combine semistructured interviewing with an ethologically derived observational technique. Details of this technique can be found in Hall *et al.* (1979). Once selected the women were seen during the seventh month of pregnancy and at four, fourteen, twenty-seven and forty-two months after the birth of their child. On each of these occasions a semistructured interview was used. Some questions were used without probes to tap attitudes, others required detailed probing to allow the interviewer to determine the presence and quality of various features of family life. For certain measures instruments designed and validated by other workers were used. Examples are the quality of the parents' marriage (Quinton *et al.*, 1976) or the behavioural problems of the young child (Richman and Graham, 1971). All interviews were recorded both on tape and on paper. Questions were used for analysis only if there had been at least 85 per cent interrater agreement on pilot testing. Weekly meetings were held to maintain the consistency of rating and interviewers were rotated so that no woman was seen consecutively and only rarely on more than one occasion by the same member of the research team.

RESULTS

The women and their backgrounds

A very first analysis of two simple but important variables, marital status and age, coded at the screening interview, showed that on these the two risk groups resembled each other and differed markedly from the women in the non-separated group. We found that 10 per cent of the women in the non-separated group were unmarried to the father of the child they were expecting. This characteristic, uncommon in the women from stable backgrounds, was in fact the norm for those in the two risk groups, 63 per cent for both the disrupted only and for those who had been in care. This very large difference was, of course, statistically significant ($\chi^2 = 48.20$, df = 2, $p < 0.001$). A similar pattern was seen when we looked at the age of the mother. Only 22 per cent of the non-separated group were in their teens during pregnancy as opposed to 51 per cent for the disrupted and 70 per cent for the in-care sample. We felt that after having had a disrupted childhood, bringing up a child in a deprived area would not be an easy task for women who were very likely to be both single and teenagers. These preliminary findings suggested that on a first view similarity in circumstances existed between the women in each of the two risk groups.

In the next interview, that taking place during the seventh month of pregnancy, we asked in detail about the woman's family of origin, both in terms of its structure and about the current relationship the woman had with family members. Some of the findings are shown in Table 4.1.

An interesting pattern is seen in terms of where the women were living during their pregnancies. Here the Group 2, disrupted-only women, stand out with the majority living with their parents. The implications of the lower rate must, however, be very different for the members of the two remaining groups. The majority of the non-separated group were with their husbands. Many of the in-care group were alone. This finding, when combined with the remaining figures shown in Table 4.1(a) suggests very different patterns of support being available during pregnancy. The majority of the non-separated group have both a husband and frequent contact and a good relationship with their family of origin. The disrupted-only group, though mainly unmarried, are generally likely to be having positive contacts with their families. The in-care group seems least supported. The majority are neither married nor likely to have a good relationship and close contact with their own parents.

This evidence of some differences between the two risk groups is heightened by an examination of various aspects of their life before their pregnancy and of certain other features of their family of origin (Table 4.1(b)). The majority of both the disrupted-only and non-separated women were brought up in the study borough. The in-care women were more likely to have moved into this deprived area. They came from larger families and from homes where the father, if present, was slightly more likely to be unskilled or semi-skilled. The commonest

Table 4.1 Family of origin and (a) current family relationships during pregnancy and (b) aspects of pre-pregnancy life

	Group 1 In Care (%)	Group 2 Disrupted Only (%)	Group 3 Intact (%)	χ^2 df = 2
(a) *Current family relationships*				
Living with parents	30	60	30	12.67**
Seeing parents at least once a week	59	89	85	8.18*
Getting on well with patients	36	76	95	28.08***
Absence of disputes with other family members	45	76	89	16.84***
(b) *Aspects of pre-pregnancy family life*				
Brought up in study borough	43	70	70	7.52*
Good relations with parents in past	27	59	86	28.32***
Father semi- or unskilled manual job	46	18	26	4.00
Last job of woman, semi- or unskilled manual	58	34	22	11.54**
Mean number of siblings	5.4	4.1	3.9	F = 4.16 $p < 0.05$

*$p^2 < 0.05$, **$p^2 < 0.01$, ***$p^2 < 0.001$.

employment amongst women in the sample was secretarial work, but the in-care group were more likely to have been doing semi- or unskilled work. We asked the women how they had got on in the past with their parents. The proportion with a good relationship rises in steps, lowest in the in-care group, highest in the non-separated and intermediate in the disrupted. We have shown elsewhere (Wolkind and Zajicek, 1983) how open questions about an individual's childhood must be treated with great caution. A depressed mood can chance an individual's perception of past relationships, but in our sample it was noticeable that this applied only to those from intact families where no separation had occurred. Those women who had been in care or came from disrupted homes tended to have a view of their early relationships which was unaffected by current mood, and which, in the case of the in-care group, was predominantly negative.

In summary, the women from both our two risk groups appear to approach pregnancy at a disadvantage compared to women from intact families. Further examination, however, suggests that certain differences exist between them. It seems at this point that not only do the in-care group start from a background of even greater social and family disadvantage, but they also appear to have far less current support than do the disrupted-only group.

Pregnancy and birth

When we look at the pregnancy itself, this initial pattern we have seen continues. With certain characteristics it is the two risk groups that are similar, with others it is the in-care group that diverges dramatically from the others. Examples of this can be seen in Table 4.2(a). On the basis of asking the women whether the pregnancy had been planned and about their feelings when they first learned they were pregnant, we rated whether at the onset it was a wanted pregnancy. If the pregnancy had been unplanned *and* the woman's main feeling had been to regret being pregnant, we described this as an unwanted pregnancy. The differences between the three groups are not dramatic, but it is the women with either category of risk who were more likely not to have wanted the child, the disrupted only having the highest rate. Attitude to a pregnancy can, and does, change and in fact a striking change has occurred by the seventh month. Fewer of the disrupted-only group are now negative towards the idea of having a baby and their rate is very similar to that of the non-separated women. In contrast, the majority of the in-care women now have restrictions. When we examine two factors which might reflect how the women were responding to medical advice, the pattern is again for the in-care women to differ from the remainder. They made slightly fewer antenatal visits during pregnancy and were more likely to have continued smoking (see Chapter 11 for effects of smoking on the child).

Table 4.2   Family of origin and (a) aspects of pregnancy and (b) aspects of childbirth

	Group 1 In Care (%)	Group 2 Disrupted only (%)	Group 3 Intact (%)	χ^2 df = 2
(a)				
Start of pregnancy—				
Unwanted baby	39	47	23	7.38*
Not positive at seven months				
of pregnancy	61	32	26	10.78**
Smoking in pregnancy	68	47	39	6.60*
Definite sex of baby wanted	78	60	36	15.13***
Mean number of antenatal visits	8.6	10.7	11.2	NS
(b)				
Discharged self from hospital	26	5	3	13.70**
Birthweight 2500 g and under	13	2	7	df = 4
Birthweight 2501–3000 g	41	28	17	$\chi^2 = 11.14*$
Mean birthweight	2950 g	3215 g	3278 g	NS

*$p < 0.05$, **$p < 0.01$, ***$p < 0.001$.

We have also asked the women whether they were hoping for a baby of a particular sex. The majority of women in the non-separated group gave a reply along the lines of 'it doesn't matter so long as it's healthy'. In contrast the majority of women in both our risk groups had definite ideas on which sex they were hoping for.

Taking the eventual outcome of the birth as the start of family building one striking finding emerged. From all three groups, five children were given up for adoption or some other form of substitute care. All five were born to women in the in-care group. It is perhaps also of interest to note the three unexpected infant deaths which occurred during the first months of life. One child was born to a mother in the in-care group, the remaining two to mothers in the disrupted-only group. With birthweight, differences between the groups are also seen (Table 4.2(b)). The mean birthweights of those babies born to the non-separated and disrupted mothers are identical, that of the in-care group babies somewhat lower. A survey of British births in 1970 (Butler and Alberman, 1978), used 2500 g as the cut off point for true low birthweight, but refers to 3000 g as 'the safe threshold'. In that year 6.9 per cent of births were of babies weighing 2500 or less, 25.7 per cent of 3000 or less. As can be seen from the table the figures for both the non-separated and disrupted groups are close to this. The in-care group are significantly more likely to have babies below this threshold for safety. Very few women in our study discharged themselves from hospital against medical advice. The proportion who did was, however, considerably higher in the in-care group. Strong feelings are held by many women about the type of care they receive in hospital and it could be argued that an early discharge was not an unreasonable course of action. Though for certain individuals this might be a sign of health independence with all we know so far of the in-care group, it is difficult, irrespective of their reasons, not to feel concern for those who did leave in this way.

Motherhood—the first stages

We are now in a position to begin to examine longitudinally the early years of motherhood of the three groups selected originally on retrospective grounds. It becomes possible to examine whether the concern felt for the in-care group and possibly to a lesser extent for the disrupted only group, is justified. Four months after the birth we asked the mothers in considerable detail about their child-rearing practices; about feeding, bathing and changing. In general, with these questions, few differences were seen. An exception, however, concerned whether or not the baby was held for its feed (Table 4.3). Not holding the baby during feed time, rare in the non-separated group, and only slightly more common in the disrupted group, was the method used by a quarter of the women in the in-care group. As the only statistically significant finding noted in this entire area of questioning this could, of course, be the result of chance. Two

Table 4.3   Family of origin and child-rearing practices and maternal attitudes four months after the birth of the child

	Group 1 In Care (%)	Group 2 Disrupted Only (%)	Group 3 Intact (%)	χ^2 df = 2
Baby not held for feed	26	13	5	8.51*
Baby enjoyable *now*	41	73	70	8.75*
Baby not seen as a person	46	31	23	4.86
Baby top priority in daily routine	38	54	63	4.56
Motherhood physically tiring	42	63	66	4.4

*$p < 0.05$.

points make us think this is not so. First, Frommer and O'Shea (1973a) in their study of young mothers, found that women from broken homes were more likely to feed their babies by propping the bottle on a pillow. Of considerable interest are certain findings from the observational side of our own study. Mention was made of the fact that as well as interviewing our subjects we also used direct observations throughout the longitudinal study. These were carried out on a sub-sample of women chosen from all our various groups. Approximately one-half of the women in each of our three groups were included in this observational study. Workers knowing nothing of the interview data observed the mothers and babies in their own homes shortly after each four-month interview was completed. Continuous-event recording was used. Amongst items recorded were the frequencies of maternal touch and vocalization. Full details of the methods and results can be found in Hall *et al.* (1979). Maternal activities, such as physical contact with the baby or vocalizations, were highest in the non-separated group, intermediate in the disrupted-only group and lowest and indeed very low in the in-care group. Though in general there is little doubt that characteristics of the baby strongly influence the amount of mother–infant interaction (e.g. Bell, 1974), in this case the differences could not be explained in this way. It does seem that a woman's early experiences were associated with the amount of her interaction with her 4-month-old infant.

The general trend of this argument is also supported by findings from a different type of question, that tapping the women's attitude to their babies and to being a mother. We must here be particularly cautious as for most of these questions differences between the groups were comparatively small. Those that were larger all point, however, in the same direction (Table 4.3). With these, it is again the in-care group that stands out. They were significantly less likely to find the four-month stage particularly enjoyable; they were either looking forward to the child being older or back to when the baby had just been born. Slightly fewer of them at four months could really see the baby as a person.

They were less likely to put the baby first in their list of priorities as they planned their day. Interestingly, fewer of them found motherhood physically tiring. One can speculate on whether this was because of their lower level of interaction with their babies! All these findings must clearly be seen as suggestive rather than conclusive. Perhaps the most crucial measure of infant–mother relationships at this early stage is a mother's sensitivity to her baby's signals (Ainsworth, 1982) a concept we have not measured directly. It seems not unreasonable, however, to suggest that the general picture could well be of the in-care women, as a group, being the least cued in to the needs of a young baby. The disrupted group are of considerable interest. Despite sharing certain important characteristics with the in-care group, they have by this stage taken up an intermediate position, if anything appearing more similar to the non-separated group. We can turn now to examine longitudinally two areas of considerable significance to family life.

Mothers' mental health and marriage

Two of the most detailed measures used during our study are an assessment of the psychiatric state of the women and of the quality of their marriage. An assessment of the women's pre-pregnancy psychiatric state was made by combining the results of a retrospective questionnaire asking about earlier symptoms with information on whether help had ever been sought for these or for similar difficulties. At all other stages a formal mental-state examination was completed, on the basis of which the woman was described as having no disorder, one with significant symptoms but no impairment (a dubious disorder) and one with both symptoms and impairment (a definite disorder). Any women with either a dubious or a definite disorder was given a clinical diagnosis; in the majority of cases this was a picture of depression with associated anxiety. In all cases, where symptoms were present, the details were discussed with the psychiatrist in the team before the final rating was made. To illustrate the type of disorder seen it is useful to give an example. Mrs A. was given a rating of a definite disorder forty-two months after the birth of her first child. The diagnosis was depression with anxiety. During the three months before the interview Mrs A's appetite had been poor. It varied a great deal but there had been weeks when she picked at food. She thought she had lost weight but was not sure. Almost every night she found it difficult to get off to sleep, lying awake for at least 2 hours. She had tried going to bed later but the same thing happened. She felt tired most of the day, she would put off jobs that needed to be done, but would feel guilty about this. She worried a great deal, mostly about her marriage which was in a bad state. She could, however, stop worrying when she wanted to, for example if there was a good television programme on. She was very frightened of the dark and, if alone, would break out into a sweat and would feel her heart beating. As far back as she could remember she had felt like this and had tried to organize her life so that she would never be alone at night. About twice a week she had similar feelings when alone during the day. She would lie on her bed for an hour until it passed. Every week she had at least two days in which she felt deeply depressed. This would last all day and she would just want to be alone. She had no time for her child on those days and would snap at her husband. She could not shake off the feeling. She used to cry a lot but this had stopped—'I think I'm past crying'. She had frequent thoughts, not only on the depressed days, about whether life was worth living, but she thought it unlikely she would ever do anything 'silly'. She could spend hours thinking of how nice it would be to live alone on a desert island. Mrs A. had been given a rating of a definite disorder by different interviewers at four and twenty-seven months after the birth and a dubious disorder (symptoms, but no impairment of activities) at fourteen months.

The rate of definite disorder at the various stages of the study for the women in all three groups is shown in Figure 4.1. As the pre-pregnancy measure involved a different form of assessment its continuity with later stages has not been noted. For each the pattern is remarkably similar, a steady decline from pregnancy to twenty-seven months, then a relatively sharp rise at forty-two months. The level at which the pattern is expressed is very similar for the women from the non-separated and disrupted groups, but those in the in-care group have at all stages a constantly higher rate. This difference is significant before pregnancy, and at four and twenty-seven months post partum ($\chi^2 = 7.59$, 6.09, 7.23 respectively, df = 2).

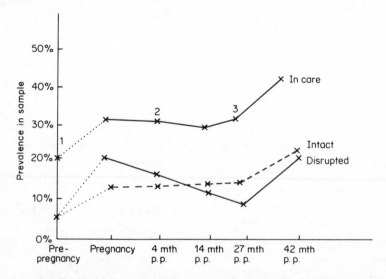

Fig. 4.1   Family of origin and prevalence of definite psychiatric disorder before and during pregnancy and 4, 14, 27 and 24 months after birth of first child. (1) $X^2 = 7.59$; (2) $\chi^2 = 6.09$; (3) $\chi^2 = 7.23$; d or f = 2; $P = <0.05$. (Note: The pre-pregnancy measure of psychiatric disorder was obtained retrospectively and direct comparisons of rate with later measures are not possible

For an assessment of the marriage we used the technique described by Quinton *et al.* (1976). The assessment was made on those who were married or cohabiting with either the father of the child or any other man who had been living with the woman for at least three months. Though many of the women had been alone at the beginning of the study, only a small minority, under 10 per cent in all three groups, were unmarried by forty-two months. A difficulty with this part of the interview was that it could not be completed if the husband was present. This occurred in approximately a quarter of cases. It does not, therefore, seem justified to submit the findings to formal statistical analysis but the pattern is so marked it seems well worth reporting. The full marriage rating was made on three occasions, at fourteen, twenty-seven and forty-two months after the birth. At fourteen months a wide range was seen, good marriages were reported for 70 per cent of the non-separated, 40 per cent of the disrupted, but only 10 per cent for the in-care group. At twenty-seven months the figures were 68 per cent, 53 per cent and 25 per cent. At forty-two months 62 per cent, 50 per cent and 20 per cent. Once again the disrupted and non-separated groups have approached one another leaving the in-care women in a position of obvious disadvantage.

The children

Certain aspects of the child have been touched upon previously, namely the lower birthweight of those born to the in-care mothers and the giving up of five children by those mothers. In addition, work from the observational sub-sample has shown that the children from both the in-care and disrupted groups were significantly below those from the non-separated group in language development (Pawlby and Hall, 1980). The main measure we will consider here, however, is the children's behaviour at forty-two months. To assess this we used the instrument designed by Richman and Graham (1971) for 3 year olds. The presence of various problem behaviour such as sleeping problems or temper tantrums is enquired about and, if present, the severity is rated. If the item is absent or mild, 0 is given, if significant but not severe 1 and if severe 2. Though not reaching statistical significance a marked trend across the three groups was seen with means of 7.04, 6.46 and 5.81 for groups 3, 2 and 1 respectively. Perhaps more important than the mean score is the cut-off point of 10 used with the scale. Scores over this are highly suggestive of behavioural disturbance. In the same order the proportion above this in each group are 31 per cent, 23 per cent and 13 per cent. Though these differences do not reach formal statistical significance, the ordering of the groups is perhaps as anticipated.

A further area of importance concerns the physical health of the children. At all stages the in-care children were more likely than those in the other two groups to have accidents requiring medical attention or to need hospital admission. The differences were not, however, very great except at fourteen months after the birth. No fewer than 52 per cent of the in-care children had been admitted by that time as opposed to 21 per cent of the disrupted and 19 per cent of the non-separated group. This difference was significant ($\chi^2 = 11.05$, df $= 2$, $p < 0.01$). For accidents the figures were 58 per cent, 23 per cent and 28 per cent ($\chi = 9.79$, df $= 2$, $p < 0.01$).

At this stage we can once again summarize the findings to date. The majority of the women from the non-separated group and their children do relatively well on all measures. Those from 'disrupted-only' families remain in an intermediate position, on most measures they eventually resemble the intact group more than they do those who had been in care. This last group do badly, not only in comparison to the other two, but also in absolute terms. The rates of a variety of psychological and social difficulties point to a distressingly high level of morbidity and suggest to us that the children of the in-care women must be viewed as highly vulnerable even if their rates of disturbance are not that high at forty-two months. These high rates of problems were reflected by subjective measures completed by the interviewers after each interview. The interviewers coded the degree of anxiety they subjectively felt for the future of the family. At every stage the in-care group were by far the most likely to cause concern. As an example, at forty-two months after the birth some concern was felt for 40 per cent of the non-separated and 41 per cent of the disrupted group but for 92 per cent of the in-care group. Severe concern was felt in 11 per cent, 12 per cent and 35 per cent of the cases. We need now to turn to our data to see if we can understand the reasons for these findings. Why do the in-care group do so badly and why do the disrupted group, starting from a point of apparent disadvantage, end up doing relatively well?

The reasons

In trying to explain our findings certain possibilities cannot be examined directly with the type of data we have collected. It could be argued that the poor outcome of the in-care group is due to a genetic effect; that those in the population with certain adverse hereditary traits are the ones most likely to go into care. Equally a physical or nutritional hypothesis could be put forward. Women whose children are admitted to care are, on average, 4 inches below the mean height of all women (Mapstone, 1969). Early nutritional deprivation of both mother and child could lead to each in turn having an impaired ability to cope with social relationships and the subtle demands of family life. It is not possible to explore these ideas in more detail here, but although the interaction between genetic and nutritional factors and the environment are of major importance in certain areas of behaviour there is little to implicate them in the areas we have been examining. Of far greater importance are psychological and social factors (for reviews see Rutter and Madge, 1976; Sameroff and Chandler, 1975;

Rutter, 1980). It is through an examination of these factors that we may find some possible reasons for the different outcomes of our two groups.

In the introduction to the chapter we referred to the emphasis placed by many workers on the way childhood experiences act as the foundation for future social development. It was these ideas that led us to use measures of childhood as one way of selecting groups at risk. There is little doubt that as far as in-care status goes, a childhood experience has proved to have considerable predictive value. However, finding an association between being admitted to care and having difficulties in early adult life does not necessarily imply a causal relationship. Two separate issues need to be examined. First, are the admission to care and the experiences while in care the crucial elements or are they merely indices of certain other more important early experiences? Secondly, do the childhood experiences, whatever they are, irreversibly affect the individual's personality or way of functioning in early life and lead directly to the adult problems, or could other rather different processes be involved? When we examine the first question the evidence allows us to come to a clear answer. Virtually all studies of children in care show them to have high rates of psychiatric disorder (e.g. Wolkind, 1974; Yule and Raynes, 1974). Equally, follow-up studies have demonstrated high rates of difficulties amongst both children (Wolkind and Rutter, 1973) and adults (Minty, 1981) who had been discharged from care. There is evidence that being brought up from birth in residential care does lead to some abnormalities in social functioning (Dixon, 1980). This applies even to a limited extent to children later removed from care and brought up in a totally different environment (Tizard, 1977 — see also Chapter 8 this volume). This type of upbringing is, however, experienced by only a small minority of children admitted to care. The majority are admitted for the first time after the toddler stage. Most experience several admissions and discharges back to their original families. For many, the first admission does not occur until adolescence. In looking at the overall data collected on these women and their families the picture that emerges is of an admission being one episode in a generally disharmonious and unsettled childhood. Perhaps, not surprisingly, the parents of children admitted to care are far more likely than the average to be having a variety of inter-personal difficulties (Schaffer and Schaffer, 1968; Wolkind and Rutter, 1973). The notion that it is this overall childhood experience of which having been in care was just one part, rather than the admission itself which relates to disturbance during childhood is supported by, for example, the apparently paradoxical finding that amongst those admitted the *longer* the child remains in care the lower its chance of having difficulties (Conway, 1957; Minty, 1982). It seems that by using an admission to care as a criterion for selecting a risk group, we were using an index of a certain extreme type of unsettled childhood. This can be well seen by briefly examining the descriptions of their childhoods given by the mothers in our in-care group.

They described a great variety of experiences. Being in care ranged from a month in an assessment centre to a whole childhood in a long-stay home; from a single short placement in a foster home to a 'career' spanning various children's homes, an approved school and a hostel. The age at entry ranged from 6 weeks to 15 years. The patterns of admission and the quality of care varied so greatly that no simple classification is possible. One woman was admitted only once following her mother's confinement. She went on to amplify this: 'Mum wasn't married when she had me. She got married when I was one, not to my father. The marriage broke up when I was four. She married him for me, and she left him for me, because he was nice to the boys but not to me.' Relationships with her mother deteriorated over the years until at the age of 17 years she was thrown out of her home because she would not give up her 'undesirable' boyfriend. As well as any, this woman's history demonstrates how, for the majority, behind even one short admission for an apparently benign reason lies a history of long-standing difficulties in relationships and of unresolved family conflicts. Each woman's history was unique both in terms of the events themselves and in her feelings about them. Our numbers are clearly too small to allow us to even begin to systematically examine any differential effects, but no one type of admission to care stands out as being more important than any other.

The second question is perhaps even more complex. Until the 1970s the weight of opinion would have been that the early experiences were having a direct and possibly irreversible effect on the child's developing personality. During the 1970s a growing body of evidence made this view far less tenable. In particular it became clear that with a change of environment many individuals could recover from even the most extreme form of deprivation and respond to more positive experiences offered to them (for reviews see Rutter, 1972; Clarke and Clarke, 1976; Chapters 8, 14 and 15 this volume). It could be that the continuity of difficulties in our in-care group is due, not to inevitable internal 'psychic damage', but rather to a continuity of difficulties in the environment. It could be that the 'disrupted only' group are for various reasons more able to escape from these difficulties, the in-care group much less so. It seems likely that unless we are dealing with a total change of environment such as occurs in adoption, attempts to differentiate the effects of the severity of the early deprivation from those of the continuing environmental difficulties will not be easy. We shall attempt to demonstrate that the more adverse the early experiences the more likely it seems that the women will have to face continuing social difficulties which will do little to increase their confidence in themselves and their ability to cope with their children. In looking at a woman's needs around the time of the birth of a first child, attachment theory can be a useful aid (Parkes and Stevenson-Hinde, 1982). Attachment has been applied to relationships which can help allay anxiety and can survive a separation. Originally used to describe the bonds established between a young child and its caretaker, it can also be a useful concept when looking at relationships between adults (Weiss, 1982).

It would seem reasonable to assume that a prime need for a young mother is the presence of someone she can have a relationship with and who can act as an attachment figure. On the whole, as we described above, originally unmarried mothers and their children seemingly fare no worse in the early years than those who are married. It has, however, been found that the exception are those who lack the presence and availability of any other adult (Kellam *et al.*, 1977). The vulnerability of young mothers to depression is increased in the absence of a spouse who can act as a confidante (Brown and Harris, 1978). We have already described marital relationships in our sample. In our study yet another key relationship may be that between the young woman and her own mother. Twenty-five years ago Young and Willmott (1957) working in the same borough, described the importance in family life of the maternal grandmother. More recently Fischer (1981) has described how the mother–daughter relationship becomes both strengthened and redefined at the birth of the first grandchild. As well as looking at the childhood experiences of the in-care and disrupted-only women we need also to look at more recent and current relationships in trying to explain the difference in outcome between the two groups.

We can start this process with a re-examination of Table 4.1. It is clear that the majority of the disrupted-only group are in regular contact with their own parents and get on well with them. The proportion from the non-separated and disrupted groups seeing their parents at least weekly is virtually identical to that found by Young and Wilmot in 1957. This pattern of contact showed only a slight fall over the course of the study. Despite many of the families in the study moving out of the borough, at forty-two months after the birth, 70 per cent of the non-separated and 61 per cent of the disrupted were still seeing the maternal grandmother weekly or more often. Only 30 per cent of the in-care group still had this degree of contact by that time. The originally poor relationships in the family of origin clearly are of major importance. They leave the in-care women without the support of their families during these crucial years. They may well also lay the seeds for various other problems that could give them little chance of succeeding. The women from this group were more likely to have moved or drifted into our study borough (Table 4.1). With a declining population it is on the whole a difficult district to move into unless there is little alternative and one is unable to afford adequate facilities. We can see these young women, having lost contact with or moving away from, their families as fast as possible, becoming pregnant and drifting into unsatisfactory marriages. Psychological difficulties will not be the only problems caused by this pattern. It could be extremely difficult for a young woman with a poor education and no family help to get into a satisfactory financial and housing position. The subsequent hardship would, of course, reinforce the psychological difficulties. The social and economic situation of the women in the various groups is examined in Table 4.4.

Table 4.4   Family of origin and social and financial circumstances during the study

	Group 1 In Care (%)	Group 2 Disrupted Only (%)	Group 3 Intact (%)	χ^2 df = 2
Early pregnancy—housing problems	45	33	19	8.06*
42 months post partum— dissatisfaction with housing	82	59	52	6.14*
Pregnancy—financial worries	50	32	21	6.75*
4 months post partum— owns washing machine	33	54	54	2.90
27 months post partum— access to car	30	63	58	6.70*
27 months post partum— has a telephone	13	40	56	12.60**

*$p<0.05$, **$p<0.01$.

We do not have detailed information on the financial situation of the women and their families but have used the possession of a car or telephone as indirect measures. We felt that possession of a washing machine was a factor which could make a great impact on the life of a woman caring for a young baby. Actual housing condition and the woman's satisfaction with this were recorded at all stages of the study. The material and housing disadvantage of the in-care group is seen throughout the study. At first the disrupted group are intermediate, worse off than the non-separated, but not as badly off as the in-care group. As the study continues, they increasingly resemble the non-separated group. In contrast, life is clearly a considerable struggle for the in-care group. The lack of consistent support from families of origin or husbands and the social and

Table 4.5   Family of origin and views of relationship between childhood experiences and later mothering capacities

	Group 1 In Care (%)	Group 2 Disrupted Only (%)	Group 3 Intact (%)	χ^2 df = 2
Close to mother in childhood	50	46	77	11.38**
Would want child to have similar upbringing as self	30	45	63	9.30**
Own experiences of being mothered a positive example for mothering	10	41	44	8.40*
Mother's child-rearing a reaction against own experiences	48	22	24	5.34

*$p<0.05$, **$p<0.01$.

financial problems would make it difficult for anyone to develop a self image as a competent mother. The in-care group are also the least likely to have any positive 'internal image' on which they can build (Table 4.5).

At forty-two months after the birth we tried to understand what early influences might have influenced the way the women were feeling as mothers. We had asked in pregnancy about which parent they had been close to and at forty-two months whether any experiences they had had were consciously affecting how they treated their children. The in-care women were least likely to have felt close to their mothers. They wanted their children to have a different childhood to that of their own and were very unlikely to be able to use their own experiences as a model of how to mother and indeed many were actually trying to use these as a negative model to be avoided. With the financial and housing problems described above it is not hard to see how they could have only a poor chance of satisfactorily coping with the complicated tasks of psychological readjustment associated with becoming a parent. With the disrupted group, the supportive contact with their own families could well have given them the breathing space they needed to adapt to their new rôles as mothers, develop satisfactory relationships with potential husbands and begin to cope. To conclude our presentation of findings we can examine whether this model holds by looking at differences within our in-care group.

Table 4.6   Women who had been in care. Factors relating to outcome for child

	Good Outcome $n = 15$ (%)	Poor Outcome $n = 14$ (%)	χ^2 df = 1
Teenager at conception	60	64	NS
Pregnancy not wanted	54	64	NS
Brought up in Study Borough	67	29	4.21*
Close to mother in childhood	64	11	5.69*

*$p < 0.05$.

In terms of the child as part of the mother's family we can divide our in-care group into two (Table 4.6). At forty-two months fourteen of the children had either high behaviour scores or were being cared for by someone else. In fifteen cases the child was being looked after by its mother and had a BSQ score of under 10. The mothers of these two groups of children are compared in Table 4.6. The mothers of both were predominantly teenagers, and equally likely to have not wanted the pregnancy. The mothers of those in the better outcome group were, however, much more likely to have reported being close to their own mothers during childhood and to have been brought up in the borough in which they were living at the time of the study. This again seems to implicate the rôle of the combination of good earlier relationships and continuing support. As further confirmation of the importance of this, a relationship has been found in our *random sample of mothers* (i.e. mainly from intact homes), between a high child BSQ at forty-two months and evidence of strain with the maternal grandmother (Ghodsian *et al.*, 1984).

In this chapter we have followed the progress over four years of three groups of women selected on the basis of certain childhood experiences. In comparing them we have, of course, been talking of probabilities or group averages. Some of the women from intact families have done badly as have their children. Some, but unfortunately relatively few of the in-care women, have done well. Though the in-care group is small, comprising only 6 per cent of those in our original sampling frame, they do make a significant contribution to the level of morbidity within the population. The data presented in the tables tells a sparse story, we also had an opportunity in our study to examine individual case histories. In looking at these histories it seemed us that the early and later experiences are inexorably intertwined. It confirmed our view that many of the poor outcome measures such as maternal depression or a bad marriage found in the in-care group can best be explained not by the direct effects of the deprived childhood as such, but rather by the inadequate material and limited social experiences open to them because of that childhood. This is not merely a theoretical point, but one of very considerable practical importance. It does suggest strongly that there is no inevitability about the process; no automatic cycle of deprivation with a passing on of bad experiences from one generation to another. Perhaps the greatest tragedy is that the one thing that our in-care group have in common is that at some time in their lives they have been the responsibility of local authority professionals. Often the problems of the families did not seem to be unsurmountable, the parents often had a commitment to the child and were conscious of the need for help. With hindsight we were often led to ask whether more could not have been done. As a research team, for many cases in the in-care group, we had to examine our consciences and question whether we should have changed our rôles. In practice, with the resources available to us, there was little we could offer. As the children got older the interlocking problems seemed so great that it is hard to see how they could easily be disentangled. Often despite many dealings with workers from statutory agencies, no one seemed to have stopped and asked the mothers what they wanted and how they wished to be helped.

We also had to ask ourselves whether individual help must not be combined with more fundamental changes in society itself. In following our in-care group over a brief but crucial period of their lives, though some have done well, we have been at times deeply distressed by the quality of the life many have been experiencing and made aware of a potential, unused and constantly frustrated.

We feel that the longitudinal approach has enabled us to look beyond a simple association. These findings have enabled us to formulate hypotheses about differences we may find at later stages amongst the children born to the in-care mothers. Of equal, if not greater, importance have been the findings from our other risk group, the disrupted-only women. The far more optimistic outcome here points to the other side of the coin. The protective factors missing for the in-care group can, if present, provide an environment which can allow the individual to cope with any residual effects of earlier difficulties. We feel that this body of longitudinal data has provided us with a variety of ideas for early intervention. The data suggests there is need for these. They should be attempted and evaluated.

REFERENCES

Ainsworth, M. D. S. (1982). Attachment, retrospect and prospect, in *The Place of Attachment in Human Behavior* (Eds C. M. Parkes and J. Stevenson-Hinde), Basic Books, New York.

Bell, R. Q. (1974). Contributions of human infants to care giving and social interaction, in *The Effect of the Infant on its Caregiver* (Eds M. Lewis and L. A. Rosenblum), Wiley, London.

Brown, G. W. and Harris, T. (1978). *Social Origins of Depression: A Study of Psychiatric Disorder in Women*, Tavistock, London.

Butler, N. R. and Alberman, E. D. (Eds) (1978). *Perinatal Problems, Vol. 2. Obstetric Care*, National Birthday Fund, London.

Clarke, A. M. and Clarke, A. D. M. (1976). *Early Experience: Myth and Evidence*, Open Books, London.

Coleman, J., Burtenshaw, W., Pond, D. A. and Rothwell, B. (1977). Psychological Problems of Pre-School children in an inner urban area, *Brit. J. Psychiat.* 131, 623–630.

Conway, E. S. (1957). The institutional care of children: a history. Unpublished PhD thesis, University of London.

Deutsch, H. (1947). *The Psychology of Women*, Grune and Stratton, New York.

Dixon, P. (1980). Quoted in Rutter, M. Attachment and the development of social relationship, in *Scientific Foundations of Developmental Psychiatry* (Ed. M. Rutter), Heinemann, London.

Fischer, L. R. (1981). Transitions in the mother–daughter relationship, *J. of Marriage and the Family* 43, 613–622.

Frommer, E. A. and O'Shea, G. (1973a). Antenatal identification of women liable to have problems in managing their infants, *Brit. J. Psychiat.* 123, 149–156.

Frommer, E. A. and O'Shea, G. (1973b). The importance of childhood experience in relation to problems of marriage and family-building, *Brit. J. Psychiat.* 123, 157–160.

Ghodsian, M., Zajicek, E., Wolkind, S. (1984). A longitudinal study of maternal depression and child behaviour problems. *J. Child Psychol. Psychiat.* 25, 97–109.

Graham, P. J. (1978). *Epidemiological Approaches in Child Psychiatry*, Academic Press, London.

Graham, P. and Rutter, M. (1973). Psychiatric disorder in the young adolescent: a follow-up study, *Proc. Roy. Soc. Med.* 66, 1226–1229.

Hall, F., Pawlby, S. J. and Wolkind, S. N. (1979). Early life experiences and later mothering behaviour: a study of mothers and their 20-week-old babies, in *The First Year of Life* (Eds D. Shaffer and J. F. Dunn), Wiley, Chichester.

Hustoin-Stein, A. and Higgins-Trenk, A. (1978). Development of female role orientations, in *Life-Span Development and Behaviour*, vol. 1. (Ed. P. B. Baltes), Academic Press, London.

Kellam, S. G., Ensminger, M. E. and Turner, R. J. (1977). Family structure and the mental health of children, *Arch. Gen. Psychiat.* **34**, 1012–1022.

Kezur, D. (1978). The development of maternal attachment. *Smith College Studies in Social Work* **48**, 183–208.

Kruk, S. and Wolkind, S. N. (1982). A longitudinal study of single mothers and their children, in *Familial Processes in Transmitted Deprivation* (Ed. N. Madge), Heinemann, London.

Lynch, M. A., Roberts, J. and Gordon, M. (1976). Child abuse: Early warning in the maternity hospital, *Develop. Med. Child Neurol.*, **18**, 759–766.

Mapstone, E. (1969). Children in care, *Concern*, **3**, 23–28.

Melges, F. T. (1968). Postpartum psychiatric syndromes, *Psychosom. Med.* **30**, 95–108.

Minty, E. B. (1981). Unpublished MSc degree, University of Manchester.

Parkes, C. M. and Stevenson-Hinde, J. (Eds) (1982). *The Place of Attachment in Human Behavior*, New York, Basic Books.

Pawlby, S. J. and Hall, F. (1980). Early interaction and later language development in children whose mothers come from disrupted families of origin, in *High Risk Infants and Children: Adult and Peer Interaction* (Eds T. Field, S. Golberg, D. Stern and A. Sostek), Academic Press, New York.

Quinton, D., Rutter, M. and Rowlands, O. (1976). An evaluation of an interview assessment of marriage, *Psychol. Med.* **6**, 577–586.

Richman, N. and Graham, P. J. (1971). A behavioural screening questionnaire for use with three-year-old children, *J. Child Psychol. Psychiat.* **12**, 5–30.

Rutter, M. (1972). *Maternal Deprivation Re-assessed*, Penguin, Harmondsworth.

Rutter, M. (1980). Attachment and the development of social relationships, in *Scientific Foundations of Developmental Psychiatry* (Ed. M. Rutter), Heinemann, London.

Rutter, M. and Madge, N. (1976). *Cycles of Disadvantage*, Heinemann, London.

Sameroff, A. J. and Chandler, M. J. (1975). Reproductive risk and the continuum of caretaking casualty, in *Review of Child Development Research*, Vol. 4., (Eds F. D. Horowitz, M. Hetherington, S. Scarr-Salapatek and G. Siegel), University of Chicago Press, Chicago.

Schaffer, H. R. and Schaffer, E. B. (1968). *Child Care and the Family*, Occasional Papers in Social Administration, No. 25, G. Bell and Sons, London.

Tizard, B. (1977). *Adoption: A Second Chance*, Open Books, London.

Weiss, R. (1982). Attachment in adult life, in *The Place of Attachment in Human Behavior*, (Eds C. M. Parkes and J. Stevenson-Hinds), Basic Books, New York.

Wolkind, S. N. (1974). The components of affectionless psychopathy in institutional children, *J. Child Psychol. Psychiat.* **15**, 215–220.

Wolkind, S. N., Kruk, S. and Chaves, L. (1976). Childhood separation experiences and psychosocial status in primiparous women: preliminary findings. *Brit. J. Psychiat.* **128**, 391–396.

Wolkind, S. N. and Rutter, M. (1973). Children who have been 'in care' — an epidemiological study, *J. Child Psychol. Psychiat.* **14**, 97–105.

Wolkind, S. N. and Zajicek, E. (1983). Adult psychiatric disorder and childhood experiences: The validity of retrospective recall. *Brit. J. Psychiat.* **143**, 188–191.

Young, M. and Willmott, P. (1957). *Family and Kinship in East London*, London, Routledge and Kegan Paul.

Yule, W. and Raynes, N. (1974). Behavioural characteristics of children in residential care, *J. Child Psychol. Psychiat.* **13**, 249–258.

Zigler, E. and Valentine, J. (1979). *Project Head Start: A Legacy of the War on Poverty*, The Free Press, New York.

Longitudinal Studies in Child Psychology and Psychiatry
Edited by A. R. Nicol
© 1985 John Wiley and Sons Ltd.

Chapter 5

Sex Difference in Outcome of Pre-school Behaviour Problems

N. Richman, J. Stevenson and P. Graham

INTRODUCTION

Clinical experience suggests that disorders in childhood often have their roots in earlier years. On the other hand one might predict that disorder occurring in the pre-school child need not be significantly associated with later problems, because the young child is changing rapidly and is likely to be very sensitive to maturational and environmental influences. The professional confronted with difficulties in the pre-school child needs to know the likely outcome later on if he is to make sensible decisions about young children. The necessary data can only be gathered in longitudinal studies.

Although there have been studied looking at individual symptoms (McFarlane *et al.*, 1954), with notable exceptions investigations into the persistence of young children's behaviour difficulties are rare, partly because there are substantial difficulties in defining behaviour disorder at this age (Minde and Minde, 1977; Kohn and Rosman, 1973; Earls and Richman, 1980b). Our follow-up study of children from 3 to 8 years enabled us to look at the natural history of pre-school disorders. We attempted to discover whether children who had problems in the pre-school period were more likely to have them at school age, and whether it was possible to identify factors indicating that a problem would continue or a new one develop *de novo*. We also looked at whether certain behaviours or symptoms were particularly relevant to outcome since in older children the persistence of problems seems to depend partly on their nature. Children showing disorders of conduct or antisocial behaviour are more likely to have difficulties in adulthood than those with neurotic disorder (Robins, 1966; Morris *et al.*, 1954).

METHOD

We decided to begin our study with 3 year olds since we thought that by this age we would be able to obtain reliable and valid methods for assessing the

At 3 years
First stage   Screening interview
($n = 705$)   Behaviour Screening Questionnaire (BSQ)

Second stage   Social interview
(Controls = 101)   Psychological assessment
(Problems = 101)

At 4 years
(Controls = 91)   Social interview
(Problems = 94)   Behaviour Screening Questionnaire (BSQ)
                               Psychological assessment

At 8 years
(Controls = 91)   Social interview
(Problems = 94)   Psychological assessment

Fig. 5.1   Plan of survey

children's behaviour and development. We examined the outcome after one year when the children were 4 years old and after five years when they were aged 8. The one-year follow-up and full details of the study are given in Richman *et al.* (1982) (Figure 5.1).

The study was carried out in Waltham Forest, an Outer London borough. This was because in this borough there was already a computerized register of families with children under 5 years, which appeared to give practically complete coverage of the pre-school population (Richman and Tupling, 1974). This enabled us to draw a random one-in-four sample which was representative of the total population of 3 year olds living in the borough. It turned out that the borough had other advantages. It was fairly representative of the country as a whole in terms of social class, and there was less mobility than in Inner London boroughs. Although there were variations in housing and social amenities, in general the population was rather homogeneous, being mainly social class III manual and III non-manual. There were more families living in high-rise blocks than in other parts of the country.

Approximately 1000 names of 3 year olds were drawn from the register in a one-in-four random sample over a twelve-month period, and we were able to interview parents of 828 children; 9 per cent were untraced and there were 3 per cent refusals (Richman *et al.*, 1975). Approximately 700 of these children were born to indigenous parents, and the findings discussed will be confined to these children; the children of immigrant parents were analysed separately (Earls and Richman, 1980a).

The initial part of the study was in two stages. In the first stage there was an interview with the parent, usually the mother, using a behaviour-screening questionnaire to decide whether the child had a behaviour problem or not. The questionnaire covers twelve items of behaviour which are rated 0, 1, or 2, depending on the severity of the behaviour difficulty. For instance, a child who takes an hour to settle to sleep or wakes three or more nights a week is rated 2 for sleeping difficulty. Scores for each item are added to give a maximum score of 24. A score of 10 or more on the behaviour-screening questionnaire is used as the cut-off point to indicate that a child is at risk of having a behaviour problem. The screening questionnaire and the cut-off point have been validated using clinic and non-clinic populations (Richman and Graham, 1971). The problem group—101 children—scored above the cut-off point. These were matched by sex and social class, with 101 children scoring below the cut-off point—the control group. A second interview with the parents and a developmental assessment by a psychologist blind to the behavioural state of the child formed the second stage. Summary ratings based on predetermined clinical criteria were made of the severity of the child's behavioural disturbance, the marital relationship, parental mental health, parental warmth and criticism to the child and family stress. All these measures were repeated when the child was 4 and 8 years old and in addition Rutter behaviour questionnaires were completed by parents and teachers (Rutter, 1967; Rutter *et al.*, 1970), and reading, spelling, and verbal and performance abilities were assessed by the same psychologist who saw them at 3 years. Interviews at each age were nearly always by different interviewers so that ratings were independent and not contaminated by previous information. At 3 years we did not categorize the type of disorder shown by the child; at 8 years we felt it was possible to make a more refined diagnosis, and all but three of the children with the problems were diagnosed as having either a neurotic or a conduct disorder. In keeping with other studies, those with mixed disorder were grouped with conduct disorder. Ninety-four children from the behaviour problem group and ninety-one from the control group were seen at ages 3, 4 and 8 years and data on these 198 children is presented here.

Although we used a clinical descriptive approach to describe the problems shown by these children this does not imply that we think they necessarily had a psychiatric disease. Their behaviour was problematic to themselves or their family and a focus of stress or tension within the family, but the nature of these problems and their meaning in the family context need further elucidation.

PREVALENCE OF DISTURBANCE

Taking into account the false negatives and false positives of our screening instrument, we estimated that at 3 years 7 per cent of the children had marked problems, and 14 per cent had mild problems. There were no significant social-class differences in boys, but girls from manual families were more likely to have behaviour problems than those from non-manual families. Boys were more likely to be described as restless, to have sphincter problems, and to show developmental delay, but the prevalence of disorder did not differ significantly between the sexes although boys tended to have slightly more problems (Richman *et al.*, 1975).

Factors associated with behaviour problems at 3 years were found in the child, the family and the environment. Compared with the control group the children with behaviour problems were more likely to have delayed language development and scored lower on neurodevelopmental testing; their families showed more tension as measured by marital disharmony, high maternal criticism and low maternal warmth, and had more stresses, for instance more financial problems and housing difficulties such as overcrowding or living in high-rise blocks. Rates of maternal depression were high in both problem and control groups but were higher in the problem group (Richman, 1977).

OUTCOME AT EIGHT YEARS

Children from the problem group continued to have more problems at 8 years. The clinical rating, the parent and teacher behaviour questionnaires, and the psychological measures all showed differences between the two groups, with significantly more marked problems in the problem group (Table 5.1). The difference between the two groups is least on the teacher questionnaire; as other studies have found, children who are difficult at home are not necessarily so at school, and our original identification of a problem used information about the child's behaviour at home.

Table 5.1   Percentage with behavioural deviance, reading retardation and low IQ in behaviour problem and control groups at 8 years

Deviant on	Controls (91)	Problem group (94)	$p*$
Teacher questionnaire	24	39	0.06**
Parent questionnaire	20	43	0.002**
Overall clinical rating of problem	22	62	0.0001***
Low full scale IQ	2.2	10.8	0.05**
Mild reading backwardness	14.3	29.0	0.05**

*significance level of chi-square test, **df = 1, ***df = 2.

Few of the families received any active intervention, these were mainly in the problem group and this could not have affected the outcome significantly. All the children but one who were lost to follow-up had emigrated. They did not differ significantly from the total group, and their loss is also unlikely to have affected the findings.

INDICATORS OF OUTCOME

We next turn to examine factors associated with good or poor outcome. We analysed a large number of variables and by chance some are bound to show

Table 5.2   Estimated rates of disturbance at 3 and 8 years

Prevalence	Boys (%)	Girls (%)	Ratio
At 3	17.7	11.4	1.5:1
At 8	34.3	20.5	1.7:1
By persistence	(12.9)	(5.4)	2.4:1
By production	(21.4)	(15.1)	1.4:1

significant associations, however, the consistency and meaningfulness of our findings does give them weight.

The sex of the child was a striking indicator of outcome. It will be remembered that at 3 years there were no significant differences in rates of disorder between the sexes. Table 5.2 shows that at 8 years boys had significantly more problems, and the ratio of disorder between boys and girls is beginning to approach that found in older children.

The ratio at which new disorders have developed in boys compared with girls (1.4:1) is similar to that at 3 years (1.5:1) but the old disorders are persisting much more commonly in boys than girls at nearly two-and-a-half times the rate.

Not only does the rate of disorder now differ between the sexes but also the type of disorder shown (Table 5.3). The rate of conduct disorder is much higher in boys than in girls whereas the rate of neurotic disorder are approximately the same, a finding similar to that in older children (Rutter *et al.*, 1970). Although fewer problems are shown in the control group the differences between the sex in rates and types of disorder are still seen (Table 5.3).

How can we explain this differential outcome? Is it because boys and girls were different to start with, because they were faced with differing stresses, or because they were sensitive to different factors? We know that at 3 years the

Table 5.3   Rates and types of disorders at 8 years in boys and girls from problem and control groups

	Boys (%)	Girls (%)	p*
Problem group (51 boys; 41 girls)			
No problem	28	54	
Antisocial/mixed	53	20	0.004
Neurotic	20	27	
Controls (49 boys; 41 girls)			
No problem	74	83	
Antisocial/mixed	22	5	0.03
Neurotic	4	12	

*Significance of chi-square test.

boys from the problem group did not differ significantly from the girls in severity of disorder or in symptomatology, although there could have been a ceiling effect with the measures used, which obscured the fact that the boys were more disturbed initially. The only significant differences at 3 years in the problem group were that the boys scored lower on developmental testing and had more sphincter problems. Thus they could have been more vulnerable because of biological factors, and it is of interest that at 4 years boys were already showing more problems in management and in concentration (Table 5.4).

Table 5.4   Differences between boys and girls in behaviour problem group

	Boys (%)	Girls (%)	p*
At 3 (57 boys, 42 girls)			
Restless	59	55	NS
Night wetting	61	36	0.05
Marked problem	57	48	NS
At 4 (57 boys, 42 girls)			
Control problem	54	21	0.01
Poor concentration	25	7	0.05

*Significance of chi-square test.

There were no differences between the sexes in family and social factors, so that if boys were subject to different social pressures these must have been of a more subtle nature than we were able to measure. We did find that different factors were associated with outcome in boys compared with girls and, although these factors apparently lay within the child, they could have been influenced by family patterns of interaction.

Whether a problem persisted or not to 8 years in a boy was related to the following at 8 years:

1 The severity of the disorder, the more marked the problem the more likely it was to persist.
2 Lower scores on developmental tests.
3 Being described as restless.
4 Having poor relations with sibs (Table 5.5).

On the other hand persistence of problems in girls was not related to any of these factors, and severity of disorder, scores on developmental testing or being restless had no influence on outcome; if anything, girls with persisting problems were brighter and had better relationships with their sibs. Thus some of the behaviour which were in general more common in boys were also related to outcome in boys.

Table 5.5 Factors associated with persisting problems in boys and girls from the behaviour problem group

	Behaviour Problem		
	Persisted (%)	Recovered (%)	$p*$
Boys at 3 years (38 persisted; 14 recovered)			
Restless	68	29	0.02
Poor relations with sibs	42	8	0.07
Marked problem	66	29	0.05
Mean score on Griffiths Scale D	97	114	0.01
Mean score on Griffiths Scale E	98	112	0.05
Girls at 3 years (20 persisted; 22 recovered)			
Restless	55	55	NS
Poor relations with sibs	29	44	0.09
Marked problem	55	41	NS
Mean score on Griffiths Scale D	113	106	NS
Mean score on Griffiths Scale E	107	109	NS

*Significance on chi-square test.

Similar differences between the sexes occurred in the development of new problems in the control group but because the numbers are small the differences are less clear cut. As shown in Table 5.2 boys were slightly more likely to develop a new problem between 3 and 8 years. These boys were duller at 3 years than control boys who remained problem free, and somewhat more restless, but not significantly so. They were also duller than the girls from the control group who developed a disorder between 3 and 8 years. Thus we see that the girls with a disorder at 8 years from both the problem and control groups are significantly brighter than the boys rated as showing a disorder at this age.

A few children from the control group were rated as having mild problems at 3 years (false negatives on the original screening) and these children, both boys and girls, were also more at risk of having a disorder at 8 years.

THE RELATIONSHIP OF SPECIFIC SYMPTOMS TO OUTCOME

We looked for associations between specific behaviours and outcome and found two symptoms which were related either to persistence and/or to type of problem—restlessness and fearfulness.

We described above the finding that restless boys' behaviour problems were more likely to persist. Restlessness has both interactional and transactional effects in boys. Boys are more likely to be described as restless in the first place (a transactional effect) and if they are restless and have a behaviour problem

Table 5.6   Outcome in restlessness, boys and girls from problem group

	Behaviour at 3		
	Not restless (%)	Restless (%)	p*
Boys (22 not restless; 29 restless)			
At 8			
No problem	46	14	
Antisocial	23	72	0.005
Neurotic	23	14	
Girls (19 not restless; 22 restless)			
At 8			
No problem	53	55	
Antisocial	10	27	NS
Neurotic	37	18	

*Significance of chi-square test.

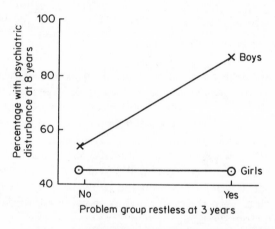

Fig. 5.2   Persistence of restlessness between 3 and 8 years in boys and girls

at 3 years the problem is more likely to persist (an interactive effect) (Figure 5.2). In girls no such relationship is found (Table 5.6).

As we have seen the type of disorder at 8 years differed between the sexes. Not only was restlessness associated with persisting disorder in boys but when the disorder persisted in a restless boy this was more likely to be a conduct or antisocial disorder at 8 years. This association between early restlessness and later conduct disorder was also present in girls but was not significant (Table 5.6).

Restlessness was also associated with the development of problems in boys from the control group in a similar manner although the numbers are too small to reach significance. Control boys who were restless at 3 years were more likely

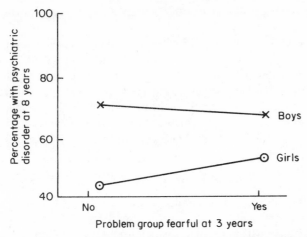

Fig. 5.3   Persistence of fearfulness between 3 and 8 years in boys and girls

Table 5.7   Outcome in restlessness, boys from control group

	Behaviour at 3	
	Not restless (43) (%)	Restless (7) (%)
At 8		
No problem	79	43
Antisocial	19	43
Neurotic	2	14
	0.09*	

*Significance of chi-square test.

Table 5.8   Outcome in fearfulness, boys and girls from problem group

	Behaviour at 3		
	Not fearful (%)	Fearful (%)	p*
Boys (41 not fearful; 10 fearful)			
At 8			
No problem	27	30	
Antisocial	61	20	0.01
Neurotic	12	50	
Girls (32 not fearful; 9 fearful)			
At 8			
No problem	56	44	
Antisocial	25	—	0.05
Neurotic	19	56	

*Significance of chi-square test.

to be rated as deviant at 8 years and to show an antisocial disorder at this age (Table 5.7).

Fearfulness did not predict whether a problem persisted or not, but if a problem did persist in a child who was rated fearful at 3 years, this was more likely to be rated a neurotic disorder at 8 years in both boys and girls (Table 5.8).

Thus although we were unable to categorize the type of disorder at 3 years, we have identified two behaviours in the pre-school period which are associated with differential outcome, although we have yet to establish that there is a *causal* relation between these early and late behavioural manifestations.

THE NATURE OF RESTLESSNESS

We have possibly made a beginning in understanding why boys show more conduct disorder at age 8 years, since restlessness in them but not in girls is associated with persisting problems which are likely to be antisocial in nature. The nature of this restlessness remains problematic. The definition used for rating its presence at age 3 years was as follows: 'Usually unable to sit still for more than five minutes at mealtimes or for other activities.' We did no observational studies and this crude definition could obviously refer to many different behaviours such as high activity level, distractibility, short attention span, impulsivity etc. The cause of the behaviour could also vary; it could be due to a temperamental characteristic, a neurophysiological deficit, a more severe

Table 5.9　Mean scores on psychological assessment in boys and girls from problem groups with antisocial and neurotic disorder at 8 years

	Clinical rating at 8 years		
	Antisocial disorder	Neurotic disorder	No disorder
Number of boys	27	10	14
Number of girls	8	11	22
Boys at 3 years			
Griffiths Scale D	100*	91**	114
Griffiths Scale E	98**	98	112
Boys at 8 years			
WISC Full Scale IQ	105*	102*	115
Girls at 3 years			
Griffiths Scale D	113	113	107
Griffiths Scale E	106	119	109
Girls at 8 years			
WISC Full Scale IQ	108	108	106

Significance of t-test comparing children with antisocial or neurotic disorder respectively and those without disorder. $*p<0.05$, $**p<0.01$.

type of disorder, a response to parental handling or an interaction between all these factors. It was not likely to be just a sign of immaturity or developmental delay, because in boys developmental delay at 3 years was equally associated with later neurotic and antisocial disorder, and if anything the neurotic boys were duller (Table 5.9).

However, since restlessness in boys was associated with developmental problems it could have been to some extent physiologically determined, although it seems likely that such constitutional tendencies only become manifest if socially reinforced. Aggressive behaviour in boys is more likely to be reinforced at home and at school and this might explain why they and not the restless girls were more at risk of persisting disorder. Similarly different academic expectations may make it easier for dull girls to cope with learning problems compared with dull boys (Serbin *et al.*, 1973). It would be of interest to examine in more detail the nature of restlessness in boys and girls. The patterns of interaction they have within their families and at school may well turn out to be different and in turn lead to quite different responses from the children themselves.

THE NATURE OF FEARFULNESS

A rating of fearfulness was made by adding together the number of mild and marked fears shown by the child at 3 years, and a child with five mild or two or more marked fears was considered fearful. As with restlessness the nature of this fearful behaviour needs elucidating. It could be based on constitutional factors, modelled on parental behaviour or a response to anxious handling. There is a striking difference in the early development of boys and girls who develop neurotic disorders, with the boys having significantly lower scores (Table 5.9). Different mechanisms seem to be at work here in the two sexes. The boys could be immature and responding with anxiety to educational pressures and the stresses of school life. The girls are brighter and it could be postulated that they are more mature and aware of family problems and stresses. It is possible that the girls are particularly sensitive to depression in their mothers, and that they develop very early on an identification with her problems and a sense of responsibility for her wellbeing. Whatever the mechanism we could be seeing here the beginning of the marked sex difference in rates of neurotic disorder which is found in adults, with women being much more prone to suffer from anxiety and depression than men, and men showing more antisocial disorder.

Our results raise a number of interesting questions about the role of constitutional and temperamental factors in the genesis of psychiatric disorder in children, and the reasons for boys apparently increased risk of developing antisocial disorder. Without further research designed specifically to answer these questions suggested causal mechanisms must remain conjectural.

The actual processes which make boys more sensitive to the effects of specific events or environmental pressures is unknown. It has been suggested that they are more at risk because of biological factors (Rutter, 1970) and in our study it was certainly the duller, less-mature boys who were likely to develop problems. Another hypothesis is that there are sex-limited temperamental traits which predispose boys to develop psychiatric disorder (Eme, 1979).

There are both conceptual and methodological problems in defining and measuring difficult temperament (Bates, 1980) but the possibility remains that temperament contributes to the development of behaviour problems. Longitudinal studies have found only limited continuity in temperamental traits themselves, but have been successful in identifying characteristics which predict the likelihood of subsequent psychiatric referral (Thomas *et al.*, 1968) or the development of a psychiatric disorder (Graham *et al.*, 1973). Dunn *et al.* (1981)—see also Chapter 2—have shown that children with certain temperamental characteristics are more likely to react adversely to the birth of a sibling. This reaction was in part related to the way temperamental differences affected the child's responses to changes in maternal behaviour.

This finding might have important implications when considering the development of behaviour problems in young children. It could be postulated for instance that certain children with a depressed mother are more likely to become restless and attention seeking as a response to her withdrawal and lack of involvement. It could also be that lack of flexibility in some children prevents improvement even though the family or environmental situation changes. Thus in our study improvement in variables like marital tension or maternal depression was not related to improvement in the child's behaviour, an unexpected finding.

Different studies of temperament have found different traits as being significantly associated with psychiatric disorder, e.g. low fastidiousness (Graham *et al.*, 1973), and negative and intensive mood (Thomas *et al.*, 1968). It is not clear whether these are artefacts of measurement, so that in fact various studies could be identifying different facets of some underlying characteristic, or whether indeed there are a number of different traits which increase vulnerability.

Whatever the child's underlying predispositions there are equally important influences from the social environment, and the two interact in such a complex manner that it is extremely difficult to disentangle causal relations. Both temperamental manifestations and outcome of behaviour problems may therefore vary in children who have similar predispositions. The social prohibition of aggressive or assertive behaviour in restless girls may diminish the likelihood of antisocial behaviour developing, whilst the latitude accorded to aggressive behaviour in restless boys may encourage antisocial responses. Thus although temperamental factors may be significantly related to the type of disorder shown by children, the relative size of their contribution may be low compared with environmental factors, and altering the child's family or social environment could have a powerful effect.

What then are the implications of our study for prevention and treatment?

First we can see that there is a considerable burden of distress in families with young children with high rates of behaviour problems and of maternal depression. The finding that women with young children are particularly prone to develop depression is borne out by a number of studies (Brown and Harris, 1978). Depression is likely to impair a woman's ability to cope with her children. This could lead to a spiralling cycle in which the child becomes ever more difficult and demanding because his needs are not being met, and his mother becomes increasingly tense and upset by his behaviour (Weissmann et al., 1972).

There are many strategies which could improve the wellbeing of parents and young children and might prevent this escalation of difficulties. Self-help groups, and adequate income, housing and pre-school facilities are basic measures which significantly affect the quality of life for children and their parents.

The possibilities of men's increased involvement in child care by means of extended paternity leave, flexible hours and so on, are now being explored in some countries (Moss and Fonda, 1980). Facilitating working outside the home may actually prevent depression or aid recovery for many women (Brown and Harris, 1978; Mostow and Newberry, 1975).

A variety of programmes are now being developed with the aim of teaching parenting skills and helping parents to understand how they influence their children's behaviour. It has to be said that there is little hard evidence to demonstrate that any preventive methods work, but there has been little research into the question. The few studies which have addressed the problem suggest that simple management advice can reduce the incidence of problem behaviour (Cullen, 1976; Chamberlin and Szumowski, 1980; Brazelton, 1962). The whole area of prevention could profitably be pursued to examine what methods would be most effective and at what point of time it is most useful to apply them.

Certainly it seems worthwhile trying to prevent or treat behaviour disorders in young children because, in addition to the current distress they cause, our study suggests that many are unlikely to clear up spontaneously. Supposing we could considerably reduce the rates of problems in pre-school children how much difference would that make to the prevalence of disorder in the early school years? We found that the rate of disorder in our control group at 8 years was 20 per cent and in the problem group 60 per cent. The control group was drawn from a much larger pool of children, i.e. 600 children from the original sample of 700, and in absolute numbers this group would contribute a larger proportion of psychiatric problems at 8 years than the original problem group. We established that only a third of all children with problems at 8 years would have been identified at 3 years, and the other two-thirds would be new problems who would not have been identified on the behaviour-screening questionnaire. Thus treatment or preventive measures directed at the problem-group alone, even if effective, would have reduced the prevalence of problems at 8 years by only one-third. It is possible that the sort of general preventive measures outlined above, available to the population as a whole would have much more impact.

We have demonstrated that there is considerable continuity in problem behaviour and that there are marked sex differences in outcome both in prevalence, type of disorder and factors associated with outcome. Although these are troubling results they do not necessarily lead to pessimism about the possibility of effective intervention. The sex differences in themselves suggest that cultural factors *might* be as important an influence as the child's individual characteristics in outcome. Change in the former, in family behaviour and child-rearing practices, and in school and social expectations generally, might override the child's predispositions to develop problematic behaviour.

On the whole those involved in the mental-health field have concentrated on working with individuals, although such work is now appropriately expanding to include the whole family. It is clear that individual children do differ in their susceptibility to develop disorder because of innate predispositions and early experiences. Families too vary in their abilities to cope. But we have seen social and cultural factors and adverse experiences have an important impact on young children and their families. However, much effort is put into helping the individual child and family, these wider influences may militate against therapeutic effectiveness. It would be logical to look for measures which might reduce the general level of adverse factors, for instance, factors affecting the levels of depression in women, of stress in families with young children, or the cultural acceptance of aggressive behaviour in boys. Certainly, it should be considered that at least as much, if not more, effort ought to be devoted to preventive measures such as these, as to more individual approaches. In the long run, working with groups, in communities and in schools, will not only reach more people, but possibly be more effective.

REFERENCES

Bates, J. E. (1980). The concept of difficult temperament, *Merrill Palmer Quart.* **26**, 299–319.

Brazelton, T. B. (1962). A child oriented approach to toilet training, *Pediatrics*, **29**, 121–128.

Brown, G. and Harris, T. (1978). *Social Origins of Depression*, Tavistock Publications, London.

Chamberlin, R. W. and Szumowski, E. K. (1980). A follow up study of parent education in pediatric office practices: impact at age two and a half. *Am. J. Publ. Hlth.* **70**, 1180–1185.

Cullen, K. J. (1976). A six year controlled trial of prevention of children's behaviour disorder. *J. Pediat.* **88**, 662–666.

Dunn, J., Kendrick, C. and MacNamee, R. (1981). The reaction of first born children to the birth of a sibling: mothers' reports, *J. Child Psychol. Psychiat.* **22**, 1–18.

Earls, F. E. and Richman, N. (1980a). The prevalence of behaviour problems in the three year old children of West Indian-born parents, *J. Child Psychol. Psychiat.* **21**, 99–106.

Earls, F. E. and Richman, N. (1980b). Behaviour problems in preschool children of West Indian born parents: a re-examination of family and social factors, *J. Child Psychol. Psychiat.* **21**, 107–117.

Eme, R. F. (1979). Sex differences in childhood psychopathology: a review, *Psychol. Bulletin*, **86**, 574–595.

Graham, P., Rutter, M. and George, S. (1973). Temperamental characteristics as predictors of behaviour disorders in children, *Am. J. Orthopsychiat.* **43**, 328–339.

Kohn, M. and Rosman, B. L. (1973). A social competence scale and symptom check list for the preschool child: factor dimensions, their cross instrumental generality and longitudinal persistence, *Dev. Psychol.* **6**, 430–444.

MacFarlane, J. W., Allen, L. and Honzik, P. (1954). *A Developmental Study of Behaviour Problems of Normal Children Between 21 Months and 14 Years*, University of California Press, Berkeley.

Minde, R. and Minde, K. (1977). Behavioural screening of preschool children: a new approach to mental health, in *Epidemiological Approaches in Child Psychiatry* (Ed. P. J. Graham), Academic Press, London.

Morris, D. P., Saroker, E. and Burruss, C. (1954). Follow-up studies of shy, withdrawn children. I. Evaluation of later adjustment, *Amer. J. Orthopsychiat.* **24**, 743–754.

Moss, P. and Fonda, N. (Eds) (1980). *Work and the Family*, Temple Smith, London.

Mostow, E. and Newberry, P. (1975). Work role and depression in women. A comparison of workers and housewives in treatment, *Am. J. Orthopsychiat.* **45**, 538–548.

Richman, N. (1977). Behaviour problems in preschool children: family and social factors, *Brit. J. Psychiat.* **131**, 523–527.

Richman, N. and Graham, P. (1971). A behavioural screening questionnaire for use with three year old children, *J. Child Psychol. Psychiat.* **12**, 5–33.

Richman, N., Stevenson, J. and Graham, P. (1975). Prevalence of behaviour problems in three year old children: an epidemiological study in a London borough. *J. Child Psychol. Psychiat.* **16**, 226–287.

Richman, N. and Tupling, H. (1974). A computerised register of families with children under five in a London borough, *Health Trends*, **6**, 19–21.

Richman, N., Stevenson, J. and Graham, P. (1982). *Preschool to School: A Behavioural Study*. Academic Press, London.

Robins, L. N. (1966). *Deviant Children Grown Up*, Williams and Wilkins, Baltimore.

Rutter, M. (1967). A children's behaviour questionnaire for completion by teachers, *J. Child Psychol. Psychiat.* **8**, 1–11.

Rutter, M. (1970). Sex differences in children's response to family stress, in *The Child and His Family* (Eds E. J. Anthony and C. M. Koupernick), Wiley, New York.

Rutter, M., Tizard, J. and Whitmore, K. (1970). *Education, Health and Behaviour*, Longman, London.

Serbin, L., O'Leary, K., Kent, R. and Tonick, I. (1973). A comparison of teacher response to the pre-academic and problem behaviour of boys and girls, *Child Dev.* **44**, 796–804.

Thomas, A., Chess, S. and Birch, H. G. (1968). *Temperament and Behaviour Disorders in Children*, New York University Press, New York.

Weissmann, M., Paykel, E. S., Klerman, G. L. (1972). The depressed woman as a mother, *Soc. Psychiat.* **7**, 98–108.

Longitudinal Studies in Child Psychology and Psychiatry
Edited by A. R. Nicol
© 1985 John Wiley and Sons Ltd.

Chapter 6

Family Pathology and Child Psychiatric Disorder: A Four-Year Prospective Study

D. Quinton and M. Rutter

ISSUES REGARDING PSYCHIATRIC DISORDER IN PARENTS AND THEIR CHILDREN

For at least the last half century there has been an awareness that mental disorder in parents may be associated with psychiatric disturbances in the children (see review by Rutter, 1966). The first reports were clinical descriptions, well exemplified by Janet's (1925) careful laying out of the issues. He noted several instances in which illness occurred in step-parents, and others where children brought up away from the family escaped the affliction. On this basis, together with his observations of family interactions, he concluded that the main effects were due to the adverse impact of mental disorders on the social life of other in the family, with parental neurosis serving to maintain psychological tensions between family members. The inference appeared plausible but systematic research was needed to test the validity of the association between parental illness and child disorder and to quantify its strength, to determine its specificity, and to test hypotheses on possible mechanisms mediating the associations.

No longer is there any doubt on the reality of the links between psychiatric disorder in parents and children. The associations have been clearly demonstrated in numerous epidemiological studies of the general population (see, for example, Buck and Laughton, 1959; Hare and Shaw, 1965; Kellner, 1963; Richman et al., 1982; Rutter et al., 1975b, 1976). It has also been shown in case-control comparisons of the parents of children with a psychiatric disturbance (Rutter, 1966), and in case-control comparisons of the children of parents with a mental disorder (see Beardslee, 1985; Cytryn et al., 1985; Watt et al., 1984). However, in most cases the associations have been of moderate strength only, with relatively weak specificity. That is, there has been only a slight tendency for children to show the *same* type of disorder as that exhibited by their parents. Moreover, the associations have not been specific to *psychiatric* conditions in parents. Child psychiatric disorder is also associated with chronic physical illness in the parents (Rutter, 1966), with parental death (Garmezy, 1983) and with parental criminality (Rutter and Giller, 1983).

A variety of alternatives have to be considered with respect to possible underlying mechanisms. First, in some cases the link might reflect genetic transmission. The suggestion is plausible because there is good evidence for the operation of genetic factors in the determination of schizophrenia (Gottesman and Shields, 1976), of major affective disorders (Gershon, 1984), of antisocial personality disorders and adult criminality (Crowe, 1983), and of some varieties of alcoholism (Bohman et al., 1981; Cloninger et al., 1981). On the other hand, genetic factors seem much less important in the emotional disorders that make up most of psychiatric out-patient practice (Torgersen, 1983). The offspring of seriously mentally ill parents have a genetically increased risk for those same conditions when they reach adult life but it is less certain that this is an important mechanism in the case of the broad run of minor depressive and anxious disorders. Also, of course, the question here is not that of the genetic transmission of psychiatric conditions in *adult* life but rather that of those arising in *childhood* in the offspring of parents with some form of mental disorder. The answer demands a knowledge on the genetic links between psychiatric conditions in childhood and those in adult life—a knowledge that is largely lacking. Of course, studies of away-adopted or fostered offspring would help answer that question. Unfortunately, although such data are available for several adult conditions, they are not available for most childhood disorders (see Chapter 7 for one example however).

A second alternative concerns the direct environmental impact of parental mental disorder. Thus, Rutter (1966) found that the parent–child association of psychiatric disorder was strongest when the parental symptoms impinged on or involved the child in some way. It appeared that the children were most at risk when they were the victims of aggressive acts or hostile behaviour, were the target of parental delusions, were neglected for pathological reasons or were involved in parental rejection. However, the findings were not prospective and relied on case-note data.

Thirdly, the sequelae for the children may stem from the indirect effects of parental mental illness. Thus, Rice et al. (1971) noted that illness might result in severe family disruptions with the children being placed in foster care or otherwise cared for outside the parental home. Other studies of depressed (Weissman et al., 1972; Weissman and Paykel, 1974) and schizophrenic women (Rodnick and Goldstein, 1974) have found that mental disorder may interfere with parenting functions. Most recently, Cox and his colleagues have shown that mothers with a recurrent or chronic depressive disorder tend to be less involved with their children, less likely to sustain positive interactions, less able to put their children's experiences into a personal context, and more often involved in unsuccessful attempts to control their children (Cox and Mills, 1983; Pound et al. 1984; Mills et al. 1984).

A fourth possibility is that the ill-effects on the children derive from correlates of parental mental disorder, rather than from the disorder itself. Thus, several studies have shown the high frequency with which mental disorder is associated with marital discord (Birtchnell and Kennard, 1983a,b). This is likely to be important because it is well established that discord is associated with a substantially increased risk of child psychiatric disorder in non-patient samples (Rutter, 1982; Emery, 1982).

There is some evidence in support of each of these broad sets of mechanisms but, at the time of planning the present study, the data were inadequate for any determination of their relative importance. Most previous studies concerned rather specialized samples and there were no prospective investigations involving both systematic assessments of disorder in the children and standardized evaluations of family functioning. The investigation reported here was designed to meet these needs. The data were gathered some years ago, and several papers have reported various aspects of the findings (Graham *et al.*, 1973; Rutter, 1970, 1971, 1977a, 1978; Rutter and Quinton, 1981). However, the present chapter provides a set of reanalyses designed to deal with issues not adequately covered in earlier reports or with questions that have arisen more recently in the light of other research.

STUDY DESIGN

Selection of sample

Because our prime objective was to study the *process* by which parental mental illness sometimes led to disorder in the children, we needed a sample of parents who had *recently* developed some kind of psychiatric condition. In order to obtain an accurate picture of the nature and extent of the associations between illness in parents and disorders in their children it was necessary to have a *representative* sample of psychiatrically ill parents, and to be able to interview the parents as soon as possible after the disorder became manifest. The Camberwell Psychiatric Register provided the kind of sampling frame we required in that it provided a comprehensive coverage of all patients living within a single inner London borough who attended National Health Service hospitals or clinics (Wing and Hailey, 1972).

As the main focus of the study was the identification of the key features of parental mental illness that put children at psychiatric risk, we undertook no parallel study of a non-patient control group. Rather, the analyses concerned systematic *within*-group comparisons according to diagnostic, family or other characteristics. Nevertheless, it was important to be able to 'calibrate' our findings by reference to general population norms. For this purpose, we used two types of controls.

1   A cross-sectional representative general population sample of the families of 10 year old children living in the same geographical areas (the 'family control group').
2   A prospective study of age and sex matched classroom controls, using teacher questionnaires (the 'classroom control group').

Patients

The criteria for selection of adult parent-patients were that:
1   The patient was living in the borough of Camberwell on the day of psychiatric contact, having had no other psychiatric contact within the previous year.
2   There was a child at home under the age of 15 years.
3   The main language spoken at home was colloquial English (in practice, at the time of the study this meant that recent immigrants from Asia and the West Indies were effectively excluded).

Our aim was to obtain a representative sample that was stratified in order to obtain adequate numbers in subgroups defined according to sex or diagnosis. For this purpose, the sample was collected in two phases during 1966–67. First, we identified a consecutive sample of all patients fitting the criteria who attended over a ten-month period—comprising a sample of 202. From within this group, a randomly chosen two-in-five sample of eighty-four was chosen for detailed study (resource limitation prevented us from studying the entire group of 202). Second, because of low numbers of male and of psychotic patients, all patients in these groups only were included in the sample over a further period. As this additional sample also comprised all consecutive cases who met the criteria it too is representative within sex and diagnosis subgroups. Altogether, 137 families with 292 children were studied ('the longitudinal sample'). From the total sample of patients selected in either sample, seventeen cases were missed because one consultant refused permission for any of his patients to be seen. In addition, one patient refused and a further four could not be traced.

More limited data were obtained on the three-in-five sample excluded in the first phase of sampling. Brief interviews in the home were undertaken to determine parental diagnosis and family characteristics and parent and teacher questionnaires were obtained on the children. The children were followed over a four-year period by questionnaire, as were the rest of the sample, but the families were not reinterviewed. The 'total sample' of 259 families with 556 children is used for certain questionnaire comparisons but otherwise it is not discussed further here.

Controls

For each child in the total sample of patients' families, the two children of the same sex nearest on the school class register, who met the criteria of having parents who spoke colloquial English at home (according to information from teachers) were chosen as controls. The method of selection was devised to ensure that no-one at school was aware which children were the offspring of patients and which were controls (see Rutter and Quinton, 1981). This comprised the 'classroom control group'.

In the final year of data collection, a sample of families with 10-year-old children was drawn from the general population of Camberwell, as part of a comparative study of psychosocial factors and child disorders in London and the Isle of Wight (Rutter *et al.*, 1975a,b). The data collection in that study deliberately paralleled that in the follow-up of psychiatric patients so that systematic comparisons of family characteristics could be made between this 'family control group' and the 'longitudinal sample' of patients' families (restricted to those who had children of approximately the same age).

In summary, the main analyses concern comparisons within a representative sample of families of patient-parents—the *'longitudinal sample'*. Between-group comparisons are made with an age and sex matched *'classroom control group'* of children and with a general population sample of families with 10-year-old children living in the same area of inner London—the *'family control group'*. For analyses using questionnaires only limited use is made of a larger representative sample of children from patients' families—the *'total sample* of patients' families'.

Data

Behavioural questionnaires

Teacher questionnaires—the Rutter 'B' scale (Rutter, 1967)—were obtained for all school-age children in the total sample, and in the 'classroom control group', at the time of initial contact and at yearly intervals over the next four years. Parental questionnaires—the Rutter 'A' scale (Rutter *et al.*, 1970)—were completed at the time of initial contact by mothers of all children 3 years of age or older. The mothers in the 'longitudinal sample' only completed the same questionnaire at yearly intervals over the next four years.

In the 'longitudinal sample' the patient and spouse were interviewed simultaneously and separately (by different interviewers) shortly after the initial psychiatric contact (year 0), again one year later (year 1) and again after a further interval of three years (year 4). The interview used non-schedule standardized techniques (Richardson *et al.*, 1965) to obtain a systematic assessment of family life and relationships and of current psychiatric disorder in both parents. The interview with the wife, irrespective of which parent was the patient, was used to obtain detailed systematic information on the behaviour of up to two children (Graham and Rutter, 1968). Details of the areas covered by the interview and of its reliability and validity are given elsewhere (Brown and Rutter, 1966;

Quinton *et al.*, 1976; Rutter and Brown, 1966). In a separate interview with the mother by a different interviewer, standardized information on the temperamental attributes of children between the ages of 3 and 7 years were obtained in year 0 (Graham *et al.*, 1973).

In the second and third years of the study, when the full family interview was not used, parents—usually the wife—were more briefly questioned to assess changes in the psychiatric state of family members and major changes in family life and relationships.

Failure rates were very low in all the major data collection phases. Only 2.4 per cent of families were not interviewed at the time of first contact, and 8 per cent were not seen at both the first-year and fourth-year follow-ups.

RESULTS

Before considering the impact of parental mental disorder on the children, and the possible mechanisms involved, it is necessary to consider the characteristics of the families concerned, the features of the parental illness, and the course of that illness over the four years of the prospective study.

Characteristics of parent-patient's families

Family circumstances

The characteristics of the parent-patient's families may be assessed by comparison with those of the general population 'family control group' living in the same inner London borough. The patient-parents tended to be slightly younger and to have fewer children; this is likely to be a consequence of the fact that the 'family control group' was restricted to families with a 10-year-old child whereas the longitudinal sample included families with children ranging from infancy to adolescence. The groups did not differ significantly in social class or in a measure of overcrowding. However, there was a marked tendency for more of the patient sample to be living in privately rented accommodation, often in a house shared with other people. This, too, may have been a function of the age of the children as by the end of the four-year period of longitudinal study the groups no longer differed with respect to shared accommodation.

Marital problems

Although most of the parents in both groups were married and living together, the proportion who were not more than twice as high (20 per cent versus 8 per cent) in the patient group. Moreover, far more of the patient's marriages showed current discord (39 per cent versus 8 per cent) or had previously broken as a result of discord (8 per cent versus 6 per cent).

Table 6.1 Parent-patients' circumstances at first contact

	Longitudinal sample (%) ($n = 137$)	Family control group (%) ($n = 97$)	Statistical significance		
			χ^2	df	p
Number of children					
1	21	6			
2–3	54	44	19.28	2	<0.001
4 or more	25	50			
Social class					
Non-manual	28	20			
Skilled manual	41	57	5.77	2	NS
Semi-unskilled manual	31	23			
Persons per room					
1.0 or less	64	49			
1.1–1.4	21	31	5.37	2	NS
1.5 or more	15	20			
Housing type					
Family house	29	30			
Shared house	35	21	6.33	2	<0.05
Flat or maisonette	36	49			
Housing tenure					
Owner	14	18			
Private rent	40	15	26.19	2	<0.001
Council	46	68			

Mean age of mother (years): longitudinal sample, 34; family control group, 37.6. Statistical significance: $t = 3.83$, $df = 230$, $p < 0.001$. Mean age of father (years): longitudinal sample, 37.7; family control group, 40. Statistical significance: $t = 2.55$, $df = 222$, $p < 0.01$.

Table 6.2 Marital problems

	Longitudinal sample (%) ($n = 137$)	Family control group (%) ($n = 97$)	Statistical significance		
			χ^2	df	p
Marital circumstances					
Married	80	92			
Cohabiting	8	2	6.20	2	<0.05
On own	12	6			
Marital problems					
None	44	77			
Some: non-discordant	7	9			
Some: discordant	39	8	33.65	4	<0.001
Broken thro' discord	8	6			
Broken: other reasons	2	0			

Psychiatric disorder in spouses

It was also clear that the patients' spouses were more likely than the spouses in the family control group to show current psychiatric disorder. However, the pattern of disorder differed markedly between husbands and wives. The higher rate of disorder in the husbands of female patients was entirely accounted for by the very high rate of personality disorder (22 per cent versus 1 per cent). Emotional disturbance, as reflected by either interview ratings or scores on the Malaise Inventory (a self-report questionnaire—see Rutter *et al.*, 1970), did not differentiate the groups. In contrast, the higher rate of psychiatric disorder in the wives of male patients was largely the result of some form of affective disturbance. High scores (7 or more) on the Malaise Inventory were nearly twice as common (42 per cent versus 22 per cent). There was also a tendency for more wives of male patients to show a personality disorder (10 per cent versus 3 per cent) but the absolute numbers were small and the difference fell short of statistical significance.

Table 6.3   Psychiatric problems and disorder in spouses

	Longitudinal sample (%) ($n = 65$)	Family control group (%) ($n = 87$)	Statistical significance		
			χ^2	df	p
Disorders in male spouses					
Total with disorder	25	12	—	—	NS
Total with personality disorder	22	1	15.17	1	<0.01
High malaise score (7 +)	11	13	—	—	NS
Disorders in female spouses	($n = 59$)	($n = 94$)			
Total with disorder	41	28	—	—	NS
Total with personality disorder	10	3	—	—	NS
High malaise score (7 +)	42	22	6.20	1	<0.025

Parent–child interaction and relationships

As parent–child relationships and interaction are likely to be affected by the age of the children, comparisons were restricted to 8–12-year-old children in the parent-patient group (the wider age range than the 10 year olds in the family control group was necessary to provide a sufficient sample size). The measures for mothers were directly comparable between the groups but those for fathers differed in that the information derived from fathers in the parent-patient group but from mothers in the family control group.

It is striking how little the groups differed in most aspects of parenting. Thus, as assessed in year 0 at the time that the parents were referred for psychiatric care, there were no differences in parental warmth or criticism of the children

Table 6.4   Parent–child relationships and interaction

	Longitudinal sample (%) (n = 45–55)	Family control group (%) (n = 92–96)	Statistical significance		
			χ^2	df	p
Mother					
Low warmth to child	14	14	—	—	NS
High criticism of child	18	11	—	—	NS
Conversations three times per week or less*	20	27	—	—	NS
Father					
Low warmth to child	25	Not rated			
High criticism of child	14	Not rated			
Conversations three times per week or less*	44	41	—	—	NS
Child's Exposure to Abnormal Behaviour (either parent)					
Moderate/marked exposure to 'hostile' behaviour*	60[†]	12	44.24	1	<0.001
Moderate/marked exposure to 'anxious/depressive'* behaviour	72[†]	13	61.08	1	<0.001

	Mean	(SD)	Mean	(SD)	χ^2	df	p
Expectations score*	17.5	(5.3)	18.1	(4.8)	—	—	NS
Prohibition score*	13.8	(4.5)	13.9	(4.9)	—	—	NS
Positive interaction mother–child*	5.8	(4.6)	6.8	(5.6)	—	—	NS
Positive interaction father–child*	3.1	(2.9)	5.1	(4.7)	3.11	135	<0.001

*Comparisons based on year 4 measures when these measures were obtained in an identical manner.
†Year 0 data on these variables based on 88–90 children as these ratings were made on *all* children in the family.

as manifest at interview. Pilot studies on patients' families had previously shown that these interview measures reliably predicted relationships as observed during conjoint sessions (Brown and Rutter, 1966; Rutter and Brown, 1966). Thus, we may conclude that the parents in the patient group were just as loving with their children as other parents. Also, at least as measured in year 4 when most of the parents still showed psychiatric problems (see below), the groups did not differ in the frequency with which the mothers played or talked with their children. The fathers too did not differ in the frequency of conversational interchange, although they did play, or do things, with their children significantly less often. The scores for 'positive interaction' were based on a detailed account of all potentially pleasurable activities between parents and their children during the week preceding the interview. The 'expectations' score was based on the activities that children were expected to do for themselves (such as travelling by bus or helping to prepare meals), and the 'prohibitions' score on those that were forbidden (such as playing with certain children or watching particular TV programmes). Thus, the former reflects the degree of responsibility allowed and the latter the extent of parental control or protectiveness. The groups did not differ on either measure.

The findings as reported here do not take into account which parent was the psychiatric patient. However, within-group comparisons showed no differences between patients and non-patients on any of these measures.

Nevertheless, it would be wrong to conclude that the children in the parent-patient group experienced the same quality of family life. As already noted, they were much more likely to experience discord between the parents. Table 6.4 shows that they were also much more likely to be exposed to 'hostile', and to 'anxious/depressed' behaviour by the parents. These ratings were based on detailed information obtained at interview on the extent to which children were exposed to abnormal behaviour that might have resulted from the parents' psychiatric condition. The 4-point scale used ranged from 'no exposure' to 'marked exposure'. In making the rating, no attempt was made to determine whether or not the behaviour was symptomatic; the criterion was simply that it had occurred in the presence of the child in question. The extent of exposure was assessed in terms of the severity of manifestation of the behaviour (e.g. violence more severe than verbal aggression), the frequency of exposure, and the degree to which the child was directly involved in the abnormal behaviour—either in terms of being a target for it or having activities restricted by it. 'Anxious/depressed' behaviour comprised all manifestations of affective disturbance such as crying, emotional withdrawal, and expressed worries or fears. 'Hostile' behaviour included both irritability/aggression shown towards the child and also quarrelling and violence between the parents in the child's presence. Both forms of these possibly symptomatic behaviours were much more likely to impinge on the children in the parent-patient sample.

Correlates of diagnostic differences

The characteristics of the parent-patients in the longitudinal sample are shown in Table 6.5. Two-thirds were out patients and, of those treated as in patients, only a handful were admitted compulsorily. Affective disorder of some kind was much the commonest diagnosis; however, over half the male patients and a quarter of the female patients showed some form of personality disorder (a diagnosis that required abnormal personality features *and* persistent social impairment for the whole of adult life). In order to allow the prospective study of newly developed psychiatric conditions, the sample had been defined in terms of disorders for which there had been no previous psychiatric care during the preceding 12 months. Nevertheless, as it turned out, two in five patients

Table 6.5   Psychiatric characteristics of patients

	Longitudinal smaple (%) (n = 137)	Consecutive sample (%) (n = 84)
Sex of patient		
Male	45	26
Female	55	74
Clinical status		
Out patient	66	76
In patient voluntary	27	19
In patient formal	7	5
Type of disorder		
Schizophrenia	10	5
Manic-depressive psychosis	10	5
Depression	47	62
Phobic anxiety state	15	17
Alcoholism/personality disorder only	15	12
Other	3	0
Percentage with personality disorders		
Male patients	56	45
Female patients	24	29
Previous psychiatric contact	42	36

(42 per cent) had received previous psychiatric care at some time in the past. Only a fifth of patients had a psychosis of some kind; nevertheless (as shown in Table 6.5) this was double the proportion found in the ten-month consecutive sample of new referrals. Although psychoses may make up a larger percentage of *chronic* psychiatric conditions, they are infrequent among new referrals. In the fully representative consecutive sample, psychiatric disorders were nearly three times as frequent in women as in men. However, because of the deliberate over-sampling of men (see above) this was not so in the longitudinal sample.

When we come to consider the effects of parental mental disorder on the children, it will be important to determine whether or not the effects vary according to diagnosis. However, in order to interpret the findings we need first to find out whether diagnostic differences are associated with variations in other aspects of family functioning. The findings are summarized in Table 6.6.

For this analysis the patients' disorders were grouped into three broad categories, (a) psychoses, including schizophrenia, paranoid states and manic-depressive disorders, (b) affective/emotional disorders, including both retarded and agitated depressions, anxiety neuroses and obsessional states, and (c) personality disorder. Patients with both personality disorders and some other

Table 6.6 Type of adult disorder and family relationships (longitudinal sample)

	Diagnosis of patient		
	Psychosis (%)	Affective disorder* (%)	Personality disorder[†] (%)
Marital relationships	(n = 24)	(n = 57)	(n = 53)
Good/satisfactory	54	54	28
Poor, not discordant	13	9	2
Marital discord	35	23	58
	$\chi^2 = 17.33$, df = 4, $p < 0.01$		
Not currently cohabiting	0	14	11
Disorders in spouses	(n = 24)	(n = 50)	(n = 49)
No disorder	83	76	47
Affective/emotional disorder	9	8	35
Personality disorder	8	16	18
	$\chi^2 = 19.51$, df = 4, $p < 0.001$		
Parent–child relationships	(n = 24)	(n = 80–82)	(n = 68)
Low warmth to child	25	27	16
High criticism of child	4	23	18
	No statistically significant differences		
Moderate/marked exposure of child to:	(n = 40–44)	(n = 102–104)	(n = 122)
'Psychotic' behaviour	43	0	11
Hostile behaviour	48	50	66[‡]
Anxious/depressive behaviour	74	61	71

*This category excluded affective psychoses and included phobic anxiety states but most disorders were depressive in type (see Table 6.5).
[†]Patients with a personality disorder *and* some other acute psychiatric condition were included here, and were excluded from the other groups.
[‡]Hostile behaviour significantly more frequent with personality disorders ($\chi^2 = 6.68$, df = 2, $p < 0.05$).
The n for children include all children in the family for whom measures were available.

more acute current psychiatric condition were included in the personality-disorder group.

Both marital discord and affective disorders in spouses were much more frequent when the patient showed a personality disorder. The spouses were *least* likely to have a psychiatric problem when the diagnosis was some form of psychosis. Parent-child relationships were not significantly associated with parental diagnosis, although again these were most likely to be good when the patient-parent was psychotic. Exposure to 'psychotic behaviour', not surprisingly, was mostly restricted to the psychotic group. However, this category included non-psychotic forms of bizarre behaviour (such as morbid jealousy or obsessional rituals) and 11 per cent of the children of parents with a personality disorder were exposed to these. Moderate or marked exposure to 'hostile' behaviour was slightly more common with personality disorders, but it was present for about half the children in the other two groups. The majority of children in all three groups were exposed to 'anxious/depressed' behaviour and there were no significant between-group differences.

Course of psychiatric and family problems

Before turning to the effects on the children over the course of the four-year prospective study, we need to determine what happened to the psychiatric problems of the parent-patients, and what happened to the families, over this same time period. The main findings are summarized in Tables 6.7–6.9.

Table 6.7   The course of psychiatric disorder in parent-patients

	Diagnosis of patient		
	Psychosis (%) ($n = 24$)	Affective disorder (%) ($n = 42$)	Personality disorder (%) ($n = 46$)
Persistence of patient's disorder			
No symptoms	13	14	6
Mild persistence (less than ⅓ time)	42	45	20
Moderate persistence (⅓–⅔ time)	33	19	15
Marked persistence (more than ⅔ time)	13	21	59

$$\chi^2 = 21.85, \ df = 6, \ p < 0.01$$

In order to allow time for recovery from the original episode leading to psychiatric referral, the persistence of adult disorders was categorized according to the patients' functioning over the three final years of the study (from year 1 to year 4). Patients were classified as having no further symptomatology associated with social impairment, or as having handicapping symptoms persisting or recurring for a third of the time or less, from over one-third to two-thirds of the period, and for over two-thirds of the time. Checks were made in order to see whether this classification misrepresented the degree of recovery because the 'continuing symptoms' groups included those whose initial episodes took longer than a year to remit. It was clear, however, that the classification was *not* misleading; the 'symptom free' group was distinct from the others, even from those with mild persistence only. For example, of the five patients with symptoms at year 1 but no handicapping symptoms beyond the second follow-up interview, three were still on medication at the end of the study, one was an alcoholic who relapsed shortly after the study finished and one was a patient with manic-depressive psychosis who was living in a sheltered environment.

At first sight, it may seem odd that the outcome of the psychotic group did not differ from the affective/emotional disorder group. However, the psychoses were quite heterogeneous, not only in type (with half schizophrenic and half manic-depressive), but also in mode of onset (with some, especially the puerperal, showing an extremely acute onset followed by good recovery). The *quality* of functioning was markedly different in the chronic psychoses from that in the chronic or recurrent affective disorders. Nevertheless, the fact remains that the two-fifths of patients with an emotional disturbance had moderate or marked persistence of symptoms accompanied by social impairment over the course of the four years following referral.

Persisting handicaps were most frequent amongst those with personality disorders where nearly three-fifths had continuing symptoms with social impairment. Only 6 per cent were symptom free for three years or longer and three-fifths remained impaired for most of the four years. Even among those patients without a personality disorder, very few (13–14 per cent) were symptom free, although far fewer showed a chronically persistent disorder. It was apparent that for the majority of patients the course of disorder over the follow-up period consisted of a fluctuating pattern with temporary remissions of symptoms and occasional or repeated recurrences of handicapping problems at various levels of severity.

Table 6.8   Duration of disorder and outcome

Duration of disorder (at initial referral)	Psychosis ($n = 24$): persistence		Affective disorder ($n = 42$): persistence	
	None/ mild	Moderate/ marked	None/ mild	Moderate/ marked
Less than 1 year	13	8	13	9
1 year or more	0	3	16	12

Differences not significant.

Although the patient sample had been chosen on the basis of no psychiatric contact during the twelve months preceding referral, it was apparent that a high proportion had had longstanding psychiatric problems. For 72 per cent of the men and 32 per cent of the women such problems were of at least five years duration at the time of referral (usually because of an associated personality disorder). As already noted, the presence of a personality disorder carried a poor prognosis. However, the duration of symptoms was of *no* prognostic value in the patients with either a psychotic or an affective or neurotic condition that was unassociated with a personality disorder. Table 6.8 gives the data according to whether or not the symptoms had lasted at least a year at the time of first hospital attendance, but the same conclusion applies to the small subgroup whose symptoms had lasted five years or longer (Rutter, 1977a). Appropriate treatment resulted in a relatively high rate of remission even among those with a longstanding disorder.

Marital relationships

The course of marital relationships in the patients' families proved to be closely associated with the patients' psychiatric condition. Marital discord and/or breakdown were twice as frequent when the patient showed a personality disorder. Also, even when this diagnostic group was excluded, marital difficulties were more likely to continue throughout the four-year follow-up period if the patient's psychiatric condition persisted. In the case of families in which the patients showed a personality disorder, that disorder (or factors associated with

Table 6.9   Patients' disorders and course of marital relationships

	Diagnosis of patient		
	Psychosis (%) $(n=24)$	Affective disorder (%) $(n=45)$	Personality disorder (%) $(n=48)$
The course of marital relationships			
No discord	67	67	35
Predominant discord	8	11	31
Breakdown	17	2	19

$$\chi^2 = 17.60, \ df = 4, \ p < 0.01$$

New spouse (none previously)	4	9	4
No spouse	4	11	10

	Persistence of disorder in patient (excluding personality disorder)	
	None/mild (%) $(n=37)$	Moderate/marked (%) $(n=22)$
Predominant marital relationships		
Good/satisfactory	92	47
Discordant	3	19
Breakdown	0	13

$$\chi^2 = 13.62, \ df = 2, \ p < 0.01$$

New spouse (none before)	0	13
No spouse or death of spouse	5	9

it) must have led to the marital difficulties rather than the other way round simply because the personality abnormalities antedated the marriage. However, when there was no personality disorder the direction of causal relationships was less easy to determine. By definition, the sample included no families with marital discord but without psychiatric disorder. There were a few families without discord when first seen who developed marital difficulties during the course of the next four years but the number was too small for statistical analysis. The data on individuals with personality disorder point to the effect of psychiatric disorder on marital relationship but the data from our follow-up of institution-reared girls (see Chapter 8) point to the opposite effect. It seems highly likely that the association represents a complex two-way interaction.

Disorder in spouses

It has already been noted that the spouses of patients showed higher rates of psychiatric disorder than spouses in the general population (Table 6.3). Table 6.10 shows the course of disorder in spouses in the patient-parent sample varied

Table 6.10 Diagnosis and course of patients' conditions and disorders in spouses

	Diagnosis of patient		
	Psychosis (%) ($n = 20$)	Affective disorder (%) ($n = 39$)	Personality disorder (%) ($n = 38$)
Follow-up of disorders in spouses			
No symptoms	55	56	37
Mild persistence	25	36	37
Moderate persistence	10	0	5
Persisting handicap	10	8	21

No statistically significant differences

	Persistence of disorder in patient			
	None (%) ($n = 11$)	Mild (%) ($n = 34$)	Moderate (%) ($n = 17$)	Marked (%) ($n = 27$)
Follow-up of disorders in spouses				
No symptoms	55	68	29	33
Mild persistence	36	24	53	41
Moderate persistence	9	0	12	4
Marked persistence	0	9	6	22

$\chi^2 = 17.05$; df $= 9$; $p < 0.05$

according to patient characteristics. There was no significant association with the diagnosis of the patient's condition, although spouses were least likely to remain free of symptoms when the patient had a personality disorder. The chronicity of the patient's disorder over the follow-up period was significantly associated with the likelihood of persistent psychiatric problems in the spouse. When the patient recovered or had symptoms for less than one-third of the follow-up period, the majority of the spouses remained symptom free. However, when the patient's disorder was persistent, only one-third of the spouses remained symptom free.

Two main alternatives may be suggested as explanations for these findings; namely 'assortative mating' (i.e. that psychiatrically vulnerable individuals chose similarly vulnerable people to marry) and 'contagion' (i.e. that illness in one person sets up maladaptive patterns of marital interaction or creates stresses that predispose to the development of disorder in the spouse). The finding that the excess of disorder in the husbands of female patients was largely accounted for by personality disorders (Table 6.3) suggests the operation of either assortative mating (in that the personality disorders must have preceded marriage) or the effect of disorder in the husbands on the wives. The possibility of a 'contagion' effect is best examined in the families in which the spouses showed *no* psychiatric disorder at the time of first interview. If there is some form of 'contagion', disorders should be most likely to develop in the spouses of patients with a psychiatric disorder that persisted over the follow-up period. The data showed that this was the case. Of twenty-four female spouses well in year 0 and living continuously with patients whose disorders remitted or showed only mild persistence, 19 per cent developed psychiatric problems during the follow-up. In contrast, 63 per cent of the wives ($n = 8$) where the persistence was moderate or marked did so (exact test $p = 0.05$). This pattern was much less marked for previously well male spouses with regard to the persistence of the wife's disorder (23 per cent versus 35 per cent). This sex difference may be due to the higher proportion of male patients with persistently handicapping personality disorders but numbers were too few to determine this point. Alternatively, wives may be more affected by illness in their husbands than the other way round.

In both sexes these disorders that developed during the follow-up period were mostly circumscribed episodes of between one and three months for men and three and six months for women. It seems clear that in these cases the spouses disorders were relatively short-term reactions to stresses associated with the patients' continuing disorder. On the other hand, the association between disorders in husbands and wives in the case of personality disorders and other more chronic conditions is likely to have included some element of assortative mating. However, it should be noted that there was no particular tendency for the disorders in husbands and wives to be similar in type. If assortative mating operated it must have involved matching on some other characteristics in the individuals or in the backgrounds in which they grew up.

Emotional and behavioural disturbances in the children

Having established the pattern of disorders in the parents, and of family relationships, during the course of the four-year prospective study, it is necessary to consider the findings with respect to possible effects on the children. For this purpose, we need initially to turn to the teacher questionnaire data—comparing the findings for children in the 'total sample' of parent-patients' families with those for children in the age and sex matched 'classroom control group'.

Teacher questionnaire findings

The 259 patients' families in the 'total sample' had 556 children aged 15 years or less at first contact (274 boys and 282 girls). Of these, 199 were less than 5 years of age at that time. By the end of the study period only 11 had not started school and 101 had reached 16 years of age, the great majority of whom had left school. Questionnaires were completed on all but four children in every year in which they were eligible (i.e. were at school).

Table 6.11 gives the case/control comparisons for each year of the study. Disturbance was operationally defined (as throughout this chapter), as a score of 9 or more on the teacher questionnaire—the score previously found to provide the best discrimination (Rutter, 1967; Rutter et al., 1970; Rutter et al., 1975a). These year-by-year comparisons show a fluctuating pattern of associations with significant case/control differences at some points but not at others, but with

Table 6.11   Child disturbance on teacher's questionnaire: total sample

	Boys		Girls	
	Cases (%)	Controls (%)	Cases (%)	Controls (%)
Disturbance by year[†]	$(n=157-186)$	$(n=308-363)$	$(n=153-197)$	$(n=300-378)$
Year 0	34	28	31	12***
Year 1	38	25**	23	17
Year 2	37	27*	25	18
Year 3	31	26	23	22
Year 4	35	28	31	20**
Persistence of disturbance[‡]	$(n=120)$	$(n=231)$	$(n=121)$	$(n=227)$
No deviance	34	47	46	57
Fluctuating	34	35	33	31
Persistent	32	18	21	11
	$\chi^2=9.78$, df=2, $p<0.01$		$\chi^2=6.42$, df=2, $p<0.05$	

Cases and controls significantly different at: *5% level, **1% level, ***0.1% level.
[†]The n on these comparisons vary from year to year because of children starting and leaving school.
[‡]Always eligible children only.

the rates always higher in the children of patients. Where significant differences occurred, there was no clear pattern regarding the type of disturbance — except in year 0 where the higher rate of disturbance among girls in the patients' families was largely accounted for by an excess of conduct disorders.

To some extent these inconsistent findings reflect differences in the children included in samples each year (as a result of children starting and leaving school), but also they reflect the high frequency of transient disturbance in children in the control group, as well as the limitations of questionnaire measures. The picture becomes clearer when persistent disturbance in those children always eligible for ratings (i.e. at school throughout the four years) is considered. Children with *no* deviant ratings during the study were rated as *non-disturbed*, those with three or more deviant scores as *persistently disturbed* and the remainder as *fluctuating*. It is apparent (Table 6.11) that the differences between cases and controls were more clear-cut for both boys and girls when this measure was used. Persistent disturbance was nearly twice as frequent in the children in the families of psychiatric patients, whereas fluctuating disturbance was equally common in cases and controls. Overall these differences were largely accounted for by an excess of conduct disturbance in the offspring of patients but this difference reached statistical significance only in boys.

The relatively high rate of emotional and behavioural disturbance in the classroom control group may seem surprising. However, not only was this an inner-city sample living in a socially disadvantaged area known for its high level of psychosocial problems (Rutter *et al.*, 1975a), but also it constituted a random sample of the population. This meant that necessarily it included many children whose parents suffered from a psychiatric disorder (Rutter *et al.*, 1975b), creating some overlap between the groups.

Psychiatric disorder

The detailed parental interview information provides a more valid estimate of clinically significant psychiatric problems than do scores on the teacher questionnaire. As on the questionnaire, about one-third of boys were judged to have current handicapping problems whereas this was true for about one-quarter of the girls — proportions that were roughly similar to those on the questionnaire. However, for both boys and girls the type of disorder at interview showed a much more even distribution than that on the questionnaire, with emotional disorders being more prominent in the interview ratings. No comparisons with general population figures are possible except within the restricted 8–12-year age band used earlier for the comparisons of family relationships (see Table 6.12). When comparison was made with the control group, no difference in rate of emotional/behavioural disorder was found. This appears to be due to the high rate of psychosocial adversity in the comparison group families (Rutter and Quinton, 1984).

Table 6.12   Child psychiatric disorder: parental interview

	Boys (%)	Girls (%)
Year 0	(n = 86)	(n = 80)
No disorder	66	76
Emotional	12	10
Conduct	12	5
Mixed	10	5
Other	0	4

$$\chi^2 = 6.02, \ df = 4, \ NS$$

	Boys (%)	Girls (%)
*Persistence of disorder**	(n = 54)	(n = 61)
Well	35	48
Fluctuating	33	41
Persistent impairment	31	12

$$\chi^2 = 6.98, \ df = 2, \ p < 0.05$$

Disorder in 8–12 year olds

	Boys		Girls	
	Cases* (%) (n = 40)	Controls (%) (n = 53)	Cases* (%) (n = 31)	Controls (%) (n = 44)
None	78	81	77	70
Disorder	22	19	23	30
Emotional type	13	6	13	14
Conduct/mixed	10	8	10	5
Other	0	6	0	11

*Year 0 data.

No control-group comparisons are possible on the persistence of disorders as the comparison sample was interviewed on one occasion only. Persistence in the cases was rated in a comparable way to the teacher questionnaire. Full psychiatric ratings were made from the mothers' account at four of the five interviews (years 0, 1, 2 and 4) for up to two children per family aged 3–15 years inclusive. For the children always eligible for assessment a rating of *no disorder* was made if there were never any periods of socially handicapping symptomatology (based on an overall clinical assessment, not on individual ratings); a rating of *persistent disorder* if handicap was present on at least two occasions with no symptom free interludes; and a rating of *fluctuating disorder* for the remaining children.

It is apparent from Table 6.12 that handicapping psychiatric problems occurred in over half the always eligible boys and girls at some time during the study period. Persistent disorder occurred significantly more frequently in boys

(31 per cent versus 12 per cent). In boys 59 per cent of these disorders were conduct or mixed problems as against 43 per cent in girls.

We may conclude that psychiatric disturbances were indeed more frequent in the children of parents with a psychiatric disorder than in the general population. The excess rate of disorder largely, if not entirely, applied to those that were persistent over time as well as pervasive over situations and was most marked in the case of disturbances of conduct. The rates of disturbance were higher in both the sons and daughters of psychiatric patients but the increased level of disorder was most evident in the boys.

Parental illness and disturbance in the children

We now move on to consider the particular patterns of relationships between mental illness in parents and psychiatric disturbances in their children. In order to eliminate artefacts due to single-parent status, or marital breakdown or disorders in spouses, many of the following analyses are restricted to children living with both natural parents and where the spouse was well. These restrictions are given with the table headings.

Type of parental disorder

Tables 6.13 and 6.14 give the findings for the type of parental disorder in year 0. In analyses restricted to children living with two parents only one of whom was ill, there were no significant differences in the rates of child disturbance or disorder according to the type of psychiatric condition suffered by the parent-patient. That is, the diagnosis of the parent did not affect the psychiatric risk for the children. However, as early analyses made clear, the restriction of the sample in this way omitted a substantial number of families, particularly those in which one or both parents has a personality disorder. This is because of the high rates of disorder in spouses in these cases. The effect of personality disorders can be examined by comparing those cases in which

Table 6.13   Parental diagnosis and child deviance and disorder year 0 (children living with both natural parents: spouse well)

| | Parental diagnosis | | |
	Psychosis	Affective/ emotional disorder	Personality disorder
Percentage deviant on teacher questionnaire	21% (14)	21% (33)	30% (27)
Percentage with psychiatric disorder	14% (21)	24% (34)	17% (23)

No statistically significant differences.

Table 6.14   Parental personality disorders and disturbance in the children (year 0)

	Personality disorder		
	No personality disorder (%)	Antisocial type (%)	Other type (%)
Teacher questionnaire	($n = 70*$)	($n = 33$)	($n = 65$)
Proportion with disturbance	19	45	37
	$\chi^2 = 10.33$, df $= 2$, $p < 0.01$		
Percentage with conduct/mixed type (of those with disturbance)	46	80	75
	$\chi^2 = 4.44$, df $= 2$, NS		
	Presence versus absence personality disorder: $\chi^2 = 3.01$, df $= 1$, NS		
Parental interview	($n = 80*$)	($n = 25$)	($n = 54$)
Proportion with disorder	21	48	47
	$\chi^2 = 7.11$, df $= 2$, $p < 0.05$		
Percentage with conduct/mixed type (of those with disturbance)	58	50	61
	$\chi^2 = 0.38$, df $= 2$, NS		

*n are numbers of children (not patients).

neither parent had a personality disorder with those in which one or both parents had such a disorder. In this analysis families were differentiated both on the presence/absence of personality disorder in either parent and also according to whether or not the disorder was of an antisocial type.

These data show that there was a significantly increased rate of both disturbance (as assessed by questionnaire) and psychiatric disorder (assessed at interview) in children where one or both parents had a personality disorder. Three-quarters of disturbed ratings on the questionnaire in families with personality disorders involved conduct problems, whereas this was the case for less than half of those whose parents showed no personality disturbance. This association was as evident when the parent had a non-antisocial personality disorder (i.e. persistently impaired interpersonal relationships and social functioning but without significant violence or delinquent activities — mostly categorized as 'inadequate' personality) as when the personality disorder was antisocial in type. In other words, the conduct disturbance in the child was associated with impaired social functioning in the parent rather than with antisocial behaviour as such. The parental interview ratings also showed that the children were most at psychiatric risk when one or both parents had a personality disorder, but there was not the same tendency for a specific link with disorders of conduct.

These two analyses suggest that features of family life associated with personality problems rather than specific types of abnormal parental behaviour or specific forms of parental mental disorder are responsible for the increased levels of children's problems. This question is considered further below.

One further issue in the linkage between the type of parental illness and the type of disorder in the child concerns the relationship between major depressive disorders in parents and depressive illness in the children. The presence of major depressive disorder in the parents was defined by the presence of manic-depressive psychosis *or* by a diagnosis of affective disorder at a sufficient severity to disrupt social or work activities, together with a score above 8 on a depressive symptoms scale involved crying, misery, suicidal thoughts or behaviour, self depreciation, loss of self confidence and feeling of reference. Depression in childhood was defined according to criteria based on those established by Pearce (1978) in a case note study of Maudsley Hospital patients. A rating of depression was made if the child had currently handicapping misery together with *two* or more of disturbances of sleep, disturbances of eating, morbid irritability, alimentary symptoms, obsessional behaviour or school refusal. The analysis on the linkage of disorders was confined to cases in which the spouse was free of personality disorder or other significant mental illness (apart from minor affective/emotional disorder only). Of the twenty-six children with some form of psychiatric disorder whose parents were free of major depressive disorder four (18 per cent) were rated as having depression whereas of the seven ill children whose parents had major depressive problems four (57 per cent) did so (exact test $p = 0.04$). This analysis lends some support to the hypothesis of a link between depressive disorders in parents and children, but the small numbers do not allow any further exploration of the nature of this link.

In summary the data show only slight links between the *form* of the parental disorder and the presence of disturbance or disorder in the children. This was to be expected if the children's problems were substantially a response to parental behaviour (rather than genetically determined) since, as Table 6.6 showed, a wide range of symptomatic behaviours were common to a number of diagnoses. The relative importance of the two main groups of parental behaviours—hostile/aggressive behaviour and expressed anxiety depression—can be assessed by fitting linear logistic models to behavioural disturbance on the teacher questionnaire.

Linear logistic modelling techniques are an appropriate multivariate method for the analysis of data in which the dependent variable is dichotomized or on an ordinal scale (Dunn, 1981). These methods are closely similar to a traditional regression analysis but with cross-classified categorical data (Swafford, 1980). The procedure is to subtract the deviance (comparable to χ^2) and degrees of

Table 6.15   Exposure to symptomatic behaviour and disturbance in the children (year 0, spouse well) linear logistic analysis

Model fitted	Deviance	df	p	model	Reduction in deviance from df	p
(A) Constant	10.73	3	0.02		—	—	—
(B) Hostile behaviour	2.10	2	NS	(from (A))	9.13	1	0.01
(C) Anxiety, depression	8.69	2	0.02	(from (A))	0.55	1	NS
(D) Hostile + anxious/ depressive	1.22	1	NS	(from (A))	9.51	2	0.01
Improvement in fit by adding (B) to (C)					7.47	1	0.01
Improvement in fit by adding (C) to (B)					0.88	1	NS

freedom (df) for a particular model from an earlier one and to decide in terms of statistical significance whether the variables included in the new model significantly reduce the overall deviance, the aim being to fit the observed to the expected frequencies in the full table with the most parsimonious model. In Table 6.15, for example, the overall deviance (Model (A) column 2) is significantly different from chance at the 0.2 per cent level showing that the model of 'no association' does not fit the data well. Fitting 'hostile behaviour' (Model (B)) gives a significant improvement in fit (10.73–2.10 = 8.63 with 1 df) and leaves the deviance (column 2) at a level not significantly above chance. On the other hand, 'anxiety, depression' on its own (Model (C)) does not reduce the deviance to a significant extent and does not fit the data well. The improvement in fit of adding 'anxiety depression' to the 'hostile behaviour only' model can be determined by subtracting the fit of the additive Model (D) from Model (B). As expected this gives no significant improvement, confirming that hostile behaviour on its own provides a satisfactory fit for the data. Large and complete cross-classified data sets can be analysed using these techniques and models including interaction terms evaluated either by forward or backward selection of models. The GLIM computer program (Baker and Nelder, 1978) was used for this analysis.

Persistence of parental disorder

Emotional/behavioural disturbance in the children that persisted through the four-year follow-up period was appreciably more frequent when the parent-patient had a personality disorder (32 per cent) than when the parental diagnosis was some form of affective disorder (13 per cent) or psychosis (0 per cent), but the difference fell short of statistical significance. The same trend was apparent on the psychiatric interview ratings of disorder in the child (38 per cent, 7 per

Table 6.16 Type and persistence of parental disorder and persistence of children's problems (always eligible children — spouse well)

	Type of parental disorder					
	Psychosis		Affective disorder		Personality disorder	
	Persistent disorders in children		Persistent disorders in children		Persistent disorders in children	
	%	n	%	n	%	n
Teacher questionnaire						
Persistence of parental disorder						
None/mild	0	6	5	20	57	7
Moderate/marked	0	5	30	10	24	21
Total	0	11	13	30	32	28

Difference by parental diagnosis: $\chi^2 = 4.49$, df = 2, NS
No significant difference by parental persistence within parental diagnostic groups

	%	n	%	n	%	n
Parental interview						
Persistence of parental disorder						
None/mild	11	9	5	20	25	4
Moderate/marked	0	6	11	9	40	20
Total	6	15	7	29	38	9

Difference by parental diagnosis: $\chi^2 = 5.98$, df = 2, $p < 0.05$
No significant difference by parental persistence within parental diagnostic groups

cent and 6 per cent respectively); the difference being statistically significant. In each case, the high rate of persistent disorders in the children occurred when the parent-patient had a personality disorder. Persistence of parental disorder was not related to persistent children's problems on either measure once parental diagnosis had been taken into account. This could mean either that the relationship between personality disorder and persistent disturbance in the children was mediated by genetic rather than experiential factors, or that parental behaviours, other than overt symptoms, were crucial in promoting persistent problems in the children. To test these alternatives the children were grouped according to whether or not the parent had a personality disorder and also according to the level of hostile behaviour they experienced (see Table 6.17).

The analysis showed that personality disorder in the parent was not associated with an increased rate of persistent disorder in the children in the absence of hostile and aggressive behaviour, whereas exposure to hostile behaviour was associated with persistent disturbance in the children irrespective of the presence or absence of parental personality disorder. The rates of persistent disturbance in the children (whether assessed by teacher questionnaire or by parental

Table 6.17   Persistence in child, exposure to hostile behaviour and personality disorder (intact families, spouse well)

	Exposure to hostile behaviour			
	None/little: Percentage of children with persistent disturbance		Moderate/marked: Percentage of children with persistent disturbance	
(1) *Teacher questionnaire* Personality disorder in patient	%	n	%	n
No	10	(21)	26	(19)
Yes	0	(12)	48	(27)
(2) *Psychiatric disorder* Personality disorder in patient				
No	0	(23)	29	(14)
Yes	0	(7)	50	(16)

Teacher questionnaire: linear logistic analysis

Model fitted	Deviance	df	p		Reduction in deviance	df	p
(A) Constant	16.09	3	0.001		—	—	—
(B) Personality disorder	14.24	2	0.001	(from (A))	2.65	1	NS
(C) Hostile behaviour	4.17	2	NS	(from (A))	12.72	1	0.001
(D) Personality + hostile	3.21	1	NS	(from (A))	13.68	1	0.001
(E) Improvement in fit by adding hostile behaviour to personality				(from (B))	11.03	1	0.001
(F) Improvement in fit by adding personality to hostile behaviour				(from (C))	0.96	1	NS

Parental interview: linear logistic analysis

Model fitted	Deviance	df	p		Reduction in deviance	df	p
(A) Constant	21.12	3	0.001		—	—	—
(B) Personality disorder	16.14	2	0.001	(from (A))	4.90	1	0.05
(C) Hostile behaviour	1.50	2	NS	(from (A))	19.62	1	0.001
(D) Personality + hostile	0.008	1	NS	(from (A))	21.11	1	0.001
(E) Improvement in fit by adding personality to hostile				(from (C))	1.49	1	NS
(F) Improvement in fit by adding hostile to personality				(from (B))	16.13	1	0.001

interview) were highest of all (48–50 per cent) when there was *both* a parental personality disorder *and* exposure to hostile/aggressive behaviour, but this interaction effect fell short of statistical significance.

Most strikingly (although the numbers were small), no children reared by parents with a personality disorder showed persistent disturbance in the absence of exposure to hostile behaviour. On the other hand, a quarter of the children whose parents did *not* show a personality disorder but who were exposed to hostile/aggressive behaviour were found to have some form of emotional/behavioural disturbance that persisted through the four-year follow-up period.

In summary, for the most part, there were few associations between the diagnosis of the parents' mental illness and the type of disorder shown by the children. One possible partial exception concerned the association between *major* (not minor) depressive disorder in the parent and depression in the child. The numbers were too small to analyse the association further but it warrants further study. The second partial exception concerned the possible link between personality disorder in the parent and conduct disturbance in the children. However, to a large extent this association was more a consequence of the children's exposure to hostile/aggressive behaviour than of the parental diagnosis per se. Nevertheless, although the effect fell short of statistical significance it is possible that parental personality disorder put the children at an additional psychiatric risk beyond that accounted for by exposure to hostile behaviour.

Marital discord

Marital discord constituted one common source of hostile behaviour; as already noted, a high proportion of patients' marriages showed marked discord at the time of initial interview or had previously broken as a result of discord. In a few further cases, discord developed during the course of the follow-up period. Table 6.18 summarizes the findings on the associations between marital discord or disruption and emotional/behavioural disturbance in the children as determined by teachers' questionnaire scores. The first comparison deals with the situation at the time of the patients' first hospital attendance (year 0). There was a strong association with disturbance in boys (57 per cent of disturbance in the presence of discord/disruption versus 0 per cent in its absence), but not girls (33 per cent versus 19 per cent).

The second comparison concerns discord/disruption at year 0 with persistent disturbance *after* year 0 (i.e. a score of 9 or more on the teachers' questionnaire on at least two occasions between years 1 and 4, ignoring the score in year 0). The same strong association is apparent for boys (57 per cent versus 18 per cent). Of the boys already showing disturbance in year 0, over four-fifths (81 per cent) showed persistent disturbance over the next four years, and of those without emotional/behavioural difficulties initially a quarter (25 per cent) went on to develop persistent disturbance. The situation was somewhat different for girls

Table 6.18   Marital discord and disturbance in the children (marital discord/disruption)

| | Marital Discord/Disruption | | | | |
| | Absent:
Percentage
disturbed
(Total n) | | Present:
Percentage
disturbed
(Total n) | | Statistical
significance | |
				χ^2	df	p
(a) *Discord/disruption at year 0 and disturbance in year 0*						
Boys	0	(17)	57	(37)	13.49	1	<0.001
Girls	19	(27)	33	(33)	1.00	1	NS
(b) *Discord/disruption at year 0 and persistent disturbance over next four years*						
Boys	18	(17)	57	(37)	5.72	1	<0.025
Girls	19	(27)	42	(33)	2.89	1	NS
(c) *Discord/disruption and disturbance in children without disturbance at year 0*						
Boys	13	(15)	22	(23)	0.05	1	NS
Girls	10	(20)	33	(24)	2.18	1	NS
(d) *Overall discord/disruption and persistent disturbance*						
Boys	13	(15)	56	(37)	6.49	1	<0.025
Girls	13	(23)	41	(37)	3.88	1	<0.05

in that although there was no association with *initial* disturbance, there was an association with *persistent* disturbance (42 per cent versus 19 per cent), albeit one that fell short of statistical significance.

A possible reason for this occurrence is evident from the findings in the third comparison, which deals with the association between discord/disruption in year 0 and/or predominant discord during the four-year follow-up period, and persistent emotional/behavioural disturbance in the children (defined as for the second comparison); the findings referring only to those children *without* disturbance in year 0. In boys, there was little tendency for disturbance to develop in the presence of discord (22 per cent versus 13 per cent), if it had not been already evident in year 0. However, in girls there was a tendency for persistent disturbance to develop if discord/disruption continued (33 per cent versus 10 per cent; exact test $p = 0.07$). It seemed that the girls were less likely to show an immediate reaction to discord, but there was a less-marked sex difference in persistent long-term disturbance in response to marital discord or disruption. Also, it should be noted that the lack of an initial effect in girls was due in part to the moderately high level of disturbance (19 per cent) in those from non-discordant homes. Presumably the disturbance in girls was associated with other family features apart from discord/disruption.

Unfortunately, small numbers prevented any adequate study of the effects on children of a change from marital discord to marital harmony. There were some families in which discord diminished (although in the majority it continued) but there were very few in which harmony resulted. The limited reduction in discord was not associated with any appreciable benefits in terms of the children's disturbance.

The last comparison summarizes the findings on long-term effects of marital discord/disruption (either in year 0 or present as a preponderant pattern thereafter) in terms of persistent disturbance in the children. There was a significant association in both sexes, although it was somewhat stronger in boys (56 per cent versus 13 per cent) than in girls (41 per cent versus 13 per cent). We may conclude that marital discord/disruption constituted an important stressor for both the sons and daughters of parents with psychiatric disorder. It seemed that the boys tended to develop disturbance *earlier* than the girls but, if the discord continued the girls also suffered in the long run.

Mental disorder in patients' spouses

The high frequency of mental disorder in patients' spouses has been noted already, as has the extent to which this was associated with high rates of family

Table 6.19 Psychiatric disorder in spouse, exposure to hostile behaviour and disturbance in the children (Disorder in spouse year 1)

	None/ mild		Moderate/ severe		Statistical significance		
	%	total n	%	total n	χ^2	df	p
Percentage disturbance teacher questionnaire	22	133	83	59	61.04	1	<0.001
Percentage disorder parental interview	20	103	38	38	3.97	1	<0.05

	None/minor				Moderate/severe			
	Low exposure		High exposure		Low exposure		High exposure	
	%	total n	%	total n	%	total n	%	total n
Percentage disturbance teacher questionnaire	13	68	31	64	80	10	84	49
Percentage disorder parental interview	11	53	31	48	17	12	46	26

Linear Logistic analyses
(a) Teacher questionnaire: For the TQ both illness in spouse and exposure to hostile behaviour significantly reduce the overall deviance at the 0.01 per cent level but both terms are needed to provide a satisfactory fit for the data.
(b) Parental interview: The table for disturbance on the parental interview is satisfactorily fitted by the inclusion of exposure to hostile behaviour on its own, although illness in spouse also gives a significant ($p<0.01$) reduction in overall deviance. The addition of illness in spouse and hostile behaviour is not significant, but the converse is at the 0.01 per cent level.

discord and disruption. Not surprisingly, therefore, the psychiatric risk to the children was greater when *both* their parents were mentally ill rather than just one (see Table 6.19). However, as Table 6.19 shows, to a large extent this was a function of the fact that the children's exposure to hostile behaviour tended to be greater when both parents had a psychiatric disorder. It may well be that the increased genetic risk was important but so too were the increased environmental hazards stemming from the high level of discord.

Gender, temperament and disturbance in the children

The final set of analyses concern the role of gender and temperament in the development of psychiatric disturbance in the children.

Sex of patient and disturbance in the children

In an earlier study (Rutter, 1966), one of us found that the ill-effects of both parental mental illness and of parental death seemed to impinge most on children of the same sex. We sought to determine whether or not that was also so in the current study. Table 6.20 shows the association between the sex of the parent-patient and the sex of the children with persistent emotional/behavioural disturbance. There was a tendency for the sons to be more likely to show disturbance when the father was the patient (40 per cent versus 25 per cent on the teacher questionnaire and 33 per cent versus 22 per cent on the parental interview ratings) and for the daughters to do so when the mother was the patient (11 per cent versus 0 per cent and 16 per cent versus 0 per cent respectively). However, the absolute numbers were necessarily small (because of the need to exclude all families in which the spouse showed psychiatric disorder) and the differences fell short of statistical significance.

Because to a substantial extent it seemed that the effects of parental illness were mediated through the children's exposure to hostile behaviour, the analysis

Table 6.20   Sex of patient and sex of children with disturbance (intact families only in which the spouse has no more than minor transient psychiatric problems)

	Female patient				Male patient			
	Sons		Daughters		Sons		Daughters	
	%	total n	%	total n	%	total n	%	total n
Percentage persistent disturbance (Teacher questionnaire)	25	12	11	18	40	15	0	16
Percentage persistent disorder (Interview assessment)	22	18	16	19	33	9	0	14

Table 6.21   Persistent disturbance in boys and girls according to which parent was hostile (intact families with children at school throughout study)

| | Girls: Hostile behaviour mother | | | | Boys: Hostile behaviour mother | | | |
| | None/some | | Moderate/marked | | None/some | | Moderate/marked | |
Hostile behaviour father	%	n	%	n	%	n	%	n
None/some	0	21	36	11	15	12	40	10
Moderate/marked	0	4	38	8	71	7	33	6

No differences significant for comparisons across diagonals.

was repeated according to which parent showed hostile behaviour (see Table 6.21). Once again there was a suggestion of a same-sex association but the differences fell short of statistical significance. The key comparisons concern the diagonals in Table 6.21, which refer to the situation when one parent, but not the other, was hostile or aggressive. When the mother, but not the father, was hostile 36 per cent of the girls were disturbed according to the teacher questionnaire scores compared with 0 per cent when the hostility stemmed from the father. The comparable figures for boys were 40 per cent and 71 per cent — i.e. the opposite trend.

Clearly, the numbers in the key cells were too small to take the matter further and, in the absence of statistically significant differences, it must remain uncertain whether or not the consistent trend for same-sexed children to be most at risk was a valid finding. The matter warrants further study.

Temperamental characteristics

At the time of the initial interview (year 0), mothers of children between the ages of 3 and 8 years were interviewed to obtain systematic information on their children's temperamental attributes. A detailed account was obtained regarding the children's behaviour in a standard list of specified recently occurring situations (such as meeting new people or adapting to changed circumstances). On this basis ratings were made on temperamental characteristics originally developed in the New York study (Thomas *et al.*, 1968) and revised and extended for the present investigation (Graham *et al.*, 1973). The data showed that the children most likely to be showing disturbance a year later were those with markedly irregular sleeping, eating and bowel habits; whose behaviour lacked malleability and who were less fastidious, being more tolerant of mess and dirt than most children.

On the basis of these findings and those from the New York study (Rutter *et al.*, 1964) the attributes of negative mood, low regularity, low malleability

Table 6.22   Temperamental adversity and persistent child disturbance

	Disturbance absent			Disturbance present	
	%	total n		%	total n
Teacher Questionnaire					
No disturbance year 0	15	13	($p = 0.14$)	67	3
	(NS)			(NS)	
Disturbance year 0	60	5	(NS)	100	6
Parental Interview					
No disturbance year 0	36	11	($p = 0.03$)	100	5
	(NS)			(NS)	
Disturbance year 0	50	6	($p = 0.12$)	100	5

and low fastidiousness were combined to form a temperamental adversity index (Rutter, 1978). The index was produced by summing the four attributes; in each case giving a score of 1 if the child's preponderant behaviour across situations was at the specified end of the dimension. Children with two or more adverse characteristics were designated *high temperamental adversity* (TA) and the remainder a *low temperamental adversity*.

Of the three children with non-deviant teacher questionnaire scores initially, but with temperamental adversity, two went on to show emotional/behavioural disturbance during the follow-up period compared with a sixth (15 per cent) of the thirteen without temperamental adversity (exact test $p = 0.14$). The comparable figures using the interview ratings for psychiatric disorder were 100 per cent versus 36 per cent (exact test $p = 0.03$). Thus, the child's temperament proved to be a better predictor of the later development of disturbance at school than was a questionnaire measure of disturbance as shown at home (see Graham *et al.*, 1973). Altogether, 89 per cent of children with temperamental adversity showed disturbance on the teacher questionnaire at some point compared with 39 per cent of those without temperamental adversity (exact test $p = 0.02$); the comparable figures for persistent disturbance were 89 per cent and 28 per cent (exact test $p = 0.003$) and for persistent disorder on the interview ratings 100 per cent and 41 per cent (exact test $p = 0.001$).

The processes that lead to disorders in temperamentally at risk children are not well understood (see Dunn, 1980; Rutter, 1977b; Porter and Collins, 1982). It may be that these children are generally more susceptible to the adverse effects of various stresses, but also it may be that their own characteristics tend to produce more negative responses in parents, especially when the parents are themselves suffering from psychiatric disorder. Because children with these attributes are more difficult to rear, they may well arouse more irritation and their parents may come to expect them to be difficult. Such expectations may become self-fulfilling.

Our numbers were rather small for a systematic test of this possibility but the data are consistent with the suggestion. Children with an adverse temperament (based on information from mothers) were somewhat more likely to come from discordant homes but, within such homes, they were more likely than other children to be the target of parental hostility and criticism (83 per cent versus 38 per cent; exact test $p = 0.18$) as assessed on the basis of an interview with the father by a different interviewer. Overall, in the sample as a whole, children with TA were twice as likely as temperamentally easy children to be subjected to maternal criticism (78 per cent versus 38 per cent; exact test $p = 0.02$). Moreover, parental criticism was strongly associated with the occurrence of emotional/behavioural disturbance during the follow-up period, especially in children with high TA. The suggestion is that the children's temperamental features in part determined the likelihood that they would be drawn into a maladaptive pattern of parent–child interaction, a pattern that in turn predisposed to the development of disturbance.

DISCUSSION AND CONCLUSIONS

Course of psychiatric disorder in parents

When we planned this prospective four-year longitudinal study we had in mind the need to study the time relationships between remissions and relapses in the parents' mental illness and the course of psychiatric disorder in the children. The hypothesis that the former *caused* the latter could be tested on the supposition that if the causal hypothesis was true, the parental condition should not only have started first but also as it remitted so should the children's disturbance lessen. The longitudinal data on the course of psychiatric disorder in the parent-patients were crucial in their demonstration that this model did not apply to the population studied. Acute onsets were the exception rather than the rule and in only about one case in ten did the patients remain symptom-free for the whole of the follow-up period starting one year after initial hospital attendance. For those who did not show a personality disorder at the initial assessment, the modal pattern was one of remissions and relapses with symptoms present for up to one-third of the time. However, two-fifths of the parent-patients *did* have a personality disorder and for them the modal pattern was for symptoms to be present for *most* of the follow-up period.

The findings emphasize the clinical importance of making an assessment of personality functioning as well as of the presenting psychiatric disorder. Other studies (e.g. Tyrer *et al.*, 1983; Weissman *et al.*, 1978) have similarly confirmed the predictive value of personality measures, although they have used rather different concepts of personality. Thus, Weissman *et al.* (1978) used the neuroticism scale of the Maudsley Personality Inventory and Tyrer *et al.* (1983) used a standardized interview appraisal designed to elicit both the presence of traits such as suspiciousness and aggression and also the extent to which they were associated with overt problems in occupational, social and interpersonal relationships (Tyrer and Alexander, 1979; Tyrer et al., 1979). The latter group of workers found that it was important to obtain data from an informant as well as from the patient, and that most personality disorders fall into the 'passive-dependent', or 'sociopathic' categories, although all types (including 'anankastic') were associated with a markedly worse prognosis (Tyrer et al., 1983). We, too, found that it was the presence of pervasively impaired interpersonal functioning that predicted a worse outcome rather than any one particular facet of personality.

The concept of personality disorder has proved elusive (Lewis, 1974) and there is justified scepticism (Shepherd and Sartorius, 1974) about the validity of the distinctions between the different subcategories of personality disorder in ICD-9 and DSM-III. Also there is continuing uncertainty regarding just what is involved in personality development and what is meant by personality (Rutter, 1984a and b). Nevertheless, the evidence from this study and from that by Tyrer et al. (1979, 1983) clearly indicates the validity of the general notion of personality disorder. Not only did it prove to be a powerful predictor of outcome but also the duration of symptoms in the absence of a personality disorder did not predict outcome in non-psychotic disorders. Similarly, as noted by others (Huxley et al., 1979), we found that the form of the acute psychiatric disorder was of little value for prognosis. The implication is that the distinction between personality disorder and other forms of psychiatric disorder is a useful one. However, the findings also suggest that what matters is the persistent impairment of interpersonal functioning at work, at home, and in social relationships. Probably, the specific traits that lead to such impairment are of much less importance.

Correlates of parental psychiatric disorder

Our results, like those of others, clearly indicate the very high frequency with which psychiatric disorders in adults are associated with a wide range of other psychosocial problems. In particular, it is very common for there to be accompanying marital discord and some form of mental disorder in the spouse. We found that this was most often the case when the patient suffered from a personality disorder but also it was a fairly common occurrence with other diagnoses. The mechanisms underlying the associations are likely to be complex. Data from other investigations suggest that to some extent the high rates of disorder in spouses reflect assortative mating. Thus, Merikangas and Spiker (1982) found that mentally ill spouses differed from those that were mentally well with respect to a family history of psychiatric disorder. That is to say, it appeared that the disorder in spouses was partially explicable in terms of their own background. However, the same study showed that in most cases neither partner had been mentally ill at the time of marriage (so that the assorting cannot have been on the basis of illness *per se*), and that the ill spouses were *less* likely than patients to have a family history of psychiatric disorder (27 per cent versus 38 per cent—Merikangas and Spiker, 1982). Our data suggest that the association between marriage partners with respect to psychiatric disorder reflects *both* assortative mating and 'contagion'. The latter is indicated by the finding that the likelihood of disorder in spouses was significantly associated with the course of the patient's disorder.

The nature of the relationship between psychiatric disorder and marital discord was even more difficult to disentangle, because both proved to be remarkably persistent over the four-year follow-up period. Cox and Mills (1983) in their six-month follow-up of depressed mothers, using a cross-lagged correlations analysis, found that depression was a better predictor of marriage at follow-up than the other way round—arguing that this suggested that depression adversely impaired marital relationships. Our own data also showed that marital difficulties were more likely to continue if the patient's psychiatric condition persisted. Obviously, then, the two are linked; the question is which leads to which. Cox and Mills's (1983) findings suggested that depression predisposed to discord. However, the findings from Brown and Harris's (1978) study of women and our own follow-up into adult life of institution-reared girls (Rutter and Quinton, 1984) indicated that the quality of marital relationships influenced the risk of psychiatric disorder. On the other hand, Bothwell and Weissman (1977), in a four-year follow-up study, found patients who had recovered from a depressive episode still showed more marital problems than normal controls. No firm conclusions on the nature and direction of the causal relationships are possible. However, there is support for at least three mechanisms, (a) a process by which marital discord predisposes to psychiatric disorder, (b) a process by which psychiatric disorder impairs marital relationships, and (c) a process by which *both* are caused by prior conditions (such as childhood adversities— Rutter and Quinton, 1984; or genetic predisposition) *and* by current circumstances (such as social disadvantage— Rutter *et al.*, 1983). The implication is that the treatment of adult psychiatric disorders needs to focus on both the acute symptoms and the accompanying social problems. It may be that different approaches are needed for these two facets of the problem.

Effects of parental mental disorder on the children

The findings from this study, like that of numerous others, show that the children of mentally ill parents have a substantially increased risk of developing psychiatric disorder during the childhood years. This is important in its highlighting of the need for psychiatrists treating adult patients to be aware that the children of their parents constitute a psychiatric 'at-risk' group. Nevertheless, it is far from inevitable that the children of psychiatric patients will suffer. We found that one-third suffered no emotional or behavioural disturbance during the whole of the four-year follow-up period, and a further third had purely transient psychiatric problems. Nevertheless, one-third of the boys and a somewhat lower proportion of the girls exhibited a persistent disorder. The difference from the controls lay almost entirely in this last persistent group. The findings re-emphasize the high frequency of transient emotional and behavioural difficulties in the general population (Rutter et al., 1970; Shepherd et al., 1971); also they show that the increased risk among the children of psychiatric patients is for the potentially more serious persistent psychiatric disorders. In addition, it is noteworthy that the disorders in the children were at least as obvious at school as they were at home. The main risk for the children did not lie in temporary situation-specific stress reactions but in disturbances that were pervasive over situations and persistent over time. Other work has shown the importance of the dimensions of pervasiveness and persistence in the assessment of children's psychiatric disorders (Rutter and Garmezy, 1983).

However, while parental mental illness constituted an important indicator of psychiatric risk for the children, the overall pattern of findings showed that in most cases the main risk did not stem from the illness itself. Rather it derived from the associated psychosocial disturbance in the family. Such disturbance may continue well after the acute symptoms abate (Bothwell and Weissman, 1977) and, hence, it is no surprise that, like previous investigators (Hobbs, 1982), we found no close connections between the ebb and flow of parental symptoms and the course of disorder in the children. The extent to which children were exposed to and involved in their parents' abnormal behaviour was relevant, but in this connection parental hostility, irritability, aggression and violence were more important than affective symptoms or psychotic manifestations. Both discord between the parents and hostility directed at the child were influential. To a substantial extent, these were consequences of the parental mental illness. However, not only were they indirect consequences for the most part, but also similar discord and hostility occurs in families without mental illness in either parent.

Of course, it is necessary to ask whether the disturbed intrafamilial relationships which *cause* disorders in the children are caused *by* the children's problems, or derive from some third set of variables. It may well be that children's difficult behaviour aggravates parental problems (indeed our findings on temperamental adversity are consistent with such a process). However, it seems unlikely that this constitutes the main explanation. Nor does it seem likely that the associations derive from some other variable. Our analyses with respect to exposure to 'hostile' behaviour showed that this was the main variable accounting for the children's emotional/behavioural disturbance *after* taking into account other measures. Moreover, it is important that family discord and disorganization has been found to provide the main effect on children's disturbance in samples as diverse as the general population (see Emery, 1982;

Rutter, 1982) and families in which a parent suffers from Huntington's chorea (Folstein *et al.*, 1983). Quarrelling, hostility and disruptive family relationships may stem from a variety of sources but it seems that, whatever their origin, they constitute a potent risk factor for the children. The implication is that preventive policies need to focus on measures designed to improve family relationships in high-risk groups.

It seems that family discord and hostility constitute the chief mediating variable in the association between parental mental disorder and psychiatric disturbance in the children. This is in keeping with the finding that the main effect was on conduct disturbances in the children; other studies have shown that children's problems of this type are commonly associated with family discord, disorganization and disruption (Rutter and Giller, 1983). Nevertheless, it would be wrong to assume that discord constituted the only operative mechanism. In the first place, our data suggested that the presence of a parent with a personality disorder may increase the psychiatric risk to the children even after taking into account exposure to hostile behaviour (although it had no effect in the absence of hostile behaviour). Stewart and de Blois (1983) found that the associations between aggression and antisocial behaviour in fathers and sons were greater when the fathers were in the home, but some association was found when fathers were absent. Both sets of data are consistent with a mainly environmental effect but a significant genetic contribution in some instances— perhaps especially in cases of pervasive antisocial disorders that persist into adult life (Crowe, 1983; Rutter and Giller, 1983).

Secondly, the mechanisms may differ according to the type of mental disorder suffered by the parent. Although, for example, parental depression and parental schizophrenia seem to carry similar psychiatric risks for the children (Cohler *et al.*, 1977; Fisher *et al.*, 1980; McNeil and Kaij, 1984; Rolf and Garmezy, 1974; Sameroff *et al.*, 1984; Weintraub *et al.*, 1978; Weintraub and Neale, 1984; Winters *et al.*, 1981; Worland *et al.*, 1984), they may well do so for different reasons. Thus, although discord constitutes the main factor involved in the association between parental depression or personality disorder and conduct disturbance in the children, Emery *et al.* (1982) found that it did not account for the increased rate of disorders in the children of schizophrenics. Our own sample included too few schizophrenics for this finding to be replicated. Nevertheless, the point is clear. The fact that the type of parental disorder is not a strong predictor of disturbances in the children does not necessarily mean that all forms of parental mental illness give rise to psychiatric risks for the children in the same way.

Thirdly, it also does not follow that discord is equally important for all types of disorder in the children. Thus, we found a more specific association between *major* depressive conditions in the parents and depression in the children. The numbers involved were quite small but other studies, too, have produced findings that point to some type of specific association in the case of major depression

(Cytryn *et al.*, 1985; Weissman *et al.*, 1984). Whether this reflects genetic or environmental transmission cannot be determined from the data but certainly the former is a possibility, at least as a partial explanation. Also, Folstein *et al.* (1983) in their study of the offspring of patients with Huntington's disease (HD) found that affective disorder (unlike conduct disturbances) was strongly associated with the presence of similar symptoms in the HD parent. They suggested that affective, but not conduct, disorders might constitute an early manifestation of the HD gene. Obviously, that is not the explanation here (as HD is a very rare condition) but the finding is important in its emphasis that different mechanisms may underlie different psychiatric disorders in children from high-risk families.

Individual differences in vulnerability

Lastly, the findings underline the extent to which children vary in their susceptibilities. We know relatively little about the basis for these individual differences in vulnerability but their existence is not in doubt. The findings on sex differences suggest that these differences are far from absolute. Thus, at the time the parent-patients first attended hospital the evidence suggested that boys were more vulnerable than girls to the ill-effects stemming from family discord—a finding in keeping with the results of much previous research (Rutter, 1982). However, by the end of the four-year follow-up period, the sex difference had greatly narrowed. It appeared that initially girls were more resilient but that, if the adverse family circumstances continued long enough, they too were likely to succumb. There is a great need for further study of the factors that underlie resistance to stress (Garmezy *et al.*, 1984); the phenomenon is of both theoretical and practical importance but already it would be wrong to suppose that any child is invulnerable.

The converse of the same issue concerns children's recovery of adaptive functioning if adversities abate. There is evidence that this occurs if environmental circumstances change for the better sufficiently (Rutter, 1981). Other data from this study (Rutter, 1971) pointed to such an effect in terms of the finding that the outcome following early stressful family disruption was better for children who subsequently were brought up in harmonious homes. Nevertheless, it is important that there was little evidence of substantial recovery during the four-year follow-up period among children in families where discord diminished. Of course, for the most part the change in families was one of degree not kind; there were very few instances of discord being followed by harmony. However, the finding (together with others like it—Richman *et al.*, 1982) emphasizes that once children have developed a marked emotional/behavioural disturbance their behaviour becomes less strongly reactive to environmental circumstances. If such circumstances change for the better *sufficiently*, there are likely to be benefits for the children, but once disorders have become well established minor improvements in the family may make little difference. The point is that children are not just passive recipients of environmental stimuli. The effects of family influences are dependent, in part, on their bringing about changes in children's self concepts and in their styles of thinking and behaving (Kagan, 1980; Rutter, 1984b). Probably it is these changes in the child that serve to perpetuate disturbance that began initially as a response to family adversity.

Our findings on the importance of temperamental differences point in the same direction. When parents became irritable, aggressive and quarrelsome this did not impinge equally on all children in the family. Parental criticism and hostility was most likely to focus on the temperamentally 'difficult' child in the family. However, it was not just that our particular child was more exposed to family discord through becoming a target for parental anger and frustration. In addition, this focusing effect served to set up maladaptive patterns of parent–child interaction that were likely to continue long after the initial stimulus for their onset had gone away. Dunn and Kendrick (1982) found much the same effect in the very much more ordinary circumstances of the birth of a sib. The firstborn's reaction to the new baby was a function of several factors (including the previous mother–child relationship and the firstborn's temperamental characteristics) but, once established, poor relationships between siblings proved to be surprisingly persistent. The implication is that the effects of family influences, such as those that are associated with parental mental disorder, need to be thought of in terms of transactional mechanisms in which both children and parents take active roles. Children's problems will not necessarily 'go away' when family circumstances improve. If they are to be successful, it is likely that interventions will need to focus as much on the children's response as on any alteration in the parents' behaviour.

ACKNOWLEDGEMENTS

This chapter is largely based on an article appearing in Psychological Medicine. I am grateful to the Editor and to the publishers for permission to use it here ('Parental psychiatric disorder: Effects on children', *Psychological Medicine*, in press).

We are grateful to both the Foundation for Child Development and the Medical Research Council for grants that supported this research. We are also indebted to numerous colleagues for help at various stages during the project but especially to Sarah Birks, John Corbett, Antony Cox, Sandra George, Philip Graham, Janis Morton, Olwen Rowlands, Celia Tupling, Stephen Wolkind, Bridget Yule and Peter Ziffo. We much appreciate the willingness of Consultant colleagues to allow us access to their cases.

REFERENCES

Baker, R. S. and Nelder, S. A. (1978). *The GLIM System, Release 3: Generalized Linear Interactive Modelling*, Royal Statistics Society, London.

Beardslee, W. R. (1985). Adaptation in children at risk: children of parents with major depressive disorder, in *Depression in Children: Developmental Perspectives* (Eds M. Rutter, C. E. Izard and P. Read), Guilford Press, New York (in press).

Birtchnell, J. and Kennard, J. (1983a). Does marital maladjustment lead to mental health? *Soc. Psychiat.* **18**, 79–88.

Birtchnell, J. and Kennard, J. (1983b). Marriage and mental illness, *Brit. J. Psychiat.* **142**, 193–198.

Bohman, M., Sigvardsson, S. and Cloninger, R. (1981). Maternal inheritance of alcohol abuse: cross-fostering analysis of adopted women, *Arch. Gen. Psychiat.* **38**, 965–969.

Bothwell, S. and Weissman, M. M. (1977). Social impairments four years after an acute depressive episode, *Amer. J. Orthopsychiat.* **47**, 231–237.

Brown, G. W. and Harris, T. (1978). *Social Origins of Depression*, Tavistock, London.

Brown, G. W. and Rutter, M. (1966). The measurement of family activities and relationships: A methodological study, *Human Relations*, **19**, 241–263.

Buck, C. and Laughton, K. (1959). Family patterns of illness: the effect of psychoneurosis in the parent upon illness in the child, *Acta Psych. Neurol. Scand.* **34**, 165–175.

Cloninger, C. R., Bohman, M. and Sigvardsson, S. (1981). Inheritance of alcohol abuse: cross fostering analysis of adopted men, *Arch. Gen. Psychiat.* **38**, 861–868.

Cohler, B. J., Grunebaum, H. U., Weiss, J. L., Gamer, E. and Gallant, D. H. (1977). Disturbance of attention among schizophrenic depressed and well mothers and their young children, *J. Child Psychol. Psychiat.* **18**, 115–135.

Cox, A. D. and Mills, M. (1983). Paper given to British Psychological Society, Developmental Section, Annual Conference, Oxford.

Crowe, R. R. (1983). Antisocial personality disorders, in *The Child At Psychiatric Risk* (Ed. R. E. Tarler), pp.214–227, Oxford University Press, Oxford.

Cytryn, L., McKnew, D. W., Zahn-Waxler, C. and Gershon, E. S. (1985). Developmental issues in risk research: the offspring of affectively ill parents, *Depression in Children: Developmental Perspectives* (Eds M. Rutter, C. E. Izard and P. Read), Guilford Press, New York, (in press).

Dunn, G. (1981). The role of linear models in psychiatric epidemiology, *Psychol. Med.* **11**, 179–184.

Dunn, J. (1980). Individual difference in temperament, in *Scientific Foundations of Developmental Psychiatry* (Ed. M. Rutter), pp.101–109, Heinemann Medical, London.

Dunn, J. and Kendrick, C. (1982). *Siblings: Love, Envy and Understanding*, Harvard University Press, Cambridge, Mass.; Grant McIntyre, London.

Emery, R. E. (1982). Interparental conflict and the children of discord and divorce, *Psychol. Bull.* **92**, 310–330.

Emery, R., Weintraub, S. and Neale, J. M. (1982). Effects of marital discord on the school behavior of children of schizophrenic, affectively disorders and normal parents, *J. Abn. Child Psychol.* **10**, 215–228.

Fisher, L., Kokes, R. F., Harder, D. W. and Jones, J. E. (1980). Child competence and psychiatric risk. VI. Summary and integration of findings, *J. Nervous Ment. Dis.* **168**, 353–355.

Folstein, S. E., Franz, M. L., Jensen, B. A., Chase, G. A. and Folstein, M. F. (1983). Conduct disorder and affective disorder among the offspring of patients with Huntington's disease, *Psychol. Med.* **13**, 45–52.

Garmezy, N. (1983). Stressors of childhood, in *Stress, Coping and Development in Children* (Eds N. Garmey and M. Rutter), pp.43–84, McGraw-Hill, New York.

Garmezy, N., Masten, A. S. and Tellegen, A. (1984). The study of stress and competence in children: a building block for developmental psychopathology, *Child Dev.* **55**, 97–111.

Gershon, E. S. (1984). *The Origins of Depression: Current Concepts and Approaches*, Springer Verlag, New York (in press). (Dahlem Konferenzen, Berlin, 1982.)

Gottesman, I. I. and Shields, J. (1976). A critical review of recent adoption, twin, and family studies of schizophrenia: behavioral genetics perspective, *Schizo. Bull.* **2**, 360–400.

Graham, P. and Rutter, M. (1968). The reliability and validity of the psychiatric assessment of the child. II. Interview with the parent, *Brit. J. Psychiat.* **114**, 581–592.

Graham, P., Rutter, M. and George, S. (1973). Temperamental characteristics as predictors of behavior disorders in children, *Amer. J. Orthopsychiat.* **43**, 328–339.

Hare, E. H. and Shaw, G. K. (1965). A study in family health. (2). A comparison of the health of fathers, mothers and children, *Brit. J. Psychiat.* **111**, 467–471.

Hobbs, P. (1982). The relative timing of psychiatric disorder in parents and children, *Brit. J. Psychiat.* **140**, 37–43.

Huxley, P. J., Goldberg, D. P., Maguire, G. P. and Kincey, V. A. (1979). The prediction of the course of minor psychiatric disorders, *Brit. J. Psychiat.* **135**, 535–543.

Janet, P. (1925). *Psychological Healing*, Vol. 1 (translated by E. and C. Paul) pp.426–427, Allen and Unwin, London.

Kagan, J. (1980). Perspectives on continuity, in *Constancy and Change in Human Development* (Eds O. G. Brim Jr. and J. Kagan), pp.26–74, Harvard University Press, Cambridge, Mass.

Kellner, R. (1963). *Family Ill Health: An Investigation in General Practice*, Tavistock, London.

Lewis, A. (1974). Psychopathic personality: a most elusive category, *Psychol. Med.* **4**, 133–140.

McNeil, T. F. and Kaij, L. (1984). Offspring of women and nonorganic psychoses: progress report, February 1980, in *Children At Risk for Schizophrenia: A Longitudinal Perspective* (Eds N. Watt, E. J. Anthony, L. C. Wynne and J. Rolf) Cambridge University Press, New York (in press).

Merikangas, K. R. and Spiker, D. G. (1982). Assortative mating among inpatients with primary affective disorder, *Psychol. Med.* **12**, 753–764.

Mills, M., Puckering, C., Pound, A. and Cox, A. D. (1984). What is it about depressed mothers that influences their children's functioning? in *Recent Research in Developmental Psychopathology* (Ed. J. Stevenson), Pergamon, Oxford.

Pearce, J. (1978). The recognition of depressive disorder in children, *J. Roy. Soc. Med.* **71**, 494–500.

Porter, R. and Collins, G. M. (Eds) (1982). *Temperamental Differences in Infants and Young Children*, Ciba Foundation Symposium No. 89, Pitman, London.

Pound, A., Cox, A. D., Puckering, C. and Mills, M. (1984). Do depressed women have an identifiable parenting style? in *Recent Research in Development Psychopathology*. (Ed. J. Stevenson), Pergamon, Oxford.

Quinton, D., Rutter, M. and Rowlands, O. (1976). An evaluation of an interview assessment of marriage, *Psychol. Med.* **6**, 577–586.

Rice, E. P., Ekdahl, M. C. and Miller, L. (1971). *Children of Mentally Ill Parents: Problems in Child Care*, Behavioral Publishers, New York.

Richardson, S. A., Dorhenwend, B. S. and Klein, D. (1965). *Interviewing: Its Forms and Functions*, Basic Books, New York.

Richman, N., Stevenson, J. and Graham, P. J. (1982). *Preschool to School: A Behavioural Study*, Academic Press, London.

Rodnick, E. H. and Goldstein, M. J. (1974). Premorbid adjustment and the recovery of mothering function in acute schizophrenic women, *J. Abn. Psychol.* **83**, 623–628.

Rolf, J. E. and Garmezy, N. (1974). The school performance of children vulnerable to behavior pathology, in *Life History Research in Psychopathology*, Vol. 3, (Eds D. F. Ricks, A. Thomas and M. Roff) pp.87–107. University of Minnesota Press, Minneapolis.

Rutter, M. (1966). *Children of Sick Parents: An Environmental and Psychiatric Study*, Institute of Psychiatry Maudsley Monographs No. 16, Oxford University Press, London.

Rutter, M. (1967). A children's behaviour questionnaire for completion by teachers: Preliminary findings, *J. Child Psychol. Psychiat.* **8**, 1–11.

Rutter, M. (1970). Sex differences in children's response to family stress, in *The Child in His Family*, pp.165–196, (Eds E. J. Anthony and C. Koupernik), Wiley, New York.

Rutter, M. (1971). Parent–child separation: psychological effects on the children, *J. Child Psychol. Psychiat.* **12**, 233–260.

Rutter, M. (1977a). Prospective studies to investigate behavioral change, in *The Origins and Course of Psychopathology* (Eds J. S. Strauss, H. M. Babigian and M. Roff), Plenum, New York.

Rutter, M. (1977b). Other family influences, in *Child Psychiatry: Modern Approaches* (Eds M. Rutter and L. Hersov), pp.74–108, Blackwell Scientific, Oxford.

Rutter, M. (1978). Family, area and school influences in the genesis of conduct disorders, in *Aggression and Antisocial Behaviour in Childhood and Adolescence* (Eds L. A. Hersov and M. Berger with D. Shaffer), pp.95–113, *Journal of Child Psychology and Psychiatry* Book Supplement No. 1, Pergamon Press, Oxford.

Rutter, M. (1981). The city and the child, *Amer. J. Orthopsychiat.* **51**, 610–625.

Rutter, M. (1982). Epidemiological-longitudinal approaches to the study of development, in *The Concept of Development* (Ed. W. A. Collins), Minnesota Symposia on Child Psychology, Vol. 15, pp.105–144, Lawrence Erlbaum, Hillsdale, N.J.

Rutter, M. (1984a). Psychopathology and development: 1. Childhood antecedents of adult psychiatric disorder. *Australian and New Zealand Journal of Psychiatry* (in press).

Rutter, M. (1984b). Psychopathology and development: 2. Childhood experiences and personality development. *Australian and New Zealand Journal of Psychiatry* (in press).

Rutter, M., Birch, H. G., Thomas, A. and Chess, S. (1964). Temperamental characteristics in infancy and the later development of behavioural disorder, *Brit. J. Psychiat.* **110**, 651–661.

Rutter, M. and Brown, G. W. (1966). The reliability and validity of measures of family life and relationships in families containing a psychiatric patient, *Soc. Psychiat.* **1**, 38–53.

Rutter, M., Cox, A., Tupling, C., Berger, M. and Yule, W. (1975a). Attainment and adjustment in two geographical areas. I. The prevalence of psychiatric disorder, *Brit. J. Psychiat.* **126**, 493–509.

Rutter, M. and Garmezy, N. (1983). Developmental psychopathology, in *Socialization, Personality, and Social Development, Vol. 4, Handbook of Child Psychology* (Ed. E. M. Hetherington), pp.775–911, Wiley, New York.

Rutter, M. and Giller, H. (1983). *Juvenile Delinquency: Trends and Perspectives*, Penguin, Harmondsworth, Middx.

Rutter, M., Graham, P., Chadwick, O. and Yule, W. (1976). Adolescent turmoil: fact or fiction? *J. Child Psychol. Psychiat.* **17**, 35–56.

Rutter, M. and Quinton, D. (1981). Longitudinal studies of institutional children and children of mentally ill parents (United Kingdom), in *Prospective Longitudinal Research: An Empirical Basis for the Primary Prevention of Psychosocial Disorders* (Eds S. A. Mednick and A. E. Baert), pp.297–305, Oxford University Press, Oxford.

Rutter, M. and Quinton, D. (1984). Parental psychiatric disorder: effects on children, *Psychol. Med.* (in press).

Rutter, M., Quinton, D. and Liddle, C. (1983). Parenting in two generations: looking backwards and looking forwards, in *Families at Risk* (Ed. N. Madge), pp.60–98, Heinemann Educational, London.

Rutter, M., Tizard, J. and Whitmore, K. (Eds) (1970). *Education, Health and Behaviour*, Longman, London. (Reprinted 1981, Krieger Huntington, New York.)

Rutter, M., Yule, B., Quinton, D., Rowlands, O., Yule, W. and Berger, M. (1975b). Attainment and adjustment in two geographical areas. III. Some factors accounting for area differences, *Brit. J. Psychiat.* **126**, 520–533.

Sameroff, A. J., Barocas, R. and R. Safer (1984). Rochester Longitudinal Study progress report, in *Children At Risk for Schizophrenia: A Longitudinal Perspective*. (Eds N. Watt, E. J. Anthony, L. C. Wynne and J. Rolf), Cambridge University Press, New York.

Shepherd, M., Oppenheim, B. and Mitchell, S. (Eds) (1971). *Childhood Behaviour and Mental Health*, University of London Press, London.

Shepherd, M. and Sartorius, N. (1974). Personality disorder and the International Classification of Diseases, *Brit. J. Psychiat.* **135**, 163–167.

Stewart, M. and de Blois, S. (1983). Father–son resemblances in aggressive and antisocial behaviour, *Brit. J. Psychiat.* **142**, 78–84; **143**, 310–311.

Swafford, M. (1980). Three parametric techniques for contingency table analysis: a nontechnical commentary, *Amer. Sociol. Review*, **45**, 664–690.

Thomas, A., Chess, S. and Birch, H. G. (1968). *Temperament and Behavior Disorders in Children*, University Press, New York.

Torgersen, S. (1983). Genetics of neurosis: the effects of sampling variation upon the twin concordance ratio, *Brit. J. Psychiat.* **142**, 126–132.

Tyrer, P. and Alexander, J. (1979). Classification of personality disorder. *Brit. J. Psychiat.* **135**, 163–167.

Tyrer, P., Alexander, M. S., Cicchetti, D., Cohen, M. S. and Remington, M. (1979). Reliability of a schedule for rating personality disorders, *Brit. J. Psychiat.* **135**, 168–174.

Tyrer, P., Casey, P. and Gall, J. (1983). Relationship between neurosis and personality disorder. *Brit. J. Psychiat.* **142**, 404–408.

Watt, N., Anthony, E. J., Wynne, L. and Rolf, E. (Eds) (1984). *Children At Risk for Schizophrenia: A Longitudinal Perspective*, Cambridge University Press, New York.

Weintraub, S. and Neale, J. M. (1984). The Stony Brook High-Risk Project, in *Children At Risk for Schizophrenia: A Longitudinal Perspective* (Eds N. Watt, E. J. Anthony, L. C. Wynne and J. Rolf), Cambridge University Press, New York.

Weintraub, S., Prinz, R. J. and Neale, J. M. (1978). Peer evaluations of the competence of children vulnerable to psychopathology, *J. Abn. Child Psychol.* **6**, 461–474.

Weissman, M. M. and Paykel, E. S. (1974). *The Depressed Woman: A Study of Social Relationships*, University of Chicago Press, Chicago.

Weissman, M. M., Paykel, E. S. and Klerman, G. L. (1972). The depressed woman as a mother, *Soc. Psychiat.* **7**, 98–108.

Weissman, M. M., Prusoff, B. A. and Klerman, G. L. (1978). Personality and the prediction of long term outcome of depression, *Amer. J. Psychiat.* **135**, 797–800.

Weissman, M. M., Prusoff, B. A., Gammon, G. D., Merikangas, K. R., Leckman, J. F. and Kidd, K. F. (1984). Psychopathology in the children (ages 6–18) of depressed and normal parents, *J. Amer. Acad. Child Psychiat.* **23**, 78–84.

Wing, J. K. and Hailey, A. M. (1972). *Evaluating a Community Psychiatric Service: The Camberwell Register 1964–1971*, Oxford University Press, London.

Winters, K. C., Stone, A. A., Weintraub, S. and Neale, J. M. (1981). Cognitive and attentional deficits in children vulnerable to psychopathology, *J. Abn. Child Psychol.* **9**, 435–454.

Worland, J., Janes, C. L. and Anthony, E. J. (1984). St. Louis Risk Research Project: experimental studies, in *Children At Risk for Schizophrenia: A longitudinal perspective* (Eds N. Watt, E. J. Anthony, L. C. Wynne and J. Rolf), Cambridge University Press, New York.

Section III

Long-term Studies
which ask a Specific Question

Longitudinal Studies in Child Psychology and Psychiatry
Edited by A. R. Nicol
© 1985 John Wiley and Sons Ltd.

Chapter 7

A Prospective Longitudinal Study of Adoption

M. Bohman and S. Sigvardsson

THE SOCIAL HERITAGE

It is common knowledge that social maladjustment, alcohol abuse or criminality are more prevalent in some families than in others. In one study of severely maladjusted and delinquent boys Jonsson (1967) found that most parents in this population also exhibited various forms of social maladjustment; often there was a greater prevalence of criminality or alcoholism with nervous or somatic disorders. It also proved possible to trace the social maladjustment back two generations to the boys' grandparents. Whilst not excluding the possible influence of genetic factors, Jonsson viewed his population mainly in terms of social pathology, interpreting the progressive maladjustment in these families as a process of social rejection over a period of several generations.

GENETIC HERITAGE

However, it has been claimed in various studies that genetic factors do play a part in the development of some forms of social and mental disorder. Robins (1966) in her, by now, classic study of the 'sociopathic personality', was somewhat reluctant to invoke definite genetic factors behind the transmission of the syndrome. But her quotation of 'When shall I be dead and rid of the bad my father did?', may illustrate her somewhat pessimistic view of the ultimate prognosis of this disorder.

The hypothesis of a genetic transmission of criminality and anti-social behaviour was earlier supported by Lange's (1931) famous twin study, *Crime as Destiny*. Lange's major conclusion that 'innate tendencies play a preponderant part among the causes of crime', has been heavily criticized because of the sampling biases of his twin series. But several decades later a large representative Danish twin study gave some support for Lange's conclusion (Christiansen, 1970). On the other hand, a more recent Norwegian twin study could not confirm the hypothesis of a genetic aetiology behind the manifestation of criminality (Dalgard and Kringlen, 1976).

It is, however, extremely difficult to distinguish satisfactorily between hereditary and environmental factors even in twin studies—children usually receive their upbringing as well as their genes from their biological parents. One way of achieving such a distinction is to study subjects who were separated from their biological parents at an early age and have been brought up by foster or adoptive parents not related to them. In this way, one can largely eliminate the influence of the social environment. Obviously adoption or fostering at an early age is a socio-legal measure that definitely breaks at least one condition for the transmission of the 'social heritage'. For *genetic research* the adoptive situation presents a ready made experimental base for testing hypotheses about the importance of heredity versus childhood environment in the development of different types of mental disorders. On the other hand, the goal of *social research* into adoption or fostering is to elucidate those factors in the child, the adoptive parents, and society which influence the adoptive process and to what extent this process can be predicted at the time of the child's placement with his new parents.

AIMS OF THE STUDY

The general aim of these two kinds of adoption research, the genetic and the social, is to work out practical models for the prediction and the prevention of mental disorders and social maladjustment. As a tool in socio-political research the 'adoption method' offers a unique opportunity to analyse the ways in which inequalities of occupational status and income are the results of genetic inheritance, family background and schooling. The lesson taught by such research may hopefully lead to changes in social and medical policies, concerning the prevention and treatment of various disorders.

THE PRESENT STUDY

In this chapter we will present some experiences and results from a longitudinal study of children born after unwanted pregnancies and registered for adoptive placement at the time of their birth. The cohort has been followed from the time of pregnancy and investigated at various periods from childhood to adulthood (11, 15, 18 and 22 years). The aim of this presentation is to discuss the social effects of adoption and fostering on the manifestation of social maladjustment among children with a negative social heritage and the implications of our results for preventive work and social policies. The specific questions we want to answer here may be formulated as follows:

1   Does early placement of children from families of antisocial, or otherwise socially handicapped families, in an adoptive or foster home protect them from social maladjustment?
2   Are outcomes different for adoption and for fostering?
3   What is the outcome for children born after unwanted pregnancies and registered for adoption, but later restored to their biological parents and reared by them?

SOME METHODOLOGICAL ASPECTS

A great deal of the knowledge about children's development has been derived from cross-sectional investigations of representative samples of different age groups. Thus, the data obtained on different occasions have not originated from the same individuals, but from groups of children of different ages. This kind of investigation has some inherent limitations when it comes to making predictions about individual development. When studying relations between previous observations and subsequent events with a view to constructing a model for *prediction* the only really satisfactory method is to make several observations of the same group of children at different points of time.

Prospective, longitudinal studies of individual development is taken to mean that the same individuals are observed in adequate studies at regular intervals during their childhood, adolescence and early adulthood.

The principle of the longitudinal follow-up, which has gained increasing practical currency in connection with preventive child care, is that progression, regression, and deviant development at certain ages is assessed in relation to the initial situation together with achievement during earlier stages (Klackenberg, 1971).

LIMITATIONS OF ASSESSMENTS

We thus have assessments of the adjustment of the children at four different stages of their development: at 11, 15, 18 and 22 years of age. However, for financial reasons we had to impose some limitations on the execution of our investigation. At 11 and 15 years of age information was collected from official records, interviews with teachers, questionnaires, school records and school health cards. For male 18-year-olds we had access to medical and psychological data from the Swedish military enlistment procedure, but no information was available for the female part of the cohort.

SUBJECTS

The investigation presented here originated in a cohort of 624 children born 1956–1957 in Stockholm, Sweden. They were all born after involuntary pregnancies, and at the time of their birth their mothers had reported to the adoption agency of the Social Welfare Board of Stockholm. Subjects, family background and so on have been detailed elsewhere (Bohman, 1970, 1971) and only a short description is given here.

Of the original cohort, 168 children were placed in adoptive homes before the age of 1 year (Group I), 208 were kept by, or returned to, their biological mothers (Group II). Finally 203 children (Group III) were placed in foster homes, most of them before 1 year of age. In these cases there were no clear decisions about the legal status of the children from the outset, because many mothers could not make up their minds about their children's future. However, almost all of these children grew up with foster parents, and after some years about 70 per cent were legally adopted. Accordingly, the three groups represent three alternative modes of placement for socially disadvantaged and unwanted children. From the very beginning of our study it was clear to us that these three groups of children provided us with an excellent opportunity to compare and evaluate the consequences of child welfare decisions on the social, cognitive and personal development of our subjects.

The adopted children in Group I were placed with families living in Stockholm or other large towns who had been thoroughly prepared for their task through a series of interviews before placement. The adoption agency took care to ensure that the children were not placed in homes where there might be marital problems or where the husband or wife had a serious illness or was registered for alcohol abuse or criminality. Among these adoptive parents, many were of good social, educational and economic standing. About 40 per cent of the adoptive fathers had professional or intermediate occupations, as compared to only 28 per cent in a representative comparison group. The children in the two other groups had less favourable placement conditions. Many of the *biological mothers*, who brought up their children themselves (Group II) were young, unmarried and lived alone. Most of them had no higher education and worked in unskilled or semi-skilled occupations. About half of them already had one or more other children to take care of. In general, their financial and social opportunities were very limited when the child was born. The biological fathers were on average a few years older than the mothers. Their situation as regards occupational training and employment was much the same as that of the mothers. Both the mothers and the fathers were heavily over-represented in the public records for criminality and alcohol abuse. Thus, about one-third of the *biological fathers* were found in the criminal records, which is a substantial over-representation, the figures to be expected for a representative group of men of the same age is about 10 per cent. Registered criminality differed somewhat between the groups (Group I, 27 per cent; Group II, 34 per cent; Group III, 40 per cent). Note that most cases concerned recurrent criminality, frequently combined with offences under the Temperance Act (abuse of alcohol). Altogether 37 per cent of the fathers were found in the Excise Board's records of offences under the

Temperance Act. This may be compared with 18 per cent in a representative group of men of the same age. The prevalence of registered fathers was significantly different between the three groups: 26 per cent in Group I, 39 per cent in Group II, and 48 per cent in Group III (p <0.01). There was also a much higher prevalence of registration for crime and/or alcohol abuse among *biological mothers* (Group I, 3.0 per cent; Group II, 1.5 per cent; Group III, 9.7 per cent) than would be expected in a random group of women.

The *foster parents* lived mostly in small communities or out in rural areas. They were stable families but did not have the high status of the adoptive parents in terms of financial means, education or occupation. The mean age was somewhat higher than that of the adoptive parents. These parents were not specially prepared for their task as non-biological parents, in the way that parents in Group I were. As a rule they were paid by the Child Welfare organization as long as the children were not legally adopted. At the time of the 11-year-old study, only 30 per cent were not adopted.

SELECTION BIAS

When we compare the outcome of the placement in these three groups, it is obvious that the process of placement itself involved a certain amount of selection. As mentioned, foster children in Group III, more often than those in Group I or II, had a negative genetic heritage: biological parents with criminal records or alcohol problems and mothers who more frequently suffered complications during pregnancy or delivery.

Also those few children whose biological fathers belonged to the upper occupational categories were preferentially placed in adoptive homes, or reared by their biological mothers, whereas children of unskilled biological fathers were more often placed in foster homes.

GENERAL DESIGN OF THE STUDY

The study was planned as a longitudinal study in combination with the adoption design, starting at the time of pregnancy. Studies have been carried out for both boys and girls at 11 and 15 years of age (in their school situation by interviews with teachers or questionnaires). Boys were studied at 18 with respect to information about the medical and psychological investigations at the time of their enlistment for military service. Controls, matched for sex and age, have been selected from school or population registers.

Finally we have obtained information about the boys and girls at 22 years of age from the criminal records and Excise Board Register for alcohol abuse. Figure 7.1 illustrates the various stages of the investigation over the years. Note that the primary aim of the investigation was to study the *social adjustment* of the subjects. Our methods (interviews, registers) have not permitted us to classify our subjects according to strictly clinical criteria.

ORIGINAL COHORT
N = 624

PLACEMENT

Adoptive homes	Biological homes	Foster homes
28%	37%	35%

LONGITUDINAL DESIGN

11 years: Data:	Adjustment and school achievement School marks Interviews with teachers and parents
15 years: Data:	Adjustment and school achievement School marks Teachers' questionnaires
18 years: Data:	(Boys only) Mental and intellectual capacity Records from military enlistment
23 years: Data:	Alcohol abuse and criminality Records from the criminal register and excise board register (for offences against the Temperance Act)

Fig. 7.1   Study design

RESULTS

Investigation at 11 years of age

The interviews with teachers during the study at 11 years showed that the adopted boys in Group I manifested a high rate of nervous and behavioural disturbance compared to class controls. Thus, 22 per cent were classified as 'problem children' compared to 12 per cent among class controls. There were, however, very few among either subjects or controls who could be classified as antisocial or delinquent at this age. The adopted girls likewise had a higher rate of maladjustment compared to controls, although not significantly (11 per cent versus 15 per cent).

The two other groups also showed a significant increase in maladjusted boys, with 20 per cent in Group II and 22 per cent in Group III (compared to 12 per cent and 8 per cent respectively among the controls). Similarly, girls in Groups II and III manifested an increased frequency of maladjustment (Group II, 9 per cent versus 6 per cent, Group III, 20 per cent versus 4 per cent). These results went against our hypotheses, as we had expected less disturbance among the adoptees in Group I, than among the children in the other two groups. However, when we looked more closely at our cases, we found that the disturbances were qualitatively more pronounced among the children in Groups II and III than in Group I. Even

Table 7.1   Adjustment at school at 11 years

	Boys		Girls	
	Probands (%)	Classmate Controls (%)	Probands (%)	Classmate Controls (%)
Adopted				
Few or no symptoms	44	70	77	84
Moderate symptoms	34	18	12	11
Problem children	22	12	11	5
With biological mother				
Few or no symptoms	54	70	65	76
Moderate symptoms	26	18	26	18
Problem children	20	12	9	6
Foster children				
Few or no symptoms	55	69	71	79
Moderate symptoms	23	23	9	17
Problem children	22	8	20	4

if the subjects were antisocial, delinquent behaviour was seldom found at this age. The results are summarized in Table 7.1. (Note: Classmates were randomly chosen as controls for each proband, however at the time of interview only 317 controls were at hand, due to reorganization between the third and fourth school years. Despite this, it was possible to randomly select a representative control series).

It is of some interest in this connection that the adjustment of the children in all three groups appeared to be independent of the various background variables, such as perinatal complications, age at placement, socio-economic status of adoptive parents, or registered criminality or alcohol abuse in the biological parents. Our conclusion at this stage of the investigation was that to be an unwanted child was an initial stressful experience which, irrespective of placement, increased the risk of maladjustment.

Investigation at 15 years of age

Four years later, when the children were attending the eighth class of the nine-year Swedish comprehensive school, we sent a questionnaire to their class teachers. The instrument used in this study was a series of rating scales, in which adjustment and various behaviour patterns of the pupils were scored on a 7-point scale. The schools also provided copies of the children's reports in different subjects. To give one example, the extremes of the rating scale for *social maturity* were defined as follows. Scale point 1: strikingly poor social adjustment,

Table 7.2   Social maladjustment (scores 1 and 2) at 15 years

	Boys		Girls	
	Probands (%)	Controls (%)	Probands (%)	Controls (%)
Adopted	(*n* = 89) 4.5	(*n* = 173) 5.8	(*n* = 71) 1.4	(*n* = 140) 2.9
With biological mother	(*n* = 108) 13.9	(*n* = 209) 5.3	(*n* = 105) 15.2	(*n* = 194) 6.7
Fostered	(*n* = 112) 12.2	(*n* = 222) 4.1	(*n* = 92) 7.6	(*n* = 180) 2.8

frequently plays truant, runs away, misuses alcohol or drugs, repeated thefts or other crimes; behaviour which has led to intervention by, for example, the Child Welfare authorities or the police. Scale point 7: mature, has further studies or an occupation in mind, reliable. Children given scores 1–2 have arbitrarily been classified as socially maladjusted. Two classmates were randomly chosen as controls for each subject.

The teachers who made the ratings, as well as other persons on the school staff who were involved in the project, did not know anything about the aim of the study. Nor did they know that some of the children were probands and others were controls.

The differences between the adopted children in Group I and their classmates were by now of little consequence. There was still, admittedly, a slight tendency to lower mean score for adjustment and lower mean grades compared to their controls, but these differences were very small and only occasionally significant.

Among the *adopted boys* 4.5 per cent were classified as socially maladjusted compared to 5.8 per cent among the controls (score 1 + 2 on the 7-point rating scale). For *girls*, the corresponding were 1.4 per cent versus 2.9 per cent (differences not significant).

In contrast, a considerable proportion of the children in the other two groups now displayed yet greater maladjustment and under achievement than was found at age 11 years. Among *boys* in Groups II and III social maladjustment was two to three times as frequent among probands as among controls: in Group II, 13.9 per cent versus 5.3 per cent; in Group III, 12.2 per cent versus 4.1 per cent. Likewise *girls* in these groups had a higher frequency for social maladjustment: in Group II, 15.2 per cent versus 6.7 per cent; in Group III, 7.6 per cent versus 2.8 per cent. Maladjustment (score 1–2 in the variable *social maturity*) is shown in Table 7.2.

Longitudinal aspects

In order to describe persistence of behaviour and symptoms over time, the results from the 15-year-old study were cross-tabulated against those of the study at 11 years. In this context only correlations concerning 'problem children' at 15 will be discussed. The two classifications do not correspond completely, since symptoms of adjustment problems change during puberty. In accordance with the study at 11 years the probands were grouped into three categories; 1 = few or no symptoms of adjustment problems, 2 = moderate symptoms, and 3 = 'problem children'. In the same way the probands have been categorized in accordance with the study at 15 years, A = good adjustment (scores 6–7), B = fair adjustment (scores 3–5), and C = social maladjustment (scores 1–2).

Group I

Twenty-seven probands in this group were classified as a 'problem child' in the 11-year-old study. Only three of them (11 per cent), plus two with moderate symptoms were given scores 1–2 (social maladjustment) at the age of 15 years. Six of the problem children at age 11 years were in fact among the best adjusted in the class (scores 6–7) in the study at 15 years.

These findings are of a certain interest in relation to our experiences of personal interviews with the adoptive parents at the 11-year-old study. In that study there were, as mentioned, significantly more 'problem children' among the probands compared to their classmates. In the interviews, the adoptive parents often expressed anxiety about the puberty of their children, anticipating a period of turmoil and crisis, which in itself might act as a 'self-fulfilling prophecy'. But, despite the fact that there had been a larger number of problem children as well as negative expectations at 11 years, there was in fact a somewhat lower percentage of social maladjustment among the adoptees compared to their classmates after puberty. It is obvious from our results so far that the high prevalence of maladjustment and nervous disturbances, which we found at age 11 years in all three groups, were to a large extent overcome among the adoptees in Group I at 15 years.

Group II

At age 11 years there were thirty 'problem children' in this group. Eight of them were classified as 'socially maladjusted' at 15 years, as also were 11 of the 52 with 'moderate symptoms' and 8 of the 122 with 'few or no symptoms' in the 11-year-old study.

Group III

Eight of the twenty-five 'problem children' at age 11 years were classified as 'socially maladjusted' at 15 years as well as five of the seventy-five who at 11 years had 'few or no symptoms'.

In summary our classification of 'problem children' at 11 years had a fairly low predictive power, lowest in Group I. On the other hand, such variables as 'aggressivity', 'ability to concentrate', and 'intellectual capacity' showed high correlations between ages, especially in Groups II and III. It is conceivable that our classification of 'problem child' at 11 years is too broad and covers too many different clinical entities to be useful for adequate prediction of social functioning.

The implication of background factors and selective placement

One of the original purposes of our study was to evaluate the effects of adoption on the development of children. It is obvious from our follow-up at 15 years that the adoptees in Group I fared much better compared with children who were reared by their biological mothers or by foster parents (Groups II and III). The next question is whether this inter-group difference is due to environmental factors in the rearing and home situation or is a reflection of selective placement.

As regards environmental factors in the children's home situation, we know from the 11-year-old study that probands in Group I grew up under better and more stable circumstances than probands in Groups II and III, a fact which in itself may explain their better school achievements and better adjustment. But we also know that, at the time of their birth and infancy, the three groups were handled and selected in a way which may have had a bearing on the differences in outcome between groups. There were, for instance, differences between groups concerning early institutional care. About 70 per cent of the probands were in infants' homes before placement, the mean duration of the stay being shortest in Group I (6 months). Perinatal complications were more common in Groups II and III than in Group I and, as mentioned, criminality or alcohol abuse were more common among parents of children reared by their own mothers or by foster parents. Finally, some children were selected and placed by the Adoption Agency and the Child Welfare Bureau according to the social and occupational status of their biological parents.

A discussion of these questions has been presented at length elsewhere in connection with the 11-year-old studies (Bohman, 1970, 1971, Bohman and Sigvardsson, 1980). As mentioned earlier the symptoms are behavioural disturbances at 11 years were by and large independent of the background factors studied, and could not explain the high frequency of maladjustment among the adoptees and their comparison groups.

We have again analysed our dependent variables with regard to those background factors in which we know that the material was selected, and which, in the light of current literature, may reasonably be suspected of having an influence on the results.

To summarize this repetition of our earlier analyses offered no explanation for the differences between the outcomes for the three groups. Perinatal complications had some influence on the performance and adjustment of some children, but did not distinguish between groups. Neither did alcohol abuse or criminality of the biological parents explain the differences, nor institutional care or age at placement. The influence of SES of biological and rearing parents could not be elucidated in this study. It is conceivable that low SES among biological parents may also reflect an inherited, genetically determined intellectual capacity which might influence their children's intelligence. It is, however, unlikely that this could account for the large differences in achievement or adjustment between the groups.

In conclusion, our results at 15 years indicate that the risks concerning the subsequent development of adopted children are in no way greater than the risks for children in the general population, provided that the adoptive homes are of a good standard and well prepared for the task of rearing a non-biological child. The prospects for these children are very good, irrespective of their social or genetic background. In contrast, our study indicated a considerable risk of maladjustment and school failure among children reared by mothers, who were originally prepared to have their child adopted. The same is true of children who, due to indecision on the part of the mothers or the social agency, were placed and reared in foster homes.

For the next two steps in our investigation we had to rely on records that were made available to us by official sources; the military enlistment procedure and registrations for criminality and alcohol abuse.

THE BOYS AT 18:
INVESTIGATION AT THE MILITARY ENLISTMENT PROCEDURE

In Sweden there is general conscription and military training for men from the age of 18 years. Before entering military training there is an enlistment procedure, to test the conscript's fitness for service in the armed forces and his suitability for training prior to posting within the military organization. Since 1968 about 90 per cent of all male youths have been required to attend a two-day, intensive medical, psychological and social examination. The results of these examinations were made available to us through the military authorities, and were used as one step in our longitudinal follow-up. The following variables of the enlistment procedure were used in the analyses of this step of our investigation.

1   Intelligence is measured on a 9-point scale and based on four tests that include logic-inductive, spatial, linguistic, and technical factors.

2   Mental capacity, is analysed during a semistructural interview with a psychologist and aims at giving a complete picture of the conscript's education, occupational experience, social background, interests, personality and social functioning. This is used as a basis for assessing his military suitability and potential for leadership. The tests took 175 minutes to administer and the results are summarized in the psychological profile.

Subjects, controls and attrition

Every subject from the original cohort of 329 boys was identified according to his date of birth, available from the official population register. For every subject, a male born on the same day and in the same town was selected as a control. When subjects and controls were checked against the military enlistment tapes, 22.8 per cent of the subjects and 15.8 per cent of the controls had dropped out for various reasons. This attrition rate was higher than was expected for both subjects and controls. Otto (1976) for instance, found that only 8.7 per cent of the 1953 cohort for military enlistment were missing, as a result of death, emigration, or exemption in advance because of illness or handicap or for other reasons. In the present series, the attrition rate was about the same for adopted boys (Group I) as for their controls (17.2 per cent versus 18.3 per cent), but was higher in Groups II and III. According to our analyses the higher attrition in these groups was due to emigration and exemption for socio-medical reasons. The somewhat higher attrition among our controls compared to the 1953 cohort may reflect currently more liberal induction practices. Thus we were left with 263 boys who had all passed the military enlistment procedure.

Results of military enlistment investigation

Intelligence was, as mentioned, assessed by four different tests, including logic-inductive, linguistic, and technical abilities. Means among subjects and controls are given for the different tests in Table 7.3.

In all four partial tests there was good agreement between subjects in Group I and their controls. In Groups II and III, however, there were highly significant differences between subjects and controls, the former having much lower means. (*Comment:* Controls in Group II had somewhat higher mean scores than the two other control groups, which reflects that the standardization of the tests was changed between 1956 and 1957. As there was an overrepresentation of boys born in 1957, which explains the higher value for the controls.)

Table 7.3 Tests at 18 years at military enlistment procedure (intelligence, means for subtests)

Subtest	Group I (Adopted)			Group II (Biol. Mother)			Group III (Fostered)		
	Subjects	Controls	p	Subjects	Controls	p	Subjects	Controls	p
	(n=79)	(n=74)		(n=90)	(n=102)		(n=87)	(n=99)	
Logic-inductive	5.24	5.46	NS	4.87	5.62	<0.005	4.44	5.28	<0.005
Linguistic	5.18	5.15	NS	4.86	5.58	<0.005	4.52	5.35	<0.005
Spatial	5.53	5.30	NS	5.34	5.98	<0.01	4.77	5.61	<0.005
Technical	4.96	4.91	NS	4.40	5.13	<0.005	4.22	4.77	<0.05

Table 7.4 Mental capacity according to psychologists assessment (means)

	Group I			Group II			Group III		
	Subjects	Controls	p	Subjects	Controls	p	Subjects	Controls	p
	(n=79)	(n=72)		(n=91)	(n=102)		(n=85)	(n=97)	
	5.19	5.15	NS	4.84	5.47	.005	4.76	5.08	NS

Table 7.4 summarizes the results of the psychological assessment of 'mental capacity' as defined above. As can be seen, there was a very good agreement in Group I between the adoptees and their controls. In contrast, subjects in Groups II and III had lower means than the controls, the differences being highly significant for Group II.

Thus interviews, intelligence tests and other investigations during the enlistment procedure confirmed our observations at 15 years of age in all three groups. The adopted boys showed much the same achievements in different tests and assessments as did their age-related controls. The drop-out rate was of the same magnitude as among controls and adoptees were also chosen and screened for military leadership as often as the controls. By contrast, subjects in the two other groups had relatively high frequencies of exemption for social or psychiatric reasons compared to controls. Their intellectual achievements in different tests fell very far behind those of their controls or of the adopted boys.

INVESTIGATION AT 22–23 YEARS OF AGE: REGISTRATIONS FOR CRIMINALITY AND ALCOHOL ABUSE

The last step to date in our longitudinal investigation of our cohort of 'unwanted children' was the search for entries in the Criminal Register and the Excise Board Register. The latter contains information about fines imposed for drunkenness, records of supervision by the Temperance Boards, and time spent in institutions for alcoholics. The incurrence of a criminal sentence of more than sixty 'day-fines' constitutes criminality. The records cover the period from the subjects' sixteenth birthdays up to 1979 when they were 22–23 years of age.

A search for entries was made for all the subjects in the cohort of boys and their controls from the 18-year-old investigation.

Results

Our findings concerning *boys* are summarized in Figure 7.2, which gives the accumulated frequencies of registrations for criminal offences, alcohol abuse and the combination of both in the three groups. The age-matched controls have been collapsed to one group, as there were no differences between controls in the three groups. It is quite obvious that for boys there was a fairly good agreement between controls (15.5 per cent) and subjects in Groups I and II (18.0 and 16.5 per cent respectively, differences not significant). Whereas probands in Group III displayed a considerable and significant increase of registrations (29.2 per cent) at this early stage of adulthood. Alcohol abuse—alone or in combination with criminal offences—seems to be a characteristic of these young men.

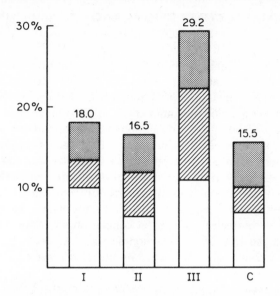

Fig. 7.2 Criminality and alcohol abuse at 22–23 years. I, adopted; II, Restored to biological mother; III, Foster children; ▨, alcohol alone; ▧, crime and alcohol; ☐, crime alone

It is obvious that the registrations for criminal offences or alcohol abuse are inaccurate instruments for the description of social maladjustment. It is well known, for instance, that registrations for criminal offences only cover a minor part of the crimes committed. Likewise, officially registered alcohol abuse does not give a true picture of alcohol abuse in a population. However, the very high frequency of registrations among boys who had lived in foster homes indicates that this group runs a great risk of developing social maladjustment.

Among *females* five probands were registered for alcohol abuse, two in Group II and three in Group III. One of the probands in Group II had eight registrations in the Temperance Board Register. The other one had only one registration but in addition was placed under supervision because of alcohol abuse. One of the probands in Group III had two registrations. There was no registered criminality in any of the three groups.

Two controls were registered for alcohol abuse, one single registration in both cases, but there was no registered criminality.

The number of cases registered for alcohol abuse is too small to permit us to draw any definite conclusions, but there was a clear tendency towards an increased prevalence of alcohol problems amongst those probands who had grown up in biological homes or in foster homes.

SUMMARY, CONCLUSIONS AND IMPLICATIONS
FOR SOCIAL POLICY

The aim of the longitudinal study presented here has been to evaluate three different placement alternatives of a cohort of children who were registered for adoption at birth. It is obvious that the rather high frequency of deviations and nervous disturbances, which we found at age 11 years in all three groups, were to a large extent overcome among the adoptees in Group I in subsequent follow-ups. The social outcome had evidently been neither better nor worse than for children in general. For adopted boys the intellectual and mental capacity, measured and classified during the enlistment procedure showed the same levels as for their age-matched controls, a validation of our findings at 15.

Regarding the high frequency of social maladjustment (criminality and alcohol abuse) among their biological parents, the conclusion is warranted that adoption largely reduced the risk of social incompetence. Accordingly, the 'genetic heritage' seems to have been neutralized by the security which a well-prepared adoption offers.

It is true, however, that the adoptive parents mostly belonged to higher occupational groups (professional or intermediate). Parents of the controls, on the other hand, corresponded to the distribution of the general population. From an environmentalistic view the adoptees could be expected to have higher means for intellectual capacity or school achievements than did their controls but this was not the case. There may be various reasons for this failure to keep up with their social-class level. It may be that the adoptive situation itself is fraught with complications and stresses (McWhinnie, 1967; Triseliotis, 1973) which have a negative impact on the general level of achievement.

One explanation could be the influence of genetic factors. The biological parents had a significantly lower SES than of comparable normal population of parents. If the SES of biological parents reflects an inherited, genetically determined, intellectual capacity (Munsinger, 1975; Scarr and Weinberg, 1976). It is conceivable that school achievement among subjects may to some extent reflect the SES of their biological parents. At present we have not sufficient data to fully elucidate this question.

A somewhat unexpected finding in our study was the negative outcome among the foster children in Group III. In the biological parents of these children the SES was significantly lower than that of the parents of the other groups, which may to some extent explain the generally low school achievements among these children (from a genetic stand-point). On the other hand, these children were placed at an early age (mean age 9 months) in socially stable foster families where, with few exceptions, they stayed permanently. The SES of these families was fairly equal to that of the general population. A majority (70 per cent) of these children were also subsequently legally adopted.

It is also true that other negative background factors, such as perinatal complications, alcohol abuse and criminality were much more common among these children. However, in our analyses at ages 11 and 15 years, such factors did not provide an adequate explanation for the unfavourable outcome amongst this group.

The unexpectedly high frequency of registration for alcohol abuse and/or criminality among boys by age 22 years may possibly reflect a genetically determined transmission. Recently published investigations concerning about 2000 adoptees of adult age (Bohman, 1978; Cloninger et al., 1981; Bohman et al., 1981) displayed a high prevalence of alcohol abuse among the grown-up children of alcoholic parents, indicating the presence of genetic factors behind alcoholism. It is conceivable that the children in the present sample have now reached an age when the drinking habits in their environment may interact with genetic factors, thus increasing the risk of alcohol abuse or alcoholism. On the other hand cross-tabulation of alcohol abuse among boys and their biological parents did not show a significant correlation in any of the three groups. As alcohol abuse or criminality was common among the parents in all three groups, it is obvious that the boys in foster homes have reacted differently and much more negatively in their social outcome.

One possible explanation for this strongly negative outcome among foster children may be connected with placement procedures. Foster parents were seldom prepared before the placement of the child as were the adoptive parents in Group I. There was also legal and psychological insecurity connected with the placement, as there was no guarantee that the child would not some day be returned to the biological mother. Many foster parents had to live with this feeling of insecurity for years, and this may have had a negative influence on the relationship with the child.

In interviews the foster parents often expressed their concern about this insecure situation, during the first few years after the placement. It is conceivable that this situation, which sometimes lasted many years, may have affected the relationship between the children and foster parents, and impaired the normal, healthy development of the former. This suggestion is supported by the findings in a recently published report on a group of British adopted and foster children (Raynor, 1980).

Our study also indicates a considerable risk of social maladjustment and school failure among subjects reared by their biological mothers. Maladjustment was common among children in this group, especially among girls, the prevalence was even higher than among boys in any other group (15.2 per cent). At 22 years of age, however, registered criminality or alcohol abuse was about the same for both sexes as among controls, indicating a less serious development than among foster children.

The general implication of our study for the policy of the care of children from disadvantaged families is of course not that adoption is always the best solution for children with social handicaps. Rather, the conclusion must be that early preventive work is important. Preparation and support should be given to everybody in charge of a child at risk. But in the best interest of the child, decisions about the child's legal status should be made as early as possible and any unnecessary prolongation of the socially, legally and psychologically insecure situation of foster care should be avoided (Goldstein *et al.*, 1973).

Finally, these studies have demonstrated the advantages of a longitudinal, prospective design. If, for instance, the investigation had been restricted to the first follow-up (i.e. if the 11-year-old study had been carried out as a single cross-sectional study), then the conclusions would have been quite different from those we have now reached.

Taken as a cross-sectional study the results from age 11 years would have indicated that the subjects, who were born of socially handicapped parents, had a less-favourable prognosis than other children—irrespective of whether they grew up in biological, adoptive or foster homes.

From a longitudinal perspective the following conclusions were drawn:

1 The risk of disturbed mental and social development was in no way greater for adopted children than for children in the general population regardless of biological background.
2 The prognosis for subjects who grew up in biological or foster homes, on the other hand, was considerably less favourable.

The different prospects for adopted children and children in biological of foster homes could not be explained by reference to biological factors or environmental variables other than possibly those concerned with placement practices.

The practical implication of the longitudinal study was consequently that preventive work in the field of adoption and foster care should to a great extent be considered in terms of placement procedures, which grant both adopting and foster parents, as well as their children, legal and psychological security as early as possible. To avoid insecurity in the rearing situation, decisions about the future of a child should not be delayed unnecessarily (Goldstein *et al.*, 1973). Another implication of the study (many times repeated elsewhere) is that much more preventive work should be undertaken with mothers who, in spite of adverse social and psychological circumstances, have decided to take care of their children themselves.

REFERENCES

Bohman, M. (1970). *Adopted Children and Their Families*, Proprius, Stockholm.
Bohman, M. (1971). A comparative study of adopted children, foster children and children in their biological environment born after undesired pregnancies, *Acta Paediat. Scand.* Suppl. 221.

Bohman, M. (1978). Some genetic aspects of alcoholism and criminality. A population of adoptees, *Arch. Gen. Psychiat.* **35**, 269–276.

Bohman, M. and Sigvardsson, S. (1980). A prospective, longitudinal study of children registered for adoptions; a 15-year follow-up, *Acta Psych. Scand.* **61**, 339–355.

Bohman, M., Sigvardsson, S. and Cloninger, C. R. (1981). Maternal inheritance of alcohol abuse, *Arch. Gen. Psych.* **38**, 965–969.

Christiansen, K. O. (1970). Crime in a Danish twin population, *Acta Gen. Med. Gemellologica*, **19**, 323–326.

Cloninger, C. R., Bohman, M. and Sigvardsson, S. (1981). Inheritance of alcohol abuse, *Arch. Gen. Psych.* **38**, 861–868.

Dalgard, O. S. and Kringlen, E. (1976). A Norwegian twin study of criminality, *British Journal of Criminology*, **16**, 213–231.

Goldstein, J., Freud, A. and Solnit, A. (1973). *Beyond the Best Interests of the Child*, The Free Press, London.

Jonsson, G. (1967). Delinquent boys, *Acta Psych. Scand.* Suppl. 195.

Klackenberg, G. (1971). A prospective longitudinal study of children, *Acta Paedat. Scand.* Suppl. 224.

Lange, J. (1931). *Crime as Destiny. A Study of Criminal Twins*, (translated by C. Haldane) George Allen and Unwin, London.

McWhinnie, A. M. (1967). *Adopted Children, How They Grow Up*, Routledge & Kegan Paul, London.

Munsinger, H. (1975). The adopted child's IQ: A critical review, *Psychol. Bull.* **82**, 623–659.

Otto, U. (1976). Male youths, *Acta Psychiat. Scand.* Suppl. 264.

Raynor, L. (1980). *The Adopted Child Come of Age*, George Allen and Unwin, London.

Robins, L. N. (1966). *Deviant Children Grown Up: A Sociological and Psychiatric Study of Sociopathic Personality*, Williams and Wilkins, Baltimore.

Scarr, S. and Weinberg, R. (1976). IQ test performance of black children adopted by white families, *Amer. Psychol.*, 726–739.

Triseliotis, I. (1973). *In Search of Origins*, Routledge & Kegan Paul, London.

Longitudinal Studies in Child Psychology and Psychiatry
Edited by A. R. Nicol
© 1985 John Wiley and Sons Ltd.

Chapter 8

Parenting Behaviour of Mothers Raised 'In Care'

D. Quinton and M. Rutter

INTRODUCTION

The possible connections between experiences in childhood and psychosocial functioning in adult life constitute a major area of interest in psychiatry and in the allied professions of psychology and social work. For clinicians working with adult patients, knowledge of the childhood antecedents of adult mental illness may throw light on its nature and causation, as well as provide the potentials for prevention and intervention. For those caring for children, an understanding of the sequelae in adult life of childhood experiences is crucial for any adequate appreciation of the developmental process as a whole—both normal and abnormal.

Nowhere are these concerns more acute than in the case of parenting. On the one hand, there is a widespread assumption that childhood experiences may serve to determine functioning as a parent when children grow up to reach adulthood. On the other hand, it is generally thought that the quality of parenting is strongly influenced by current living conditions, by the marital relationship, and by the mental state of the parents. At first sight this seems a choice between influences from the past and those in the present, but that constitutes a misunderstanding of the alternative explanations. Thus, we need to ask whether the apparent effects of childhood experiences are just an artefact of genetic background or rather of continuities between adversities in childhood and adult life. Perhaps there are no persisting sequelae from deprivation in early life, it is simply that individuals living in poor circumstances in childhood tend to be living in equally disadvantageous conditions in adulthood. Conversely, we may ask whether the apparent effects of current environmental circumstances are no more than a consequence of the types of individuals who land up in them. Maybe it is not that overcrowded housing or a discordant marriage impede a mother's or father's ability to parent well but rather that individuals with longstanding personality problems fail to cope socially, financially and personally so that the parenting difficulties are just one facet of a much broader psychosocial disability.

157

Of course, these competing hypotheses, do not necessarily constitute alternatives. It is apparent that continuities and discontinuities in development can arise through many different mechanisms (Rutter, 1984) and that the interactions between individuals and their environments can take many forms (Rutter, 1983). It is necessary that we seek to understand the various processes involved. If we are to succeed in doing so it will be crucial to test different types of explanations one against the other, and to use some imagination in considering how things may have come about in the ways that they have.

In this chapter, we use data from a follow-up study of girls who spent part of their childhoods in institutions to examine the factors influencing parenting. The hypothesis that there are substantial continuities between adverse experiences in childhood and poor parenting behaviour in adult life raises a variety of different issues that require systematic tackling (Rutter and Madge, 1976; Rutter. et al., 1983).

First, it is necessary to determine whether such links exist at all, and if they do to specify how the links apply to different features of parenting and to different types and degrees of parenting problems. If some level of continuity *is* found, the next question concerns the *interpretation* of the statistical associations. On the one hand they may reflect causal mechanisms such that the experience of poor parenting as a child may cause a person to become a poor parent herself. If causal links of this kind do exist it is necessary to ask whether the effects are on parenting *per se* or whether they have an impact on personality development more generally, with parenting affected only in so far as personality disorders involve problems in parenting. On the other hand the associations may reflect either genetic factors or continuities mediated by some third variable such as social disadvantage or stressful experiences in adult life. However, unless continuities are complete there is a further question to be considered; why do some individuals become normal well-functioning adults in spite of severe adversities in childhood? It may be that such discontinuities are to be explained by a weaker exposure to the adverse factors in childhood that predispose to maladaptive outcomes. But, equally, it may be that discontinuities are determined by the presence of compensating or mitigating factors of a positive kind.

Finally there is the question of the extent to which the ill effects of seriously adverse experiences in childhood are modifiable or reversible once adulthood is reached. It is now widely accepted that a substantial degree of recovery *in childhood* is possible if bad experiences are followed by good ones (Rutter, 1981b), but as yet little is known about the extent to which major changes in social functioning can occur as the result of beneficial experiences in adult life.

In our examination of these issues in this chapter we focus on three main variables (see Quinton *et al.*, 1984). We use disrupted parenting and institutional rearing as our chief measures of adverse childhood experiences; the qualities of the girls' marriage and of their marriage partners constitute the prime measures of adult experiences and the women's quality of parenting comprises the principal dependent variable. Our purpose is to delineate the patterns of connections between these three sets of measures in order to suggest possible processes and mechanisms. Finally, we attempt to draw some clinical lessons from the empirical findings derived from this segment of data analysis from one longitudinal study.

STUDY DESIGN

Choice of independent variables

Childhood

The admission of a child into the care of the local authority, together with admission into a children's home, has been found to be a good index of adverse experiences. Several studies have shown the very considerable difficulties in relationships and in child rearing experienced by the parents of children admitted into care—even when the ostensible reason for admission is the mother's confinement or physical illness (Quinton and Rutter, 1984a,b; Schaffer and Schaffer, 1968; Wolkind and Rutter, 1973); about 2 per cent of 7-year-old children in Britain have been 'in care' for some period in their lives (Mapstone, 1969); and follow-up studies have had the consistent finding of a marked increase in emotional and behavioural problems among the children taken 'into care' (Lambert *et al.*, 1977; Roy, 1983; Wolkind and Rutter, 1973; Yule and Raynes, 1972) with differences persisting into adulthood (Wolkind, 1977). Social-service records allow a rapid identification of all families living in a defined geographical area who have a child admitted into care, and an earlier study of children currently in care by King *et al.*, 1971 and Yule and Raynes, 1972, provided a sample of adults who had the experience of institutional care when young.

Of course, it would not be sensible to isolate admission to institutional care from children's other life experiences; moreover the empirical findings showed important continuities between different forms of stress and adversity. Accordingly, more limited attention is paid to other happenings in childhood in order to understand the possible processes involved. (Other experiences are discussed in Rutter *et al.*, 1983.)

Adulthood

Our choice of the marital relationship as the main measure of experiences in adult life was an obvious one in the circumstances. To begin with, for many young people it constitutes the greatest change of circumstances in early adult life, and, moreover, a change that might be thought to constitute a major discontinuity with childhood. Accordingly, it provided the opportunity to test the hypothesis that a radical alteration in environmental conditions, even in adult life, could do much to modify the long-term effects of childhood experiences. Secondly, parenting takes place within the family and is a shared endeavour between husband and wife. Many studies have shown that parenting is best considered from the broader perspective of family functioning, with the marital relationship one key feature of that functioning (Belsky, 1981; 1984). Thirdly, a variety of investigations have suggested the importance of social supports in modifying adult behaviour in conditions of stress (Henderson, 1982; Rutter, 1981a), with a close confiding marital relationship as the most powerful of such supports (Brown and Harris, 1978).

Parenting

Although parenting qualities constitutes our key dependent variable, the results show that it is closely associated with the women's overall psychosocial functioning. It has, therefore, seemed appropriate to discuss findings in relation to social functioning generally as well as parenting as a specific 'outcome'. Because the numbers are smaller for the parenting analyses (only a minority of the women had children by the time of follow-up), in some cases we have preferred to give the findings for social functioning when presenting multivariate analyses with several variables. However, when we have done so, the pattern of findings from parenting has been found to be similar, unless we specify to the contrary (there are some differences; see Rutter *et al.*, 1983).

Sample

The study consisted of a follow-up into early adult life of ninety-four girls who, in 1964, were then in one or other of two children's homes run on group cottage lines. The girls had been admitted to institutional care because their parents could not cope with child-rearing, rather than because of any type of disturbed behaviour shown by the children themselves. The regimes in the cottages were studied systematically by Tizard and his colleagues (King *et al.*, 1971) and the children's behaviour at school was assessed by means of a standardized questionnaire (the Rutter 'B' scale—Rutter, 1967). Both sets of data were made available to us. The sample was restricted to children identified as 'white' (on Tizard's original record sheets); and was defined in terms of those aged between 21 and 27 years on 1 January, 1978. Of the ninety-four, 'ex-care' women, five had died by the time of the follow-up (the deaths were caused by: kidney failure, leukaemia, one road traffic accident, one drug overdose, one death by fire in a club associated with drug trafficking). Of the eighty-nine women still living, eighty-one (91 per cent) were interviewed (including one in Germany and three in Australia).

The contrast group of fifty-one, comprised a quasi-random general population sample of individuals of the same age, never admitted 'into care', living with their families in the same general area in inner London, and whose behaviour at school was assessed at approximately the same age by means of the same questionnaire. The group was originally studied because it constituted the control group for a study of the children of parents with some form of psychiatric disorder (Rutter and Quinton, 1981; see also Quinton and Rutter, Chapter 6 of this volume). The contrast sample was similarly followed to age 21–27 years using methods of assessment identical to those employed for the 'ex-care' sample. Of the fifty-one controls, forty one (80 per cent) were interviewed; five could not be traced and five did not agree to be seen.

Methodology

Data were collected by interviews with subjects and their spouses, lasting 2½–4 hours using a non-schedule standardized approach based on methods established in earlier investigations (Brown and Rutter, 1966; Graham and Rutter, 1968; Quinton et al., 1976; Rutter and Brown, 1966). The interview covered the person's recall of their childhoods; their later family, peer and work experiences; and their current circumstances, functioning and adjustment. Parenting skills were rated by interviewers on the basis of detailed parental accounts of what they did in dealing with recent episodes concerned with disruptive behaviour, difficulties in peer relationships and distress. In addition, questions were asked on the amount and nature of parental involvement in play. Summary ratings included those on overall style of parenting, effectiveness and consistency in control, parental sensitivity to the child's needs, and the amount of expressed warmth towards and criticism of the child. The prospective design also included direct home observations of the interactions between mothers and their 2–3½-year-old children (Dowdney et al., 1984a; Mrazek et al., 1982).

RESEARCH FINDINGS

Circumstances in childhood

The great majority of the 'ex-care' sample in the prospective study had experienced prolonged periods of institutional care from an early age. According to the children's homes records, over one-third had been admitted before age 2 years and over two-thirds before age 5 years. On their own accounts nearly 90 per cent spent at least 4 years in institutional care and over half remained there until age 16 years or later. On the other hand, many returned to their families for greater or lesser periods of time (over one-third were with their families for at least one year between the ages of 5 and 11 years). Three-quarters of those who returned to their parents experienced persistent family discord.

Thus, it may be seen that the 'ex-care' group's experiences were a mixture of severe discord and dysharmony with their own families and the more harmonious but less intense and less personal multiple caretaking of the institution.

King et al., (1971) have described the staff organization and pattern of care provided in the two children's homes where the 'ex-care' group spent their early years. Each home contained about 350 children, the great majority of whom were of school age. The homes were divided into living units, known as cottages, which held some fifteen to twenty children each under the care of a housemother together with her deputy and assistant. King et al. (1971) felt that 'the cottages provided a system of care geared very closely to the individual needs of those for whom it existed' (p. 94). Overall, their measures showed that the two children's homes had a very high level of child-oriented practices—at least as compared with long-stay hospitals. Nevertheless, although they gave no quantitative data, their descriptions strongly suggest that most of the children who spent several years in the homes are likely to have had a substantial turnover of houseparents—although this would not be so with all.

It was striking that most of the subjects' memories of their life in the institution were rather more negative than would be suggested by the King et al. (1971) report. Half said that their relationships with staff had been poor and only a minority reported developing any strong personal attachments to any of them. Nearly two-thirds had generally negative memories of their relationships with peers and sibs and only 6 per cent recalled *clearly* supportive relationships. Many of the interviews were characterized by rather undifferentiated descriptions of relationships in which neither adults nor other children were remembered as individuals. It was *not* that they experienced the regime as harsh, punitive or excessively restrictive (in that, most agreed with King et al., 1971), but rather that their life lacked personal meaning or affection.

All studies of children in long-stay institutions have shown a high prevalence of emotional and behavioural problems (Pringle and Bossio, 1960; Wolkind, 1974). Our findings provided no exception to this picture. As judged by scores on the teachers' questionnaire (obtained in the mid-60s when the girls were aged 7–13 years), six times as many of the 'ex-care' girls as their controls (35 per cent versus 6 per cent) showed disturbed behaviour at school—a statistically significant difference. The 'ex-care' girls also showed high rates of disturbance on questionnaires completed by houseparents (26 per cent had deviant scores) but no comparison data were available for these. In all, over half of the 'ex-care' girls (53 per cent) were rated as disturbed on one or both questionnaires.

Outcome in adult life

Parenting

The outcome of the two groups of women may be considered first in terms of their parenting histories, in which there were marked differences. Nearly twice

Table 8.1   Pregnancy and parenting histories of women

	Ex-care women (%) (n=81)	Comparison group (%) (n=42)	Statistical significance		
			χ^2	df	p
Ever pregnant	72	43	8.50	1	0.01
Pregnant by 19 years	42	5	16.75	1	0.001
Had surviving child	60	36	5.85	1	0.02
Of Those with Children	(n=49)	(n=15)			
Without male partner	22	0	Exact test p=0.039		
Any children ever in care/Fostered	18	0	Exact test p=0.074		
Temporary or permanent break-down in parenting	35	0	Exact test p=0.009		
Living with father of all children	61	100	6.52	1	0.02

as many of the women reared in an institution had become pregnant and given birth to a surviving child by the time of the follow-up interview; moreover whereas none of the control group had become pregnant before their nineteenth birthday, two-fifths of the 'ex-care' sample had. It is also apparent that the institution-reared women with children were less likely to be in a stable cohabiting relationship; only 61 per cent were living with the biological father of all the children compared with all those of the comparison group; and 22 per cent were without a current male partner compared with none of the comparison group. Serious failures in parenting were evident only in the institutional sample; nearly a fifth of the children had been taken into care for fostering or placement in a children's home and there had been one case of infanticide. Altogether, for one reason or another, 18 per cent of the 'ex-care' mothers had children who were no longer being looked after by them, compared with none in the control group. Moreover, just over one-third (35 per cent) had experienced some form of transient or permanent parenting breakdown with at least one of their children; this occurred with *none* of the comparison-group mothers. Parenting breakdown, in this context, meant that the children had been looked after by someone other than the mother for a period of at least 6 months. In eight cases this involved some form of fostering or institutional care, in three cases care by some adult other than the parents, and in five cases care by the father (plus the one case of infanticide). From the child's point of view, of course, the parenting may not have 'broken down' if the father was providing good care. Here, however, the figures refer solely to the *mother's* parenting.

An overall assessment of parenting for women with children aged 2 years or more was made on the basis of our interview measures of current parental

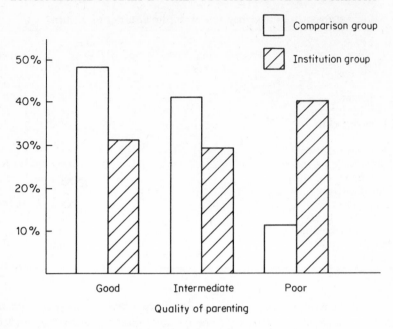

Fig. 8.1 Women's parenting qualities. □, comparison group; ▨, institution group

functioning with respect to the one selected child. 'Poor' parenting was rated if there was a marked lack of warmth to the children (score of 0–2 on a 6-point scale) or low sensitivity to children's needs (score of 1–2 on a 5-point scale) *and* difficulties in at least two out of the three areas of disciplinary control (consistency, effectiveness and style). Conversely, 'good' parenting was rated if there were no difficulties on any of the scales of current parenting. An intermediate rating meant some current problems that fell short of the criterion for 'poor'. Because so few of the comparison group had children aged 2 years or more, for this analysis the data for the comparison group are based on both the women in that group (*n* = 13) *and* the female spouses of the men (*n* = 14). The findings for the comparison women and the female spouses were generally similar.

Two-fifths of the 'ex-care' sample had a rating of poor parenting compared with only about one in nine of the comparison group—a nearly four-fold difference. A further six (13 per cent) 'ex-care' women, but no women in the comparison group, had had children taken into care but were not currently parenting. On the other hand, nearly one-third (31 per cent) of the women reared in institutions showed good parenting. It is clear that in spite of the fact that *all* of them had experienced an institutional rearing for part of their childhoods and that most had experienced rather poor parenting when with their own families, there was great heterogeneity of outcome in the 'ex-care' sample, with

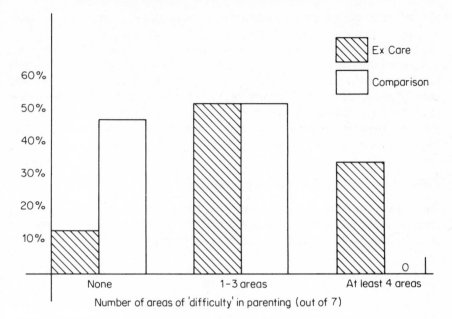

Fig. 8.2   Observation measures of parenting. ▨ , ex-care group; ☐ , comparison group

a substantial minority showing *good* parenting. It is evident also that a surprisingly high proportion (just over half) of the comparison group mothers showed some problems in parenting, although far fewer showed severe difficulties.

The validity of the finding that poor parenting was significantly more common in the 'ex-care' group could be tested in several different ways. First, the difference between the groups was very marked even when analyses were restricted to purely objective measures of parenting breakdown, such as the children being taken into care (see Table 8.1). Secondly, the women who had experienced temporary or permanent breakdown in the past were more than twice as likely to show currently poor parenting on the interview assessment. Of the seventeen women who had experienced parenting breakdown, ten had children in the age group currently with them at home. Of these ten women, eight showed poor parenting compared with nine (29 per cent) out of the remaining thirty-two women (exact test $p = 0.01$). Thirdly, the group differences were similarly evident on the direct observational measures of mother–child interaction in the home. Figure 8.2 gives the findings for the overall observational assessment of parenting based on seven different aspects of parenting (positive affect, negative affect, frequency of distress, frequency of control episodes, ignoring of child initiations, amount of child initiations, amount of joint play). A third (35 per cent) of the 'ex-care' women fell into the lowest quartile on at least four out of these seven areas of parenting—compared with none of the comparison group. Conversely, over two-thirds (71 per cent) of the comparison group were in the top quartile on at least one parenting area, compared with only one in nine in the 'ex-care' sample. The highly significant difference between the groups on the observational measures once again confirms the validity of the finding that poor parenting was more frequent among the 'ex-care' mothers. The individual observational measure findings are reported more fully elsewhere (Dowdney *et al.*, 1984b).

Other aspects of psychosocial functioning

We may conclude from these findings that there is some continuity (as well as substantial discontinuity) in parenting across two generations. It is next necessary to consider whether these continuities apply to parenting *as such* or whether

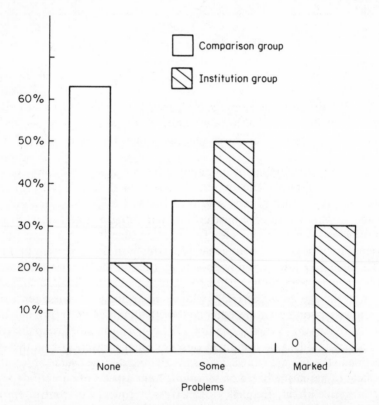

Fig. 8.3 Overall psychosocial assessment (women). □, comparison group; ◨, institution group

they reflect the intergenerational persistence of overall psychosocial functioning (of which parenting was but a part). The 'ex-care' and comparison groups differed markedly in all aspects of psychosocial outcome. Many more of the former showed current psychiatric disorder, or had a criminal record, or had substantial difficulties in their sexual or love relationships (Rutter et al., 1983). Overall, 25 per cent were rated as showing a personality disorder as evidenced by persisting handicaps in interpersonal relationships since their early teens or before (compared with none in the control group).

An overall assessment of psychosocial outcome was obtained by combining these measures. 'Marked problems' were rated if there was a personality disorder or severe and longstanding difficulties in sex/love relationships, or if there were definite current problems in *at least* three of six areas of marriage, broken cohabitation, social relationships, criminality, psychiatric disorder or living in hospital/hostel/or sheltered accommodation. A good outcome was rated if there were no problems on any of these measures. On these criteria, 30 per cent of the 'ex-care' women but none of the controls had a poor outcome. Indeed, nearly two-thirds of the latter showed good functioning, a rating made for only one-fifth of the institution-reared group.

Parenting and psychosocial outcome

The next issue is how far the parenting and psychosocial outcome measures overlap (see Figure 8.4). Four main conclusions may be drawn. First, there was no association between the two measures in the comparison group. The implication is that parenting difficulties need not be a consequence of overall psychosocial impairment. Secondly, the two measures overlapped to a very considerable extent in the 'ex-care' group. As a consequence, there are very few 'ex-care' women with poor parenting but a good psychosocial outcome on non-parenting measures (2/42), and scarcely any with good parenting but a poor psychosocial outcome (2/42). Thirdly, the main differences between the two groups applied to the proportions with both or neither set of difficulties. There was little evidence of parenting links across the two generations if parenting difficulties *occurring in isolation* are considered. Indeed, intermediate-level parenting difficulties shown by women with generally good psychosocial functioning were largely a feature of the comparison group (8/28 versus 5/42 in the 'ex-care' group). That observation suggests the inference for the fourth conclusion — namely, that the explanation for isolated parenting difficulties of mild to moderate degree may well be different from that for severe and generalized psychosocial problems that include parenting difficulties as one of many areas of concern.

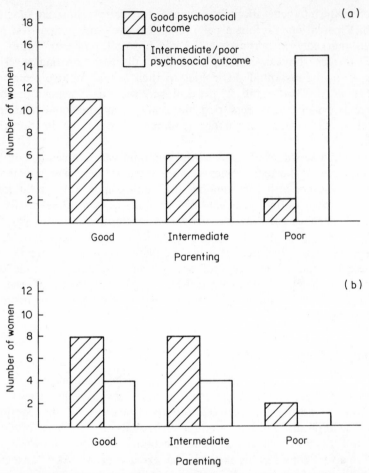

Fig. 8.4   Associations between parenting and psychosocial adjustment. (a) Ex-care women; (b) comparison women. ▨ , good psychosocial outcome; ▢ , intermediate/poor psychosocial outcome

Behavioural precursors of parenting difficulties

Another aspect of the question of the extent to which parenting difficulties are just part of a broader spectrum of psychosocial problems concerns the role of emotional and behavioural difficulties during childhood and adolescence. As noted above, about half of the institution-reared women were already showing problems during the pre-adolescent years. It is necessary to determine the extent to which these problems constituted precursors of later parenting difficulties. Figure 8.5 shows that to an important extent they did. Of the women without any evidence of emotional/behavioural problems when young, 41 per cent

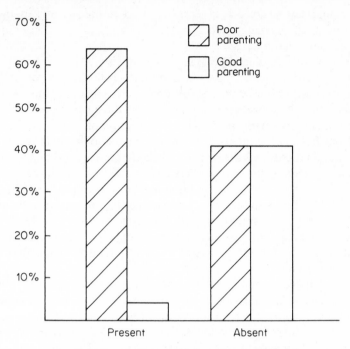

Fig. 8.5   Girls teenage behaviour and later parenting (ex-care group). □ , poor parenting, ▨ , good parenting

showed poor parenting compared with 64 per cent of those with such problems. Nevertheless, it is apparent that the 'ex-care'–comparison group difference on parenting was not wholly explicable in terms of emotional/behavioural functioning before maturity. Even among those without overt problems when young, the outcome for the 'ex-care' women was substantially worse (41 per cent poor parenting) than that for the comparison group (only 10 per cent of whom showed poor parenting).

Ordinal position

It might seem to follow from the very substantial overlap in the 'ex-care' group between severe parenting difficulties and generally poor psychosocial functioning that the parenting problems were an intrinsic and unmodifiable aspect of maladaptive personality functioning. However, it is apparent that this was not necessarily the case. Thus, the detailed observational measures of parent–child interaction (Dowdney *et al.*, 1984b) showed that the difficulties in parenting rarely amounted to neglect or abuse; rather they comprised somewhat subtle (although marked) problems in sensitivity and responsiveness to the child, together with an increased tendency to show negative affect outside of disciplinary interchanges.

At first sight that finding appears inconsistent with the high rate of parenting breakdown. Accordingly, we sought to determine whether or not parenting might have improved with experience. The first approach to that question was to assess what happened with subsequent children where there had been some form of parenting breakdown with the first born. Adoption of infants in the early or middle teens from two mothers were not considered to be breakdowns for this analysis since in these cases the young women did not parent the children before the adoptions. One of the two mothers had two children adopted at this time and went on to have four further children with no subsequent breakdowns. She was assessed in the intermediate current parenting groups on both interview and observation. The second mother subsequently had her next child in temporary foster care and was currently parenting poorly on both assessments. The first parented child of these two women is treated as the first child in subsequent analyses.

There were fifteen women who had parenting breakdowns with their first-parented children. Examination of those who went on to have second children who were over 2 years of age at follow-up showed that most, but not all, still experienced considerable parenting difficulties, both with regard to parenting breakdowns and on assessments of current parenting (Dowdney et al., 1984b).

Thus, we may conclude that of those with the most severe parenting problems in the past many, but not all, still experienced considerable parenting difficulties. Equally, however, it was evident that many of the women with the worst overall social functioning were not currently parenting for one reason or another. It should be added that there was only one woman who experienced a breakdown in parenting with later children who had not experienced a breakdown with her first born.

The second approach to the question of whether parenting improved with experience was to compare the parenting of first- and subsequent-born children in women who had had at least two children. Of the twenty-seven first-born children seven (25.9 per cent) had experienced parenting breakdown compared with six (28.6 per cent) of the twenty-one subsequent-born children. The interview assessments of current parenting (confined to the twenty-two first-born children and the twenty with subsequent born) also provided no evidence of any improvement in parenting with experience (poor parenting was rated in 36 per cent and 45 per cent respectively). In sharp contrast, the observational data (Dowdney et al., 1984b) showed a marked difference in the extent of parenting difficulties according to ordinal position. Of the eight women with difficulties in at least four out of seven areas of parenting, seven were assessed on first-born children (the difference between seven out of eleven and one out of twelve being highly significant).

It is not entirely clear why the observational measures should show an ordinal position effect whereas the historical and interview data did not; however, there are possibly relevant differences in the nature of the data. First, it is apparent that some of the most socially impaired women who had experienced breakdowns of parenting were no longer parenting children aged 2 years or more (this applied to five of the sixteen mothers with an overall rating of 'poor' social functioning but only one of the remaining thirty-one mothers). Secondly, the parenting breakdown measure referred to the past and hence did not necessarily reflect the current situation. Thirdly, the interview rating applied to parenting as it ordinarily took place rather than in the (usually) one-to-one situation used for home observations. This may have been relevant here in that, obviously, the mothers of subsequent-born children were having to deal with several children whereas those of first born were not. It may be, therefore, that the mothers of subsequent-born children were having to parent in more difficult family circumstances. If that is so, the observational data would suggest that their parenting skills may have been improved but that they remained vulnerable to the effects of social stressors and pressures. We must conclude that the evidence is ambiguous on whether or not parenting improves with experience in these circumstances but, probably, it does so in some women (although clearly not in all and perhaps it is less likely to do so in those with the greatest initial social impairment).

Genetic factors and disrupted parenting in early childhood

The next issue is whether the worse outcome of the 'ex-care' group was a function of their genetic background or their experiences in childhood. The study was not designed to differentiate between these two types of risk factors and obviously both are likely to have been operative. Nevertheless, it was possible to obtain some leverage on the question of possible genetic factors by means of

Table 8.2 Parental deviance and psychosocial outcome (ex-care women)

	Parental Deviance		
	Absent (%) ($n = 13$)	Present (%) ($n = 27$)	Statistical significance (exact test)
Behavioural disorder (childhood)	54.5	58.3	NS
Delinquency (childhood)	23.1	14.8	NS
Criminality (adult and child)	23.1	29.6	NS
Personality disorder (adult)	7.6	40.7	0.03
Poor overall psychosocial functioning	23.0	40.7	NS
Poor parenting	42.9	41.7	NS

Note: The sample size is substantially reduced here because of the number of social services case records that were missing from the files or not made available to us.

further analyses within the 'ex-care' group—dividing the sample according to the presence or absence of parental deviance. Using the contemporaneous social-services records this was rated as present if either of the girls' parents had a criminal record in adult life, or had been treated for a psychiatric disorder, alcoholism or dependency on 'hard' drugs. Parental deviance was recorded for two-thirds of the girls. The presence or absence of parental deviance was then assessed in relation to the various outcome variables. As shown in Table 8.2, parental deviance showed a significant association with adult personality disorder and a non-significant association with poor overall psychosocial functioning, but no association with the other outcome variables. Because personality disorder was rated on the basis of overall psychosocial functioning, the two ratings necessarily overlapped. However, they differed in that the former required persistently impaired functioning over many years, although not necessarily significant handicap at the point of follow-up. Conversely, the overall psychosocial outcome rating was based *solely* on current functioning without reference to persistence over time. As it happened, four of the fourteen women with poor overall functioning did not show a personality disorder and two of the twelve women with a personality disorder did not show current poor overall functioning at the follow-up assessment.

Table 8.3   Disrupted parenting in infancy and psychosocial outcome in adult life

	Personality Disorder		Poor social Functioning		Poor Parenting	
	%	n	%	n	%	n
Disrupted early parenting	32	59	39	59	59	34
Non-disrupted early parenting	5	21	5	21	29	14
Exact probability	0.01		0.01		0.06	

Comparable within-group analyses were undertaken with respect to whether or not the 'ex-care' children experienced disrupted parenting during the first 4 years of life. Disrupted parenting was rated as having occurred if there had been short-term admissions into care, multiple separations through parental discord or disorder, persistent familial discord, or admission into long-term care before the age of 2 years. As Table 8.3 shows, the adult outcomes (with respect to personality disorder, poor social functioning and poor parenting) were all substantially worse in the case of women who experienced disrupted parenting in infancy.

As was to be expected, disrupted parenting in infancy occurred more frequently in the subgroup of 'ex-care' women with deviant parents. Accordingly the next question was which had the greater effect on outcome—parental deviance or disrupted parenting. Figure 8.6 presents the overall pattern of

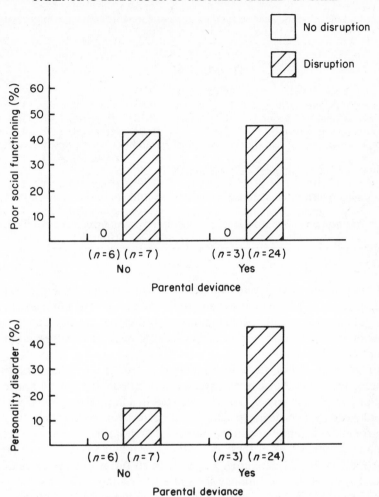

Fig. 8.6   Parental deviance, disrupted parenting and adult outcome. □ , no disruption; ▨ , disruption

findings for the outcome measures of overall social functioning and personality disorder and Table 8.4 presents the results of the linear logistic analyses (a form of multivariate analysis broadly comparable to the more familiar parametric multiple regression analysis—see Swafford, 1980).

Ideally, it would have been desirable to consider separately the child's age at the time of admission to the children's home in that the disrupted parenting that resulted from multiple caretaking in the institution was rather different in quality from that which stemmed from discord and disorder in the biological findings. The findings showed that the outcome for children admitted to the

Table 8.4   Linear logistic analysis for the effects of parental deviance, disrupted parenting and age on adult personality disorder

Model fitted	Deviance	df	p	Reduction in deviance	df	p
(a) Initial model fitted	16.05	5	0.01			
(b) Parental deviance only	10.73	4	0.05	(from (a)) 5.32	1	0.05
(c) Disrupted parenting only	8.56	4	0.10	(from (a)) 7.49	1	0.01
(d) Age of admission only	12.66	4	0.02	(from (a)) 3.39	1	0.10
(e) Improvement on parental deviance model by addition of disrupted parenting				(from (b)) 4.70	1	0.05
(f) Improvement on parental deviance model by addition of age				(from (b)) 4.08	1	0.05
(g) Improvement on parental deviance model by addition of disrupted parenting and age				(from (b)) 7.24	1	0.01
(h) Improvement on parental deviance plus disrupted parenting model by addition of age				(from (e)) 2.54	1	NS

institution in the first 2 years of life and who remained there throughout childhood was as bad as that for any other subgroup. The numbers involved were rather small for the examination of the effects of the child's age of admission to long-term care after taking account of other variables but this was attempted in Table 8.4.

As Figure 8.6 shows, there was a massive effect of disrupted parenting on the outcome variable of overall psychosocial functioning but no appreciable effect of parental deviance. This was reflected in a linear logistic analysis which showed a highly significant ($p < 0.01$) main effect for disruption but no main effect for either parental deviance or age of admission, and no significant effects from any combinations of these variables after taking into account the effect of early disruption in parenting. In short, in so far as our measures allowed a test of the matter, the findings showed an important effect from early life experiences that was not explicable in terms of biological parentage.

The findings for personality disorder (see Table 8.4) were more complicated in that there was a significant main effect for both parental deviance and disrupted parenting, with a further significant effect from the combination of these variables. The best model for the data was provided by the addition of the child's age at admission to long-term care, but the improvement thereby gained was not statistically significant.

We may conclude that, in so far as we can use parental deviance as a proxy measure for genetic background, the results suggest the influence of *both* genetic background and early life experiences. Little can be concluded regarding age of admission *per se* in that admission under the age of 2 years was taken as one of the several indices of parental disruption. There was no suggestion that very early admission to an institution in these circumstances was protective but, equally, there was no suggestion that it made matters worse. We return to this issue later in the chapter.

Mediating and ameliorating factors

The analyses thus far have shown that disrupted parenting in the early years followed by institutional rearing in middle and later childhood significantly predisposed to poor psychosocial functioning in early adult life, of which poor parenting constituted one important facet. Nevertheless, we have commented on the finding that many of the 'ex-care' women did *not* show poor parenting and a substantial minority showed good parenting. It is necessary now to consider possible mediating and ameliorating factors that might explain that heterogeneity.

Positive experiences at school

It has been shown already (Figure 8.5) that the girls' behaviour in middle childhood and early adolescence constituted an important link between infancy and adulthood. The outcome was significantly worse for those girls already delinquent or showing disturbed behaviour at home or at school at that time. Positive experiences at school exerted a somewhat parallel protective effect.

School experiences were rated as positive if the subject had two or more of: CSE or 'O' level success, a markedly positive assessment of school work and/or relationships with peers, and a clearly positive recall of three or more areas of school life (e.g. academic work, sport, drama, arts and crafts). Thirty-one per cent of 'ex-care' women were rated as having positive school experiences compared with 37 per cent of controls. Positive experiences amongst the controls were more likely to involve examination successes (in the control group 35 per cent of the girls had exam success compared with 7 per cent in the 'ex-care' group) but the presence or absence of positive experiences was not related to adult functioning among the control girls. The picture was different in the 'ex-care' sample. In their case, 43 per cent of those without positive experiences had poor social functioning in adult life compared with 6 per cent of those with positive experiences. This pattern was also true for parenting where 62 per cent of those without positive experiences showed poor parenting as against 21 per cent of those who reported their schooling positively. It is important to consider whether these effects are simply artefacts of an association between poorer schooling experiences and behavioural deviance as indicated by the teachers questionnaire.

Table 8.5 shows that this is not the case. Although behavioural deviance was strongly related to the presence of positive school experiences, these experiences appeared to have a protective or an ameliorating effect when deviance was taken into account. However, since such positive school experiences were relatively

Table 8.5   Teacher questionnaire, positive school experiences and social functioning

| | Positive School Experiences | | | | |
| | No | | Yes | | |
	Percentage poor functioning	Total n	Percentage poor functioning	Total n	Statistical significance (exact test)
Teacher's questionnaire					
Non-deviant	35	31	8	13	0.06
Deviant	55	20	0	4	0.07

infrequent in both deviant and non-deviant children, the overall beneficial contribution of schooling to more satisfactory adult outcomes was relatively small. Nor can it be concluded that such experiences were necessarily having an effect on adult functioning irrespective of the circumstances in which the women later found themselves. As we consider in greater detail below, it is more likely that the effects of positive experiences in school arose through their impact on subsequent life chances by virtue of their initiating or perpetuating chains of more positive or rewarding circumstances. The same applies to other experiences during the teenage years (see Rutter *et al.*, 1983). Accordingly we need to turn now to the women's circumstances in adult life.

Family relationships on return home

In considering such trains of events, it is appropriate first to consider what happened when the girls left the children's home. The findings with respect to family experiences subsequent to discharge from residential care are summarized in Table 8.6. In most cases this involved a return to one or both biological parents but eight long-term fostering placements were also included. About half the girls returned to some kind of family environment, with the remainder staying in the institutions until they left to live independently. Although the numbers involved were quite small, a poor psychosocial outcome seemed less likely if the girls returned to a harmonious family setting or one with no more than parent–adolescent disagreements. Of those going to a home with pervasive quarrelling and disharmony, half showed poor social functioning; a substantially worse outcome than that for those remaining in care. But this did not apply to the quality of parenting. The outcome was much the same whether or not the girls returned to their families and there was no consistent association with the characteristics of the home to which they returned.

Table 8.6   Circumstances on return home and parenting

	Poor social functioning		Live births		Poor parenting*	
	%	Total n	%	Total n	%	Total n
Remained in care	26	39	51	39	55	20
Characteristics of home life on return						
Non-discordant	10	10	30	10	0	3
Arguments with parents only	33	18	72	18	54	13
General family discord	50	14	93	14	46	13
Statistical significance of home life trend (df = 1)						
χ		4.15		12.46		NS
p		<0.05		0.001		

*Includes parenting breakdown.

Pregnancy

However, one further point requires to be taken into account. As evident from Table 8.6, those who returned to a discordant family environment were much more likely to become parents than those who returned to a harmonious family or those who remained in the institution until they achieved independence. Altogether, 93 per cent of the discordant family subgroup gave birth to a child (often as a teenager) compared with 51 per cent of those remaining in the institution and 30 per cent of those going to harmonious families. Of the women returning to a discordant environment who had living children five had children adopted or in care and three had children living with the father. Also, the *timing* of the first pregnancy was associated with the quality of parenting as assessed at the time of follow-up. Nearly two-thirds (64 per cent) of the women who became pregnant by the age of 18 years were rated as showing poor parenting compared with one-third (32 per cent) of those who did not have their first baby until later.

Disrupted parenting in infancy and circumstances on leaving care

As we have discussed already, the children's experience of parenting during the infancy period showed a significant association with the women's social functioning in adult life. It might be thought that the finding implies that experiences during the early years have some sort of critical impact on personality development — perhaps as a result of influences on children's first acquisition of selective social attachments. However, the results summarized in Table 8.7 indicate that that would be an unwarranted assumption. They show that

Table 8.7   Disrupted parenting in infancy and return home on leaving institutional care

	Return to Non-discordant family (%)	Return to discordant family (%)	No return (%)
Admitted under 2 years ($n = 18$)	6	34	61
Disrupted parenting and admission over 2 years ($n = 41$)	5	49	46
Non-disrupted parenting and admission over 2 years ($n = 21$)	33	29	38

$\chi^2 = 12.67$, df = 4, $p < 0.025$

disrupted parenting in infancy is significantly associated with what happens when the young people leave institutional care in late adolescence. Of the girls who did *not* experience disrupted parenting in infancy many (33 per cent) left the children's home to return to a non-discordant family environment. In sharp contrast this happened with a mere 5 per cent of those who had had disrupted parenting during their early years. Most (61 per cent) of the girls admitted to the children's home under the age of 2 years did not return to any type of family when they left the institution (not surprisingly, because few had a family to which they could return). In contrast, although this also applied to many of those who experienced disrupted parenting but were not admitted until after age 2 years, also many (49 per cent) returned to a discordant family, usually the one from whence they had been taken many years before. It is apparent that the measure of disrupted parenting could not be considered solely in terms of what happened in infancy because what happened then served to influence the girls' circumstances on leaving the institution more than a dozen years later.

It should be added that these circumstances also helped to determine what happened next. Thus, for example, as we have seen, it was strongly associated with the chances of having a teenage pregnancy. It was also, as one might expect, linked with the likelihood of the girls' marrying for a negative reason (i.e. to escape from stressful circumstances or because an unwanted marriage was forced by pregnancy). Of those returning to a harmonious family one-fifth married for a negative reason; of those going to a discordant family 53 per cent did so; and of those not returning to a family at all 46 per cent did so. The effects of adverse circumstances need to be seen in terms of chains of events and happenings, rather than any one single decisive stressor.

Characteristics of the spouse and of the marital relationship

The next point to consider is whether the characteristics of the women's spouses and current marital situation at the time of follow-up were associated

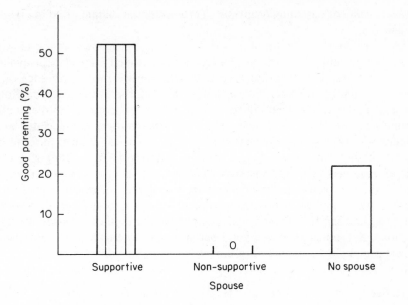

Fig. 8.7   Mothers parenting and support of spouse

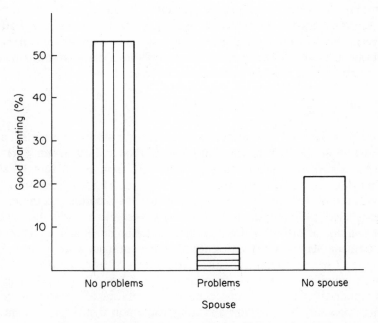

Fig. 8.8   Mothers parenting and problems of spouse

with the quality of parenting behaviour. Three aspects are summarized in Figures 8.7 and 8.8.

First, over half (56 per cent) of the small group ($n = 9$) without a spouse showed poor parenting and only a quarter showed good parenting. Secondly, the quality of parenting was significantly associated with the presence or absence of a supportive marital relationship (this was rated if there was a harmonious marriage, and if the women talked warmly about her spouse or said that she definitely confided in him). Thirdly, parenting was significantly associated with whether or not the spouse showed psychosocial problems (defined in terms of psychiatric disorder, criminality, a drink or drug problem, or long-standing difficulties in personal relationships). This last association is the more striking because the two measures largely came from different informants (parenting from the women and psychosocial problems from her spouse). It is apparent that over half of the women with supportive spouses or spouses without psychosocial problems showed good parenting—a rate as high as that in the general population comparison group.

Protective effect of marital support—causal influence or artefact?

The findings suggested that the spouses' good qualities exerted a powerful ameliorating effect leading to good parenting. There was a substantial overlap between whether the spouse had problems and whether he provided a supportive relationship and, with the sample size available, it was not possible to determine which feature made the difference. However, the data suggested that both had an effect. But before concluding that the spouses' support constituted an ameliorating feature it is necessary to ask whether the statistical association merely reflected the women's own characteristics.

Assortative mating

The first possibility to consider is that of assortative mating. Perhaps the girls who were non-deviant themselves during childhood and adolescence were the ones to choose better functioning supportive men to marry. Figure 8.9 shows that this was not the case to any significant extent. The female subjects were subdivided into 'deviant' and 'non-deviant' groups according to their parent and teacher questionnaire scores in childhood. As shown already, those women deviant on one or other (or both) of these questionnaires had a substantially worse outcome. However, the presence of behavioural deviance did not predict the women's spouses' characteristics. Nearly two-fifths of both groups were without a cohabiting partner at the time of follow-up. About half the spouses of the remainder showed substantial personal problems of one sort or another but there was only a very slight and statistically non-significant tendency for the deviant women to select men with problems as their spouses. The lack of

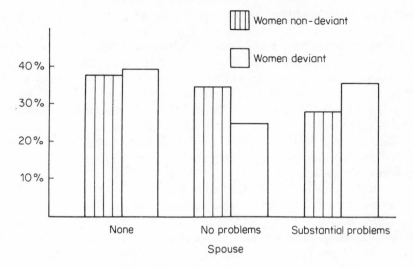

Fig. 8.9   Childhood deviance of female subjects and spouse characteristics. ▥ , women non-deviant; □ women deviant

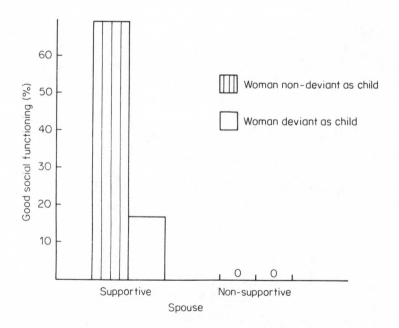

Fig. 8.10   Women's social functioning, own childhood deviance and support of spouse. ▥ , woman non-deviant as child; □ , woman deviant as child

assortative mating within the 'ex-care' group may be a function of the fact that, in leaving the institution, the girls were scattered to a variety of settings different from those in which they had been reared — a circumstance that contrasts sharply with that of girls brought up in their own families and one likely to introduce a greater degree of randomness in the pool of men available.

Whether or not this was the case, the findings indicate that the protective effect of a non-deviant supportive spouse still applied after taking account of the women's own behaviour in childhood. The protective effect was most marked, however, for those women not already showing behavioural disturbance as children or adolescents.

Nevertheless, it should be noted that although there was no indication that the 'ex-care' women's behaviour matched that of their male spouses, there was a marked tendency for the group of institution-reared women as a whole to be more likely that the comparison group to marry men with problems (51 per cent versus 13 per cent; $\chi^2 = 11.32$, df $= 1$, $p < 0.001$). Moreover, as already noted (Table 8.1), the 'ex-care' women with children were much more likely at follow-up to be without any kind of spouse (22 per cent verus 0 per cent). For both these reasons, the 'ex-care' women were much less likely to *experience* the protective effect of a supportive spouse (26.6 per cent versus 74.1 per cent).

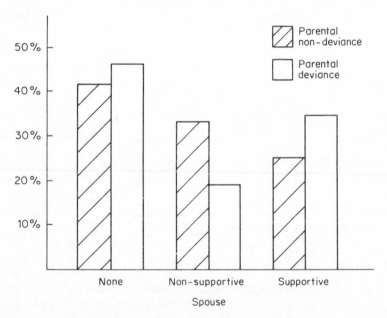

Fig. 8.11 Parental deviance and marital support (ex-care women). ▨ , parental non-deviant; □ , parental deviance

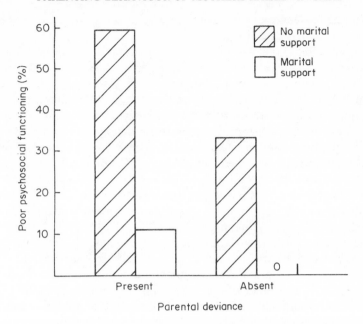

Fig. 8.12   Parental deviance, marital support and poor psychosocial functioning (ex-
care women). ▨ , no marital support; □ , marital support

Genetic factors

A second possibility to consider is that the choice of spouse was influenced,
not by the women's own behaviour, but rather by their own genetic background.
However, we found no evidence that this was the case. There was no association
between parental deviance and choice of spouse. Indeed, if anything, the trend
was in the opposite direction; the women with deviant parents were *more* likely
to have a supportive spouse. Figure 8.12 shows that the protective effect of
marital support applied in the case of both women who did and those who did
not have deviant parents. The findings, then, showed no evidence that the
benefits of marital support were an artefact of assortative mating in terms of
either the women's behaviour or the women's parents' deviance. The pattern
for parenting was closely similar.

'Planning' for a good outcome

It is important next to consider whether the choice of spouse was merely a matter
of chance and circumstances or whether the women play a more active part
in determining or 'planning' their own future. No direct measures of their
intentions in mate selection were available but the matter could be approached

by considering the length of time they knew their first spouse before they began to live with them, together with the reasons for the cohabitation. In this context, 'planning' was rated if they knew their future spouse for over six months before cohabitation *and* if the reasons for living together were positive—that is, they involved a clear positive decision without outside pressures (such as pregnancy or an unhappy home) affecting their choice or timing. 'Non-planners', on the other hand, included all those who had known their spouses for six months or less and/or who had clearly negative pressures that influenced their decision.

The first question is whether 'planners' chose less-deviant spouses. This was indeed the case. Seventy-six per cent of them had non-deviant first spouses compared with only 35 per cent of non-planners ($\chi^2 = 8.17$, df $= 1$, $p < 0.001$). Nor was planning merely a reflection of earlier adjustment. Forty-seven per cent of 'planners' were previously rated as deviant on one or both questionnaires compared with 64 per cent of 'non-planners' ($\chi = 1.78$, df $= 1$, NS).

The second question concerns the overall parenting outcome for those in both groups according to the kind of marital support that they were *currently* experiencing. This was a test both of whether 'planning' simply stood for a generally better level of adjustment and of the effects of marital support on later psychosocial functioning and parenting. For this analysis lack of marital support was rated if the woman was a single parent, has an overtly discordant marriage or if her husband had psychiatric, drink or drug problems or current criminality.

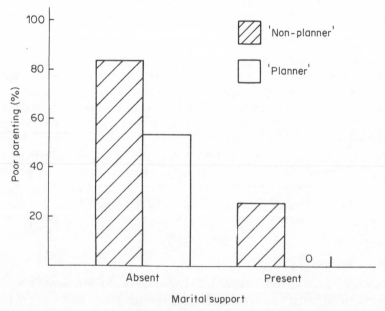

Fig. 8.13 Planning, marital support and poor parenting (ex-care women). ▨ , non-planner; ▢ planner

Table 8.8   Planning, marital support and parenting (linear logistic analysis)

Model fitted	df	Deviance	p	Reduction in deviance	df	p
Initial model fitted	3	23.69	0.001	—	—	—
Planning only	2	15.68	0.001	8.01	1	0.01
Marital support only	2	6.24	0.05	17.45	1	0.001
Planning and support	1	0.97	NS	22.72	2	0.001

The results of this analysis are clear-cut (see Figure 8.13). Both planners and non-planners were less likely to show poor parenting in the presence of marital support. It was particularly striking that this effect applied to women who were non-planners. They were less likely to have a supportive spouse but if, by good fortune, they happened to do so, the protective effect still applied. This was true when the analysis was confined to those currently parenting only. Among planners marital support was also associated with an increase in the proportion showing good parenting (80 per cent versus 8 per cent) but this was not apparent in non-planners (20 per cent versus 14 per cent). This suggests that marital support reduces the likelihood of poor parenting in all women but that the personal limitations associated with non-planning meant that relatively few achieved really good parenting. Unsupported non-planners had the highest rates of problems on both the parenting and psychosocial outcome measures. Taken together these data imply that lack of planning may have been associated with generally poorer psychosocial adjustment in the late teens and early twenties which led to persisting vulnerabilities. If this was so, however, it makes the beneficial impact of supportive spouses even more impressive.

The extent to which the factors used in this analysis really represent a more considered plan for the future cannot be determined from these data. Nor is it possible to assess the extent to which 'planning' was a consequence of foresight on the part of the spouse. However, we may conclude that both the choice of a non-deviant spouse and the chance of a better outcome were related to a courtship long enough for the couple to be able to form some assessment of each other's characteristics, and to a decision to cohabit that was not forced by circumstances. These conditions may relate to a more conscious plan on the part of some women to escape from adversity. The evidence suggests that they are not simply reflections of prior or subsequent adjustment and that actions or chances that lead to more satisfactory circumstances may constitute major breakpoints in the continuity of adversity across generations.

Positive school experiences and planning for marriage

Of course, that raises the crucial question of why some of the institution-reared women seemed to plan their lives whereas others did not. If this was not simply

Table 8.9   Positive school experiences and planning for
marriage

	Positive experiences	
	0/1 (%) ($n = 49$)	2 or more (%) ($n = 22$)
Planner	47	77
Non-planner	53	23

$\chi^2 = 4.51$, df = 1, $p < 0.05$

a function of a lack of behavioural deviance (and, as we have seen, it was not), perhaps it arose as a result of some type of ameliorating *positive* experiences. As shown in Table 8.9, the findings strongly suggested that this may well have been the case. The girls who reported having had positive experiences at school were significantly more likely to have planned their marriage (as operationally defined—see above), and hence more likely to make a harmonious relationship with a non-deviant spouse. Obviously, we cannot know precisely how this came about, but other research has suggested the importance of feelings of self-esteem and self-efficacy (Bandura, 1977; Harter, 1983). It may be that the girls acquired a sense of their own worth and of their ability to control their destinies as a result of their pleasure, success and accomplishments in a few specific areas of their lives. Certainly, it is a common observation that many people with multiple psychosocial problems feel at the mercy of fate and hence do not act in any decisive way to resolve their difficulties. The findings suggest that the experience of some form of success, accomplishment, or even just pleasure in activities, may be important, not so much because it dilutes the impact of unpleasant or stressful happenings, but because it serves to enhance confidence and competence to deal with the hazards and dilemmas of life.

The effects of spouses: direction of causal influences

The next issue is a rather different one. It is clear that the association between marital support and good parenting is not an artefact but still we have to ask in which direction the causal effect operates. Was the effect from the woman to her husband rather than the other way round? In other words could the 'lack of support' be a consequence of the effect of poorly functioning women on their husbands? In order to test that proposition it was necessary to examine the association of the women's social functioning with those adverse characteristics of spouses that could not have been subject to this influence (namely those present before they knew one another). For this purpose we used criminal, drink, drug or psychiatric problems occurring in the spouse's teens *before* he met the subject. Both current and most recent spouses were included

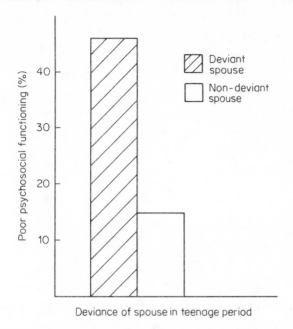

Fig. 8.14   Spouse's teenage deviance and subject's current social functioning. ▨ , deviant spouse; ▢ , non-deviant spouse

in this analysis. As Figure 8.14 shows, there was still a substantial association between the spouse's *teenage* deviance and the 'ex-care' women's social functioning at follow-up. Obviously, the effects are likely to have been two-way (i.e. both from and to the husbands) but it is clear that any effects from the women to their husbands could not account for the protective effect of spouses with respect to the women's parenting and social functioning generally.

Figure 8.15 puts together the findings on the spouse's teenage deviance with the earlier findings on the women's own teenage behaviour. It is clear that there was still a large and statistically significant effect of the spouse's teenage characteristics on the women's overall psychosocial functioning, including parenting (the details of the multivariate analyses are given in Quinton *et al.*, 1984).

Lastly, it is necessary to return to the comparison of outcomes between the 'ex-care' women and the comparison group after taking into account the presence or absence of marital support. The results are summarized in Figure 8.16. Three main conclusions derive from this analysis (see Quinton *et al.*, 1984 for statistical details). First, almost all instances of poor parenting (seventeen out of twenty) occur in the 'ex-care' group, but to a large extent this is a consequence of the fact that most instances of lack of marital support (twenty-six out of thirty) also occurred in the 'ex-care' group. Second, provided that marital support *was*

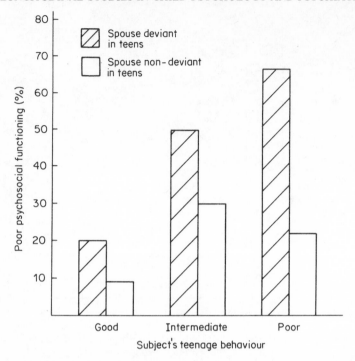

Fig. 8.15   Subject's teenage behaviour, spouses's teenage deviance and poor psychosocial functioning (ex-care women). ☒ , spouse deviant in teens; ☐ , spouse non-deviant in teens

available, poor parenting was a rare occurrence (less than 5 per cent of women), irrespective of the pattern of rearing. The inference to be drawn is that childhood adversities had a powerful *indirect* influence on parenting as a result of effects on the choice of spouse, but very little direct influence provided that marital support was present. Third, poor parenting was more frequent in the 'ex-care' group if such support was lacking (65 per cent versus 29 per cent of the comparison-group women without support). This suggests that the pattern of rearing exerted an effect on parenting above and beyond that mediated through lack of marital support.

The overall pattern of findings suggests that childhood adversities led to poor parenting through two rather different mechanisms. On the one hand, there was a process by which they set in motion a train of events that predisposed the women to experience both poor social circumstances and lack of marital support (the data reported here referred only to the latter but the same general pattern also applied to social disadvantage— see Quinton *et al.*, 1984). This chain of maladaptive experiences often began with marked deviance or disorder in the girls' parents (reflecting probably a genetic risk as well as an environmental one); this led to disrupted parenting in infancy followed by institutional rearing

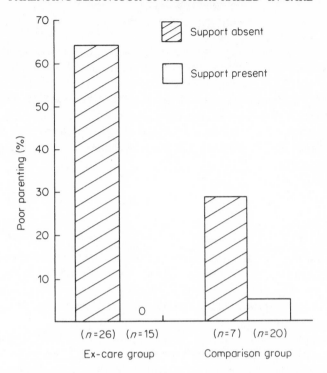

Fig. 8.16   Marital support and current parenting. ▨ , support absent; □ , support present

and later return to a discordant family or alternatively a lack of family to which
to return on leaving the institution; these circumstances in late adolescence
predisposed to teenage pregnancy, early marriage to escape a stressful home
environment, and marriage to a man with similar psychosocial problems from
an equally disadvantaged background; finally, these adverse circumstances in
adult life predisposed to poor parenting.

   On the other hand, childhood adversities also seemed to lead to some kind
of increased vulnerability or decreased coping skills which made it more likely
that the women would *succumb* when faced with poor social circumstances or
lack of marital support. Only a minority of women with a stable harmonious
pattern of upbringing exhibited poor parenting when subjected to chronic stress
in early adult life; in contrast, a *majority* of those who lacked a good upbringing
with continuity in parenting did so. It seemed that the experiences in childhood
had no *necessary* effect on parenting (as shown by the good parenting of the
'ex-care' women with a supportive spouse) but the early adversities left the
women less-well prepared to deal with stress and disadvantage in adult life.

   It follows from the same set of findings that compensatory good experiences
could set off a train of events that led to good outcomes in spite of early

adversities. Thus, positive experiences at school were associated with an increased likelihood that the girls would plan their lives; in turn their tendency to plan made it more likely that they would make a harmonious marriage with a well-functioning man; then, *seriatim*, the presence of marital support was associated with better parenting and improved social functioning more generally. At first sight, the beneficial impact of a 'good' marriage seems to represent discontinuity in development, a change resulting from a new and different experience in adult life. But the discontinuity is to an important extent misleading. The likelihood of making a successful marriage was itself influenced by prior experiences in childhood.

CONCLUSIONS AND CLINICAL IMPLICATIONS

Children's homes

The follow-up findings clearly document the worse adult outcome for the women who spent much of their childhoods in institutions. The validity of the outcome difference between the groups was shown in a variety of ways. Thus, the substantially higher crime rate in the 'ex-care' group was equally evident on the official statistics and on self-report data. Similarly, the much greater parenting problems were shown by the proportions of children being taken into care, by interview ratings and by direct observations in the home.

Perhaps the first question with respect to this finding is whether the worse outcome reflects the girls' adverse experiences in childhood or rather their adverse genetic background. The demonstration that the association between early disrupted parenting and poor social functioning in adult life could not be accounted for in terms of disorder or deviance in the biological parents suggests the importance of experiential factors. This inference also derives from a parallel study by Roy (1983) in which she used both questionnaire and observational data to compare the behaviour of two groups of 5–8-year-old children, one of which had been reared in foster families and one in institutions. The rates of parental deviance were very high and closely comparable in the two groups but the children in the institution-reared group were more likely to show overactive, socially disruptive behaviour. Taken together, the findings of the two studies provide a strong indication of the likely importance of adverse experiences, especially disrupted parenting, in the early years of childhood.

The poor outcome for the girls who experienced disrupted parenting in their own biological families and who were admitted to residential nurseries or children's homes after the age of 2 years points to the harm stemming from serious family discord and disruption—a finding that is in keeping with the results of numerous other studies (see Emery, 1982; Rutter, 1982a). What may be more surprising, and certainly a cause for concern, is the equally poor outcome for girls admitted to institutions in infancy and who remained there for the duration of their upbringing. The concern arises from the fact that they had been taken from their parents by social services to *protect* them from the likely damage of discordant, neglectful, or abusive rearing by their own parents—and yet this protective policy seems to have been associated with an equally bad outcome. We need to ask ourselves whether this implies that the harm stemmed from institutional care; in other words that a 'good' institution was as harmful as a 'bad' family.

A degree of caution is needed before drawing any such conclusion. In the first place, we cannot know what would have happened to the girls if they had remained with their parents—perhaps they would have fared even worse. Also, however, it is necessary to recognize that the girls had both an institutional rearing *and* an adverse genetic background. It would not be warranted to assume that an institutional upbringing would lead to an equally unfortunate outcome if the children were otherwise normal—say those orphaned as a result of a parental car accident. It may be that the ill-effects of an institutional rearing largely apply when the children are constitutionally disadvantaged as well. In addition, we cannot be sure that the poor outcome derived from the institutional rearing as such rather than from the girls' experiences in early infancy before admission. Nevertheless, the findings from other studies strongly indicate that it is unlikely that adverse experiences in the first year or so *per se* could influence adult behaviour in the absence of other adversities in later childhood (Rutter, 1981b). On the other hand, it is quite possible that disrupted parenting in the girls' own families during the first two years predisposed them to be more susceptible to the ill-effects of an institutional upbringing.

The next question is *which* aspect of the girls' institutional experience led to the worse outcome in adult life. Direct study of the particular children's homes in which these children grew up (King *et al.*, 1971), as well as parallel studies of other institutions (Tizard, 1975, 1977; Tizard and Hodges, 1978), showed that in many respects they provided high-quality conditions for the rearing of children. The one feature that stands out as quite different from ordinary family life concerns the very high turn-over in caregivers. Whereas we do not have exact figures on the turn-over experienced by these girls, Tizard's data on good residential nurseries shows that fifty or more parent-figures during the first five years is not at all unusual. It seems probable that this constituted an important limitation in the girls' pattern of rearing. If that supposition is accepted, two implications for practice follow. First, we need to seek to change the arrangements in residential nurseries so that there can be much greater stability in parenting. Of course, there are practical difficulties in ensuring that just one or two staff provide personalized care for each child. Nevertheless, it should be possible to arrange that one or other of a small number of staff is always available to care for a child at key times (such as getting up, mealtimes, going to bed, times of sickness, etc). Probably, children can cope with three, four or five caregivers; what very young children find very unsettling is a roster of ever-changing caregivers so that there is no-one on whom they can rely to be available at times of distress or discomfort. Secondly, Roy's (1983) finding on the better outcome (at least in the short term) for family-fostered children suggests that foster-care may be preferable to residential nurseries for very young children, provided that the child can stay throughout with the same foster parents.

However, it would be quite wrong to see the effects of institutional care solely, or even mainly, in terms of what happens during the early years of childhood. Our results showed that the experience of disrupted parenting in infancy also predicted what happened at the time the girls left the institution in late adolescence. Moreover, the findings strikingly demonstrated the importance of the period of transition after leaving the institution—in terms of family experiences at that time, careers, and whom they married. All too often the girls returned to unhappy discordant homes, to parents with whom they had largely lost touch and with whom they did not get on. Frequently, too, the girls married men whom they had only recently met in order to escape from what they experienced as an intolerable family environment. Both our interviews with the women, and the social-service records, showed that very few of the girls had had much advice or support after they left the children's home in spite of that being the time when they experienced the greatest change of environment and when often they were most in need of help. Of course, it may well be that some would not be very receptive to help at that time but still there is the clear implication from our findings that much more needs to be done to provide social work support and guidance during the critical period of transition of the couple of years or so after leaving the institution.

Marriage

The research findings provided a dramatic demonstration of the major ameliorating effect on adult social functioning of a harmonious marriage to a non-deviant spouse. Particularly because the effect appeared so powerful, we undertook an extensive range of analyses (see also Quinton et al., 1984) to determine whether or not it constituted some form of artefact, deriving perhaps from the characteristics of the women themselves. After all, it might well be supposed that the best-functioning women were the ones most likely to make a successful marriage to a well-functioning man. We were able to identify a variety of predictors of the marital relationship but, equally, the findings were clear-cut in their demonstration that the protective effect of a 'good' marriage was indeed real, and not in any way artefactual. The finding is important in terms of its indication both that experiences in *adult* life can have a massive effect on social functioning, and also that marriage constitutes an environmental factor of major importance. The first conclusion shows that the process of development continues well past the childhood years and that good experiences in adulthood can do much to reduce the ill-effects of serious and prolonged adversities in childhood. Clearly, the potential for change remains for a long time; notions that 'it's too late to do any good' are rarely justified. The finding is also important in its demonstration of the power of 'good' experiences to counteract the ill-effects of 'bad' ones (Rutter, 1979b). So far, the evidence mainly points to two types of protective experiences: a close harmonious relationship and accomplishments that enhance self-esteem. The marital relationship provides an example of the former but our previous research has shown also the protective effect of a warm parent–child relationship (Rutter, 1971; 1982a). Positive experiences at school constitute an example of the latter. However, too little is known on protective factors for any conclusions that these are the only kinds of experience with an ameliorating effect. The topic as a whole is greatly in need of further research.

It might be thought that the finding of the importance of the marital relationship has few practical implications for services. After all, we can scarcely prescribe good husbands for our clients! But that constitutes much too narrow a view of the matter. Our longitudinal data are important in showing the factors associated with a good marriage. Perhaps the most important feature concerns the value of 'planning'. One of the characteristics of a deprived unhappy upbringing, and perhaps even more so of an institutional rearing, is that it is liable to engender a feeling that one is at the mercy of fate with key life decisions always being taken by someone else. It would seem likely to be helpful to do all possible to ensure that young people acquire the belief that they *can* control what happens to them (see Bandura, 1977), and that they gain the social problem-solving skills to enable them to do so (see Pellegrini, 1984). This has implications both for the ways in which children's homes are run and for the goals and approaches used in psychological and social therapies more generally (see Rutter, 1982b).

A further aspect of preparation for a successful marriage, however, concerns the range of opportunities available. One of the aspects of a deprived, or unhappy childhood is a tendency for social contacts to be restricted to individuals from a similar disadvantaged background and for early marriage and pregnancy to occur at a time when individuals are still emotionally immature and uncertain about their futures. The implication is that experiences that widen people's horizons and social opportunities are likely to be helpful (the benefits of scholastic success to some extent operate in this fashion) and that it may be advantageous for young people to postpone both marriage and childbearing until they are ready and able to accept the responsibilities that they entail. Contraceptive advice is necessary but that is not likely to be sufficient in itself. Many unwanted pregnancies arise against the background of a general feeling of hopelessness and inevitability, of a pervasive lack of foresight in the planning of all aspects of life (see Rutter, 1979a). Family planning must form part of a wider community service that is educational in the broadest and best sense (DHSS, 1976; WHO, 1977).

Parenting

A third area in which the findings of this study have implications for practice is that of parenting. The data on associations with overall social functioning showed a marked difference in pattern between the 'ex-care' group and the comparison group. In the former, poor parenting was usually associated with widespread psychosocial problems, whereas in the latter it was not. This implies that adverse childhood experiences and genetic predisposition are likely to be much more important in the origins of parenting problems that constitute part of a broader social impairment than in the origins of isolated parenting difficulties in the context of generally satisfactory social functioning. Our results are relevant only for the first of these. In short, the intergenerational continuities largely apply to poor social functioning rather than to parenting *per se*. By the same token, however, this means that it would not be appropriate to view parenting simply as a set of skills that apply to the upbringing of children. It involves such skills, of course, but also it constitutes a specific type of social relationship; admittedly one with its own particular characteristics but nevertheless part of a broader set of social qualities (Rutter *et al.*, 1983). But also parenting must be considered in terms of resources—social, emotional, and practical; that is there must be an ecological perspective that recognizes the family as a functional social system, the operation of which will be influenced by its internal composition and external forces (Belsky, 1981; Belsky, 1984; Bronfenbrenner, 1979; Rutter *et al.*, 1983). This was shown, for example, by the extent to which parenting qualities were effected by both the marital relationship and by social circumstances generally. The findings indicate that we must be concerned with these aspects of the family, as well as with parent–child interaction, when we seek to facilitate better parenting.

The same implication derives from the findings on parenting breakdown. Although this occurred with women who lacked good parenting skills, also it tended to happen in the context of lack of marital support, severely discordant marital relationships and/or poor living conditions and social disadvantage. The breakdown in parenting was as much a reflection of these widespread personal and social difficulties as of any specific problem in caring for the children. The findings from our earlier study of families at the time children were admitted into care showed exactly the same (Quinton and Rutter, 1984a,b). However, the observational findings highlighted another feature; namely that parenting difficulties were most prevalent with the first child and that the parenting of the second child tended to be somewhat better than that of the first. The interview data did not show this ordinal position effect and it may be that although parenting skills improved, the vulnerability to social stressors did not change. Certainly, it seems unlikely that the gains occurred solely as a result of the passage of time; both the experience of parenting *per se* and improved family/social circumstances seemed to play a part in this improvement.

Moreover, not all women improved to the same extent; gains were least with the most handicapped. However, very few women had the benefit of any kind of therapeutic intervention so that we do not know how much could be achieved.

An early pioneering study by Sheridan (1959) into the rehabilitation of seriously neglectful mothers showed that many improved and came to cope satisfactorily. Her finding that the best results were obtained with women who had a steady and affectionate husband is closely in line with our own results. We need further research into the best methods of helping both mothers and fathers with severe parenting problems but the implication is that important improvements are possible and that the therapeutic endeavours need to focus on both parents, on marital as well as parenting functions, and on the practical learning experiences that stem from parenting as such. Holbrook (1978) has described how these concerns may be applied in practice.

The substantial overlap between parenting problems, social impairment and personality disorder in the 'ex-care' group should not, of course, be held to mean that these difficulties all have the same origins or are influenced by the same developmental factors. Our findings show both similarities and differences. In all three cases, disrupted parenting in infancy constituted an important risk factor and a good marriage constituted an important ameliorating factor. However, parental deviance was of much predictive value only in the case of personality disorder. The implication is that, although genetic factors probably play a significant role in the origins of personality disorder (Schulsinger, 1972) they are less influential in the genesis of social impairment and parenting difficulties. Also there was some suggestion (see Rutter *et al.*, 1983) that good relationships during adolescence were of some benefit with respect to later social functioning but had little impact on parenting *per se*.

Another point to emerge from the findings on parenting derives from the observational data (see Dowdney *et al.*, 1984b). These suggested that many of the parenting difficulties derived from serious, but quite subtle, deficits in sensitivity and responsiveness to the infants. Moreover, many of the problems in discipline and control stemmed from interactions *outside* disciplinary confrontations, from what was done to prevent disruptive behaviour arising, rather than from interventions after it occurred. The finding carries implications for concepts of parenting and for the need to observe parent–child interaction directly if we are to identify specific problems in parenting—a necessary step in planning therapeutic procedures.

Schooling

The finding that positive school experiences had a protective effect in the 'ex-care' group raises several rather different issues. First, it implies that it may be important for all young people to have positive experiences that create a sense of worth, accomplishment, self efficacy. The observation that positive school experiences did not predict adult outcome in the control group may be a consequence of the fact that the girls in that group had ample *other* sources of self-esteem in their family and in their peer group. Secondly, it seems that good experiences *outside* the family may go some way in the amelioration of adversities within the home. It is necessary that we broaden our horizons with respect to the areas of influence on children—the family is important but not all-important. Thirdly, the finding that most of the protective positive experiences at school in the 'ex-care' group did *not* involve academic success serves to remind us that schooling constitutes a rich source of *social* experiences as well as an instrument for scholastic instruction. We need to use schooling to ensure that all children have a range of opportunities for success and pleasure—scholastic accomplishments should not be the only goal of a good education. Fourthly, schools should be organized to ensure that they constitute social environments that are conducive to good behaviour, harmonious relationships and high accomplishments. While this particular study was not designed to assess the qualities that make for successful schools, other investigations have provided useful leads on some of the important features that facilitate pupil success (Rutter, 1982a; Rutter *et al.*, 1979).

Concepts of development

Finally, our findings carry implications for concepts of personality development. The results undoubtedly show important continuities over time and indeed some consistency in behaviour; the girls already showing emotional or behavioural disturbance in middle childhood were the ones most likely to be showing social impairment or parenting problems in adult life. Nevertheless, the results are equally clear in their demonstration that even the most severe childhood adversities do not have a once-and-for-all effect on psychosocial functioning. At first sight, the finding that disrupted parenting in infancy had substantial measurable effects on adult functioning seems to suggest very long-term sequelae stemming from experiences in the first few years of life. However, that inference does not flow from the data. In the first place, the disrupted parenting was followed by institutional rearing, often combined with further experiences of family discord. Thus, the adversities in infancy, not only were not followed by normal parenting which might be expected to have recuperative effects, but also were succeeded by other adversities that may well have intensified the ill-effects.

Secondly, the experiences in infancy were associated with systematic differences in what happened to the young people when they left the institution in late adolescence. The events of the first two years of life to some extent predetermine the events of later years. It is not justifiable to regard the disrupted parenting as if it were an experience confined to the infancy period. Equally, however, it may well be the case that disrupted parenting is most likely to be seriously damaging if experienced during the age period when young children are first establishing selective attachments. That would be consistent with our data as well as with expectations stemming from what is known about early social development (Rutter, 1980). Moreover, it is noteworthy that no social experiences in middle childhood were found to have effects of the same strength—although this may reflect no more than the relative lack of variation in the children's life at that time.

Nevertheless, what is clear is that our findings offer no support for conventional theories of development in terms of the 'structure' of personality or in terms of 'fixation' at particular developmental points. Rather, our findings portrayed a much more fluid view of the developmental process with both continuities and discontinuities in socio-emotional development, but with most links indirect rather than direct (Rutter, 1984). Some continuities stemmed from linkages between different environments rather than from a lack of change. Thus, we found that childhood experiences had a powerful effect on the choice of spouse and that the characteristics of the spouse then had a strong effect on the quality of parenting. The environments change but the experience of one sort of 'bad' environment makes it more likely that the individual will go on to experience other sorts of 'bad' environment.

A further mechanism concerns the effects stemming from the opening up or closing down of opportunities. Thus, institutional rearing was associated with an increased risk of teenage pregnancies which in turn made a poor social outcome more likely. It seems that early pregnancies tended to tie the women to the same disadvantaged environment, as well as making it less likely that they would go on with further education or occupational training. The effect is to much increase the likelihood of poor living conditions in adult life. The sequelae in late adolescence of a disrupted parenting in infancy reflected a similar mechanism in that the break-up of the family in early life meant that often the teenagers did not have a family, or at least not a harmonious family, to which they could return when they left the institution.

The substantially worse parenting of the institution-reared women than the comparison-group women in the presence of marital difficulties and lack of support from the spouse suggests that the adverse childhood experiences had left the women without the necessary resilience, emotional resources or social coping mechanisms to deal successfully with later life hazards. The finding that they coped equally well if they *had* marital support indicated that there was no direct effect leading to poor parenting; rather the pattern of findings suggested some kind of indirect effect that operated through influences on vulnerability to stress, or on social problem-solving skills, or on adaptability.

Yet another set of processes involved effects on habits, attitudes and self-esteem. Both the effects of positive school experiences and the benefits of 'planning' in relation to the choice of marriage partner may operate in this way.

The practical implications of these suggested mechanisms come from the many opportunities presented for the bringing about of change. Sometimes, therapeutic interventions are thought of in terms of the need to bring about some basic change in personality functioning. Our results suggest that this view rests on a rather misleading view of personality development. Alternatively, some behaviourists may see the main need as the elimination of maladaptive deviant behaviours as they manifest themselves in childhood. The findings indicate that this constitutes an unduly narrow view of therapeutic goals. Rather, there is a need to focus on personal changes that will enhance self-esteem, self-efficacy and confidence, and increase coping skills (as well as those associated with a reduction in maladaptive behaviours); and on environmental changes that will increase opportunities and make it more likely that later social circumstances will be beneficial.

Continuities in development involve linkages within the environment as well as within the child (see Rutter, 1984; Rutter *et al.*, 1983). In some circumstances the indirect effects of early adverse experiences may be quite long-lasting. Even so, such long-term effects are far from independent from intervening circumstances. The continuities stem from a multitude of links over time. Because each link is incomplete, subject to marked individual variation and open to modification there are many opportunities to break the chain. Such opportunities continue right into adult life.

ACKNOWLEDGEMENTS

The research was supported by grants from the DHSS/SSRC Working Party on Transmitted Deprivation and the William T. Grant Foundation, New York. We are indebted to the late Ms Freda Sklair, Ms Gerrilyn Smith and Ms Margaret Winkworth for their help with the interviewing; to Ms Christine Liddle for active partnership in the research from start to finish, to Dr Graham Dunn for statistical advice; and to Ms Linda Dowdney and Dr David Skuse for permission to refer to their observational data findings. We are grateful also to the Social Services Departments for their assistance throughout the project. This chapter is based on an article by us, together with Ms Christine Liddle, in *Psychological Medicine*; we thank Cambridge University Press for permission to quote from it.

REFERENCES

Bandura, A. (1977). Self-efficacy: Toward a unifying theory of behavioral change, *Psychol. Review*, **84**, 191–215.
Belsky, J. (1981). Early human experience: a family perspective, *Develop. Psychol.* **17**, 3–23.
Belsky, J. (1984). The determinants of parenting: A process model, *Child Development* **55**, 83–96.
Bronfenbrenner, U. (1979). *The Ecology of Human Development: Experiments by Nature and Design*, Harvard University Press, Cambridge, Mass.

Brown, G. W. and Harris, T. (1978). *Social Origins of Depression*, Tavistock, London.

Brown, G. W. and Rutter, M. (1966). The measurement of family activities and relationships: A methodological study, *Human Relations*, **19**, 241–263.

Department of Health and Social Security (1976) *Fit for the Future*. Report of the Committee on Child Health Services. Chairman: Professor S. D. M. Court. HMSO, London.

Dowdney, L., Mrazek, D. A., Quinton, D. and Rutter, M. (1984a). Observation of parent–child interaction with two-to-three year olds, *J. Child Psychol. Psychiat.* **25**, 379–407.

Dowdney, L., Rutter, M., Skuse, D., Mrazek, D. and Quinton, D. (1984b). Parenting qualities—Concepts, measures and origins, in *Recent Research in Developmental Psychopathology*. (Ed J. Stevenson), Pergamon, Oxford (in press).

Emery, R. E. (1982). Interparental conflict and the children of discord and divorce, Monograph 4. *Psychol. Bull.* **92**, 310–330.

Graham, P. and Rutter, M. (1968). The reliability and validity of the psychiatric assessment of the child. II. Interview with the parent, *Brit. J. Psychiat.* **114**, 581–592.

Harter, S. (1983). Developmental perspectives on the self-esteem, in *Socialization Personality and Social Development,* vol. 4, *Mussen's Handbook of Child Psychology,* 4th edn (Ed. E. M. Hetherington), 275–385, Wiley, New York.

Henderson, S. (1982). Social relationships, adversity and neurosis: an analysis of prospective observations, *Brit. J. Psychiat.* **138**, 391–398.

Holbrook, D. (1978). A combined approach to parental coping, *Brit. J. Social Work*, **8**, 439–451.

King, R. D., Raynes, N. V. and Tizard, J. (1971). *Patterns of Residential Care: Sociological Studies in Institutions for Handicapped Children*, Routledge & Kegan Paul, London.

Lambert, L., Essen, J. and Head, J. (1977). Variations in behaviour ratings of children who have been in care, *J. Child Psychol. Psychiat.* **18**, 335–346.

Mapstone, E. (1969). Children in care, *Concern*, **3**, 23–28.

Mrazek, D. A., Dowdney, L., Rutter, M. and Quinton, D. (1982). Mother and preschool child interaction: A sequential approach, *J. Amer. Acad. Child Psychiat.* **21**, 453–464.

Pellegrini, D. (1984). Training in social problem solving, in *Child and Adolescent Psychiatry: Modern Approaches 2nd edn* (Eds M. Rutter and L. Hersov), Blackwell Scientific, Oxford (in press).

Pringle, M. L. K. and Bossio, V. (1960). Early prolonged separations and emotional adjustment, *J. Child Psychol. Psychiat.* **1**, 37–48.

Quinton, D. and Rutter, M. (1984a). Parents with children in care. I. Current circumstances and parenting skills, *J. Child Psychol. Psychiat.* **25**, 211–229.

Quinton, D. and Rutter, M. (1984b). Parents with children in care. II. Intergenerational continuities, *J. Child Psychol. Psychiat.* **25**, 231–250.

Quinton, D., Rutter, M. and Liddle, C. (1984). Institutional rearing, parenting difficulties, and marital support, *Psychol. Medicine*, **14**, 107–124.

Quinton, D., Rutter, M. and Rowlands, O. (1976). An evaluation of an interview assessment of marriage, *Psychol. Med.* **6**, 577–586.

Roy, P. (1983). Is continuity enough?: Substitute care and socialization. Paper presented at the Spring Scientific Meeting, Child and Adolescent Psychiatry Specialist Section, Royal College of Psychiatrists, London, March, 1983.

Rutter, M. (1967). A children's behaviour questionnaire for completion by teachers: Preliminary findings, *J. Child Psychol. Psychiat.* **8**, 1–11.

Rutter, M. (1971). Parent–child separation: psychological effects on the children, *J. Child Psychol. Psychiat.* **12**, 233–260.

Rutter, M. (1979a). *Changing Youth in a Changing Society: Patterns of Adolescent Development and Disorder*, Nuffield Provincial Hospitals Trust, London. (Harvard University Press, 1980, Cambridge, Mass.)

Rutter, M. (1979b). Protective factors in children's responses to stress and disadvantage, in *Primary Prevention of Psychopathology*, vol. 3, *Social Competence in Children* (Eds M. W. Kent and J. E. Rolf), 49–74. University Press of New England, Hanover, New Hampshire.

Rutter, M. (1980). Attachment and the development of social relationships, in *Scientific Foundations of Developmental Psychiatry* (Ed M. Rutter), pp.267–279, Heinemann Medical, London.

Rutter, M. (1981a). Stress, coping and development: Some issues and some questions, *J. Child Psychol. Psychiat.* 22, 323–356.

Rutter, M. (1981b). *Maternal Deprivation Reassessed*, 2nd edn. Penguin Books, Harmondworth, Middx.

Rutter, M. (1982a). Epidemiological-longitudinal approaches to the study of development, in *The Concept of Development*. Minnnesota Symposia on Child Psychology, Vol. 15, (Ed W. A. Collins), pp. 105–144, Lawrence Erlbaum, Hillsdale, New Jersey.

Rutter, M. (1982b). Psychological therapies: Issues and prospects, *Psychol. Medicine*, 12, 723–740.

Rutter, M. (1983). Statistical and personal interactions: Facets and perspectives, in *Human Development: An Interactional Perspective* (Eds D. Magnusson and V. Allen), 295–319, Academic Press, New York.

Rutter, M. (1984). Continuities and discontinuities in socio-emotional development. Empirical and conceptual perspectives, in *Continuities and Discontinuities in Development* (Eds R. Emde and R. Harmon), 41–68, Plenum, New York.

Rutter, M. and Brown, G. W. (1966). The reliability and validity of measures of family life and relationships in families containing a psychiatric patient, *Social Psychiatry*, 1, 38–53.

Rutter, M. and Madge, N. (1976). *Cycles of Disadvantage: A Review of Research*, Heinemann Educational, London.

Rutter, M., Manghan, B., Mortimore, P. and Ouston, J. (1979). *Fifteen Thousand Hours*. Open Books, London.

Rutter, M. and Quinton, D. (1981). Longitudinal studies of institutional children and children of mentally ill parents (United Kingdom), in *Prospective Longitudinal Research: An Empirical Basis for the Primary Prevention of Psychosocial Disorders* (Eds S. A. Mednick and A. E. Baert), pp.297–305, Oxford University Press, Oxford.

Rutter, M., Quinton, D. and Liddle, C. (1983). Parenting in two generations: looking backwards and looking fowards, in *Families at Risk* (Ed N. Madge), pp.60–98, Heinemann Educational, London.

Schaffer, H. R. and Schaffer, E. B. (1968). *Child Care and the Family*, Occasional Papers on Social Administration, No. 25, Bell, London.

Schulsinger, F. (1972). Psychopathy: heredity and environment, *Int. J. Ment. Health*, 1, 190–206.

Sheridan, M. D. (1959). Neglectful mothers, *Lancet*, i, 722–725.

Swafford, M. (1980). Three parametric techniques for contingency table analysis: a nontechnical commentary, *Amer. Sociol. Review*, 45, 664–690.

Tizard, B. (1975). Varieties of residential nursery experience, in *Varieties of Residential Experience* (Eds J. Tizard, I. Sinclair and R. V. G. Clark), pp.102–121, Routledge & Kegan Paul, London.

Tizard, B. (1977). *Adoption: A Second Chance*, Open Books, London.

Tizard, B. and Hodges, J. (1978). The effect of early institutional rearing on the development of eight-year-old children, *J. Child Psychol. Psychiat.* 19, 99–118.

Wolkind, S. N. (1974). The components of 'affectionless psychopathy' in institutionalized children, *J. Child Psychol. Psychiat.* **15**, 215–220.
Wolkind, S. N. (1977). Women who have been 'in care' — psychological and social status during pregnancy, *J. Child Psychol. Psychiat.* **18**, 179–182.
Wolkind, S. N. and Rutter, M. (1973). Children who have been 'in care' — an epidemiological study, *J. Child Psychol. Psychiat.* **14**, 97–105.
World Health Organization (1977). *Child Mental Health and Psychosocial Development: Report of a WHO Expert Committee*, WHO Technical Report Series no. 613, WHO, Geneva.
Yule, W. and Raynes, N. V. (1972). Behavioural characteristics of children in residential care in relation to indices of separation, *J. Child Psychol. Psychiat.* **13**, 249–258.

Longitudinal Studies in Child Psychology and Psychiatry
Edited by A. R. Nicol
© 1985 John Wiley and Sons Ltd.

Chapter 9

Down's Syndrome in the First Nine Years

A. Gath

Down's syndrome is the most common and most easily recognized single cause of mental retardation. The incidence is 1 in 660 live births and about one-third of the children in a reception class at a special school can be seen to have the characteristic features of the condition. Unlike other medical causes of mental retardation, Down's syndrome is usually recognized at, or shortly after, birth by the medical attendants or midwives and not infrequently by the parents or other relatives. As has been described in many papers, the impact of the news is traumatic and is experienced as a crisis during which there is much emotional distress but which can also offer an opportunity for personal growth as well as a period of danger to physical and mental well being. Although most parents are content to let time elapse before any judgement is made about their offspring's capabilities, the facial appearance of the Down's syndrome child which has led to the label of 'mongol' and the well-known association of these features with mental retardation impels the parents to ask the paediatrician for a detailed prognosis. How long will the child survive? When will he walk? Will he be able to read? Will he be able to hold a job down and manage to look after himself in adult life? Twenty years ago, parents were given a very gloomy picture and were advised frequently to put the child in an institution and even to forget his existence. Attitudes to people with mental retardation have changed and it is now assumed that most parents will take their child with Down's syndrome home and bring him up with support from the medical, educational and social services. Nevertheless, parents, still shocked by the discovery that their newborn child is so different from what they had confidently expected, want a lot of information from those immediately on hand following the birth on which to base their decisions and to help them come in time to a healthy adaptation following the initial crisis. Too pessimistic or too glib and superficial forecasts may affect attitudes for years to come, causing resentment at insufficient warning or regret at missed opportunities.

Paediatricians who usually make the diagnosis and first discuss the possible outcome with the parents may base their prognosis upon their clinical experience, which is often restricted to the Down's syndrome children whom they see in their out-patient clinics without being aware of the bias towards those with serious health problems, such as congenital heart disease and those whose parents are particularly persistent in seeking medical help. Thus the hospital doctor will have had less experience in dealing with those Down's syndrome cases who are physically well and who are being brought up successfully by their families.

Surveys of children with Down's syndrome and their families are valuable in providing information about the lives of such children in the community, the services they use or need and do not have and the health of the affected children themselves and their immediate relatives. The positive aspects of living with such a handicap become apparent. There are families with problems, some with serious and seemingly intractable difficulties, but the majority of families do well with no serious repercussions on the lives of the other family members, who are often very attached to the handicapped child and derive much pleasure from him, in the same way as other people enjoy sons or daughters or younger siblings.

Cross-sectional studies of whole populations do give a more balanced view of the lives of handicapped children and their families than can be obtained from impressions gained from clinical experience alone. However, although associations may be found between various factors in cross-sectional studies, it is difficult if not impossible to deduce causal relationships. For example, in research on Down's syndrome and other forms of mental retardation, there are many studies linking institutional care with low scores on intelligence tests, as compared with home-based control subjects (Centerwall and Centerwall, 1960; Lyle, 1959, 1960; Stedman and Eichorn, 1964), but longitudinal studies are needed to exclude the possibility that this difference can be explained by the brighter children being kept at home while the more severely handicapped are admitted to hospital. At least two assessments must be made with data collected concerning the children, their families and background social factors, first before or at the time of the child's departure from the home, and then later so that home-reared children can be compared with those initially comparable but who have since been reared away from home, for example, in a long-stay unit.

There are particular problems arising from cross-sectional studies concerning the cognitive development of children with Down's syndrome. The early studies, largely of institutionalized subjects, showed that the majority of patients, nearly two-thirds of the total, scored between 25 and 49 on intelligence tests and a third scored below 25. Only a very small minority, 2–3 per cent, produced intelligence quotients above 50 in the so-called 'educable' range. A frequent finding in the research on the intelligence of patients with Down's syndrome was that higher scores were found in the younger cases in both hospital and community studies. Gibson (1978), reviewing this research suggests that a possible explanation could be that brighter children are more frail and are the first to die. There has been a high mortality in Down's syndrome so the cross-sectional studies are prone to bias by sample depletion. A longitudinal study is required to answer the question: Does the more intelligent child have a tendency to die younger? From those studies which are able to provide the answer, there is no evidence that brighter children do have an increased mortality. The second possible reason why younger children with Down's syndrome have higher scores on intelligence tests is that the finding is the result of an artefact caused by the mode of construction of the tests themselves. Some tests have been modified for use with subjects with specific handicaps but most tests are standardized on samples of children who are essentially normal.

PREVIOUS LONGITUDINAL STUDIES

Evidence has accumulated from a number of prospective studies in which serial testing of the same group of children has been carried out over a number of years to confirm that there is a decline in intelligence quotients achieved with age (Cornwell and Birch, 1969; Dicks-Mireaux, 1972; Carr, 1975). Considering the results reported in these studies and from work of his own, Gibson (1978) concluded that psychological growth in Down's syndrome does not follow a linear pattern but is more likely to develop in stages interspersed by plateaux. Early experience in a well-designed pre-school programme may have some effect in preventing the decline in scores on intelligence testing (Hayden and Haring, 1977).

The study of different age groups of children within the same cross-sectional study is limited by the impossibility of keeping constant certain key variables. Close matching of groups in every aspect except age is rarely possible. In the past twenty years there have been a number of changes in the families of children with Down's syndrome. The comparison of three age groups of children in the same cross-sectional study shows a decline in maternal age with each successive younger group. Similarly, there is a decline in the mean family size. The second finding could be explained by the families not yet being complete in the younger group. However, the trend is a mirror of a change in the general population in which mothers are having smaller families over a shorter period in their reproductive life with a particular decline in the numbers of babies born to the women aged 40 years or older. This change in reproductive pattern has altered the social characteristics of the mothers of Down's syndrome children. The cause of 95 per cent of the chromosome anomaly, trisomy 21, is non-dysjunction, which is the failure of the chromatids to separate during the first or second meiotic division during the formation of the ova, which is more common in older mothers. Such older women could be producing a child after a number of previous births, so there is a bias towards a large family size and lower social class or, less frequently, they are women who have delayed marriage and child bearing for educational and career reasons with a bias towards the upper social classes.

One of the longest, in terms of length of follow-up, and the largest, in terms of sample size, of longitudinal studies of Down's syndrome is that of Oster and van den Tempel (1975). They took as their sample all known cases of Down's syndrome living in one area of Denmark in 1949. Adults and children were include so there was a wide variation in age from birth to 50 years of age. Initially there were 524 cases but, of course, the sample was depleted by death over the twenty-one years of the follow-up. Seventy-three died in the first ten years and a further fifty-six before the final contact in 1971. Most of the deaths occurred in the youngest age group, from birth to 4 years. Over the years there was a decrease in the mortality from infections, due presumably to the increased use and efficacy of antibiotics over this period. Also Oster and van den Tempel noted that the difference in mortality between those at home and those in institutions also diminished. By the end of the study, there were many more people with Down's syndrome in the older age groups than had been found twenty-one years before. Initially, just under half (47 per cent) the cases were patients in an institution. This proportion increased to 58 per cent by 1959 and by the end of the follow-up period was 63 per cent, when the last contact was made with the families in 1971. More detailed information was obtained by interviewing twenty-seven families where the child with Down's syndrome had been kept at home and thirty-two families whose child had been admitted to an institution. These intensive interviews took place after the main longitudinal study had been completed and the data collected from them are largely retrospective. The families had been largely unsupported professionally at the start of the study and some of the parents felt that they had been driven to the decision to arrange admission for their child as a last resort having failed to obtain any other form of help. These findings concerning the families are typical of the results of early research on families of retarded children (Holt, 1957; Schonell and Watts, 1957; Tizard and Grad, 1961).

Another large and long follow-up study was of 612 patients with Down's syndrome who had been seen over a period of twenty years in an out-patient clinic for retarded children (Melyn and White, 1973). The findings indicate the wide variation found in Down's syndrome, such as the age of walking unassisted from 7 months to 74 months, and the previously noted point that younger children appeared to have higher intelligence quotients.

Since Oster and van den Tempel began their study, there have been significant changes in attitude towards the mentally retarded and, in many countries, changes in social and educational policy, with a deliberate move, particularly for children, from services centred in the institutions to care in the community with the presumption that the handicapped child will, like the majority of normal children, live with his or her parents and attend a local school on a daily basis. More recent studies which follow the development of children from shortly after birth show that some attempt has been made to support the families so that they are not forced to request institutional care. Carr (1975) followed a group of children with Down's syndrome who were born in 1963 and 1964 and who had been the subjects of a neurological study in their first year by Cowie (1970). Carr saw the children in the original group up to 4 years of age, visiting them at the ages of 1.5 months, 6 months, 10 months, 15 months, 2 years, 3 years and 4 years. Interviews concerning the family and child-rearing practices took place at the same time as the first and last of the visits, at 1.5 months and at 4 years of age. The study is an important one concentrating on the mental development of the children showing that the scores on the developmental tests did decline with increasing age. At this time, there were few sources of help for the families. It was presumed that the children by virtue of the diagnosis would not be eligible for school, but would be sent to a 'training centre', a day-care unit run by the Health Authority rather than by the Education Service. Health visitors called and the families attended paediatric out patients but little effective help was forthcoming. At 4 years, nine children were not living with their families but had been boarded out since birth. Carr was able to compare the progress of these nine with that of the children reared in their own homes, finding that developmental scores were similar at the first two visits, at 1.5 and 6 months but thereafter the boarded-out group diverged from the home-reared children and were 'consistently and significantly below' those reared by their families. After four years, forty-five children were still in the study, thirty-nine at home and six boarded out.

The children in Carr's study have been seen again at the age of 11 years (Carr and Hewett, 1982). Of the original forty-five, thirty-five are still living with their families, one has died and three boys who had been at home when they were 4 years, had, by the age of 11 years, been admitted to a subnormality hospital. Of the six children who had been boarded out since birth, three were in children's homes, two in long-term foster homes and the last went to a boarding school, returning each holiday to the foster mother who had cared for him all his life. Comparing Carr's study with the previous longitudinal studies, there is clear evidence of a change in attitude to give the handicapped child without a family and home of his own the same sort of alternatives that are given to normal children, rather than the previous automatic admission to an institution. The decline in scores on intelligence tests had continued but was not as marked as in the first four years. The difference between the home-reared and the boarded-out groups had disappeared except on language testing using the Reynell Language scales, which showed that the boarded-out group were particularly behind in expressive language. Some preliminary data are available from postal questionnaires sent to the same children at 16 years of age. The overall impression is an encouraging one, although two more boys are in a subnormality hospital but return home each weekend, another boy has moved from home to a children's home and one girl has died. Most of the children had good health, could occupy themselves on their own initiative and were capable of helping with housework. Eighty-eight per cent were continent day and night and two-thirds could look after their own physical needs adequately. Some had surprising skills, for example in carpentry and several enjoyed taking part in dancing and sport. The families had managed to cope with rearing a handicapped child and many had derived joy from doing so.

THE PRESENT STUDY

The prospective study to be discussed in this chapter was begun in 1970. All children with Down's syndrome born in one administrative region of the National Health Service between 1 January 1970 and the 31 December 1971 were eligible for inclusion. Forty children in whom the diagnosis was established were born in that period. Four babies died shortly after birth before they could be enrolled in the study, two of congenital heart disease, one of congenital leukaemia and one of duodenal atresia. Four children were not taken away from the hospital where they were born by their parents, three of them were taken into local authority care and eventually fostered and one was admitted to the children's ward of a subnormality hospital. One baby was born to a private patient who also did not take the child home. It is known that this baby was cared for by a charitable organization but no further details were available. Thirty-one children with Down's syndrome fulfilled the main criterion for inclusion in the study of living at home as part of the family. One family refused to take part because they had conscientious objections to being interviewed and to completing questionnaires, even the National Census form.

A control group of normal babies was found by matching each Down's syndrome child. The control child was selected as being the child born on the same day, or as near as possible to that date, who was the same sex; the same ordinal position in the family; from the same socio-economic group; had a similar home neighbourhood, rural urban or small town, and, as far as possible, with a mother of the same age.

These two groups of thirty families were visited six times over a period of two years. Data were collected on the babies themselves and on the other members of the family, with special emphasis on mental and physical health and on interpersonal relationships. Unlike Carr's study, no systematic investigation of the development of the children was attempted because it was considered that detailed and repeated examinations of the children, which could emphasize the degree of handicap, would interfere with the data being collected on the emotional impact of a handicapped child upon the family, which was the main aim of the study. The children were all examined physically near the start of the study at the second interview. Evidence of congenital heart disease was found in 14 (47 per cent) of which three were seriously incapacitated, becoming dyspnoic and cyanotic, particularly during feeds. The other common finding was of abnormality of muscle tone, six had mild hypotonia, thirteen moderate hypotonia and six a severe degree of loss of muscle tone. At subsequent visits to the family, the developmental milestones were noted. Although some of the babies with Down's syndrome were not significantly behind the normal controls in the first year, the gap between them grew in the second year. No Down's syndrome child could walk before the age of 20 months. Speech too, although showing a wide variation in the rate of development also clearly lagged behind that of normal babies of the same age. An assessment of the quality of the marital relationship between the parents was carried out about eighteen months after the birth of the baby and used the method devised by Brown, Rutter and their colleagues, (Brown and Rutter, 1966; Quinton et al., 1976). All interviews throughout the study were recorded on tape with the exception of one family of a Down's child who requested that the tape recorder was not used. Nine marriages were rated as poor in the Down's syndrome families but none of the marriages of parents of normal babies (Gath, 1978).

THE NINE-YEAR FOLLOW-UP

The families were visited again in 1979 when the children were aged from 7.5 to 9 years. Once more the families were interviewed in their homes and the child was also seen by a clinical psychologist. Data were collected concerning the family health, the present state of the siblings and the marital relationship with a repeat of the marital interview referred to above. By now all the children were in school and each school was visited, the child being seen in the school setting with the teacher who was asked to complete rating scales concerning behaviour and adaptive behaviour. Three main outcome measures concerning the child were the intelligence quotient as assessed by the psychologist, the score on the American Association on Mental Deficiency Adaptive Behaviour Scale and the overall judgement from data from home and school on the presence of significant behaviour or emotional disorder. Outcome measures of the family functioning included the quality of the parent's marital relationship, the parents' physical and mental health and the health and general adjustment of the siblings.

Table 9.1 shows the deaths which occurred in the original forty who were identified in the region over the two-year period. Four had died before enrolment and six were not enrolled in the study, leaving thirty who were seen during the first two years, but five of the children who had taken part had died before the end of the initial period of study in 1973. Two children died within the next five years. Nine years after the start of the prospective study, twenty-three children with Down's syndrome were traced and reinterviewed, including one who had gone with his family to New Zealand. A large cross-sectional survey of children with Down's syndrome which was carried out at the same time as the follow-up of the prospective study group showed that two of the children taken into local authority care were still in the same area and in foster care, the little girl in the family who had declined to take part was found to be alive and well in one of the special schools visited, leaving two untraced of the original

Table 9.1   Forty children with Down's syndrome born in one region from 1 January 1970 to 31 December 1971. Deaths before January 1979

Died in first two months of life before enrolment	4
Congenital heart disease 2	
Congenital leukaemia 1	
Duodenal atresia 1	
Died during first two years of life in course of first study	5
Congenital heart disease 4	
Acute leukaemia 1	
Died after original study completed, before follow-up	2
Bronchopneumonia 1	
Meningococcal meningitis 1	
Total deaths	11
Enrolled in study, families and children seen in 1979	22
Emigrated to New Zealand; taped interview only	1
Not enrolled in study, known to be alive and well	3
Not enrolled in study, not traced in 1979	3
Total	40

forty Down's syndrome children born in the region in the two-year period (Table 9.1). Congenital heart disease was the most common cause of death. Leukaemia killed two children, one in the neonatal period and one aged 3 years. Most of the deaths occurred early in the first year of life. Twenty-six (65 per cent) of the forty babies born with Down's syndrome in a two-year period were thus known to be alive when the follow-up visits were done, nine years after the start of the study.

Of the thirty children enrolled in the prospective study, twenty-three (77 per cent) were followed up in the latest interviews. Only two children seen in 1979 had health problems giving rise to serious concern. One of these, a boy with a ventricular septal defect, had had a systolic murmur with palpable thrill when first examined and had been to The Hospital for Sick Children, Great Ormond Street, as an out patient, when he was 1 year old, and under the care of the cardiologists since. The other child had appeared robust in early childhood, no murmur having been heard until age 5 years.

Death is clearly an obvious outcome variable. This study confirms the findings of Oster and van den Tempel that the first four years have a higher mortality than age 4–9-years age range. Three of those thirty whose parents had been interviewed died between the ages of 3 months and 1 year so that seven (14 per cent) had died in the first year, if those who died before they were able to be taken home to be part of a family are included. Two more died in the third year and the other two at 4 years and 6 years of age. The accuracy of any prediction as to which infant is likely to die in childhood may be judged from these data which are only available for those children whose parents took part in the study, that is for the thirty of whom seven died before the second follow-up.

PREDICTIVE FACTORS

Birth weight was not a good predictor of death in infancy as four children with a birth weight over 6 pounds died, and nor was the clinical condition at birth (Table 9.2). The muscle tone as found at the clinical examination at the second interview does appear a better predictor since only one child of the eleven judged to have normal tone or only a mild degree of hypotonia died. He was the boy who developed acute lymphoblastic leukaemia at the time of his third birthday, dying within 3 weeks of the diagnosis. Previously, he had been one of the most healthy and advanced in both motor and cognitive development of the group. Fourteen children (47 per cent) were found to have a heart murmur at the clinical examination and four of the deaths occurred in this group. Two babies were particularly difficult to feed in the first six months because of cyanotic attacks and dyspnoea. One died at 7 months, the other was alive and showing minimal disability from her heart condition at 8 years. Another girl was examined in the course of the study, by her general practitioner and by a paediatrician during the first two years and no signs of heart disease found. She, at 8 years, is suffering severely from the heart condition first noted at 4 years of age and her parents have been told that her expectation of life is now poor. Two more babies were admitted more than six times in the first year of life with respiratory infections and problems with breathing and again, one had died just before his first birthday and the other is alive and with no symptoms. Thus, after the babies with Down's syndrome have survived long enough to leave the hospital to go home to their parents it is extremely difficult to tell which child will survive early childhood and which will not.

Twenty-three children thus survived and were traced at the follow-up nine years after the beginning of the longitudinal study. One child had gone with his parents to New Zealand where the family was seen and an interview recorded

Table 9.2 Clinical condition at birth and survival to 8 years

	Good	Moderate	Poor	
Special Care	None	Less than 1 month	More than 1 month	
Alive at 8 years	4	14	5	23
Died before 8 years	1	4	2	7
Total	5	18	7	30

$\chi^2 = 0.1508$, df = 2, NS.

on tape. The teacher was able to complete some of the questionnaires but it was not possible to arrange for the child to be seen by a psychologist or to obtain any results from psychological testing done by the educational services. The families of the remainder were all interviewed at home. Three children spent a large proportion of their lives away from the parental home. One boy was fostered during the school week and for some weekends by a teacher at his special school. Another boy was at a hostel for mentally handicapped children run by the local authority, attending a school near the hostel and returning home for weekends and holidays. The parents of both these boys had been young, in their early twenties, at the birth of their handicapped children and had severe marital problems in the first two years. Although the marriages had not broken down in the interceding years, they still had many difficulties which were compounded by unemployment. A third boy had behaviour difficulties at home. Although no such problem was seen at the special school he attended locally, he was sent to a boarding school to relieve the situation at home.

COGNITIVE DEVELOPMENT

The children were tested at school, using either the Merrill Palmer or Stanford Binet tests of intelligence and, where appropriate, the Reynell Language Scales. All the children were assessed by the same clinical psychologist. The parents and the class teacher both completed the American Association on Mental Deficiency Adaptive Behaviour Scales in the 'Public School' version (Nihira et al., 1974; Lambert et al., 1974).

The intelligence quotients were very varied, ranging from below 20 to 79. Two girls scored in the normal range of intelligence with scores above 75. Seven were classified as mildly retarded, with scores between 50 and 74; six were moderately retarded, with scores between 35 and 49; three were severely retarded scoring between 20 and 34 and the remaining two were profoundly retarded with scores below 20. There was no significant difference between the scores of the eight girls and fourteen boys. No relationship was found between the intelligence quotient and maternal age, the clinical condition at birth, ordinal position, social class or the marital relationship, either soon after birth or at follow-up. However, birth weight and muscle tone, as determined at the physical examination at the second interview, were both related to the scores on intelligence tests at the follow-up when the children were aged 8 and 9 years. The heavier children at birth tended to be brighter later in childhood. Children with a moderate or severe degree of hypotonia were likely to be more handicapped at 8 or 9 years of age.

The scores on the Adaptive Behaviour Scale, taking the higher scores of the two completed by parents and class teacher, were found to have similar correlations to those of the scores on intelligence tests (Table 9.3), with a strong relationship to birth weight and a somewhat weaker one to the quality of muscle

Table 9.3   Birth weight and muscle tone in infancy related to outcome
measures of IQ and adaptive behaviour score

| Factors found in infancy 1970/1971 | Outcome measures at follow-up in 1979 | |
	IQ	Adaptive behaviour
Birth weight	r = 0.56	r = 0.57
	p < 0.01	p < 0.01
Quality of muscle tone	r = 0.50	r = 0.36
	p < 0.05	p < 0.05

Spearman rank-order correlation (Siegel, 1956).

tone. Similarly, the age and parity of the mother at birth and the clinical condition of the child were found to have no significant effect upon the Adaptive Behaviour scores, as determined at 8 or 9 years of age.

The Adaptive Behaviour Scales are a good measure of the degree of handicap. The children with the highest scores were very little different from normal children of the same age in self-help skills, social functioning and ability to communicate. At the other extreme, the lowest scorers were very dependent, requiring help with all toilet functions, feeding and dressing, had poor communication and little play repertoire. The Adaptive Behaviour Scales were related to the scores on the intelligence tests (r = 0.44, p < 0.05) (Figure 9.1). Particularly interesting are those children who did much better on the scales than would be expected from their scores on intelligence tests. One such child had been fostered with his teacher while his mother did her training for state enrolment as a nurse. Two children who did poorly on the Adaptive Behaviour Scales, having much lower scores than might be expected from their scores on intelligence tests, had both got congenital heart disease and suffered symptoms

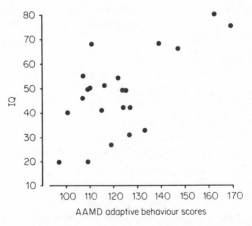

Fig. 9.1   Down's syndrome prospective study, IQ versus AAMD

such as dyspnoea and cyanosis. This finding suggests that anxiety about a child's health may prevent a child from functioning practically at a level in keeping with his or her potential.

The quality of the relationship between the parents in the first two years after the birth of their handicapped child bore no relationship to the outcome as measured by intelligence or adaptive behaviour at 8 and 9 years. Nor was the marital relationship at follow-up at 8 and 9 years a factor influencing the achievement of the Down's syndrome child.

EMOTIONAL DEVELOPMENT

It might be thought likely that the emotional atmosphere in the home would be an important influence on the development of emotional or behavioural disorders in the Down's syndrome children. Eleven children were judged as being additionally handicapped by disturbances of behaviour or emotions which could not be explained by the fact of retardation alone. One child had a conduct disorder, one child had a neurotic disorder and one child had a mixed neurotic and conduct disorder. Three children were very active, highly distractable and with very short attention span. Two of these children also had problems in communication and their behaviour was difficult to control particularly by mothers who relied on gentle verbal prompts and correction. Although it could be seen that the parents' usual ways of controlling the child were not very effective in two of the cases, there is no indication from either the data collected when the children were young or from the family interview conducted when the children were 8 and 9 years that bears any relation to the development of the condition characterized by distractability, diminished attention span and hyperactivity. Two children had been found to be hyperactive in the second year of life, (Gath, 1978), one of whom was now regarded as having a behaviour disorder which was specific to one situation, being evident only in the home and not at school, while the other child was found to be a well-socialized little girl with no problems of behaviour or of ability to concentrate on a task either at home or at school.

The child whose problems were only in evidence at home showed behaviour which fitted the criteria for the diagnosis of a conduct disorder and there was ample evidence of family stress in the family interview at the follow-up and some indication of these difficulties in the first two years. One of the other two children had a mixed disturbance of behaviour and emotions which was an understandable reaction to stress, both at home due to a crisis in her parents' marriage and at school where she, although the brightest of this group, was only grudgingly tolerated in the local village school. This child was moved to a more congenial school and her parents managed to solve their own difficulties. The child's misery and aggression abated. A similar adjustment reaction closely related in time to a specific stress was seen in a boy who became withdrawn and mute when he lost the companionship of his younger brother. Recovery occurred after six months. The problems seen in these last three children are similar to those described by Chess (1977), and classified by her as reactive behaviour disorder.

Five more boys had severe problems in communication, accompanied by behavioural problems both at home and at school. With these small numbers, a full clinical picture of each child can be built up. At the same time as the longitudinal study is being carried out, a cross-sectional study of 200 children with Down's syndrome has taken place with attention being specially paid to the incidence of behaviour disorders. Data from this larger study are more amenable to statistical analysis but the small study over a number of years provides richer detail.

MARITAL RELATIONSHIP

An important finding in the study of the first two years following the birth of the children in this study was the greater number of unsatisfactory marriages in the group of parents of Down's syndrome children as compared with control parents with a normal child of the same age. The sample, as has been described, was depleted by death and deaths tended to occur more often in the more unhappy families. When the parents of the survivors were seen again at the follow-up, the marital relationship could be compared again with that found in the control families (Figure 9.2). The changes have not been striking. One separation has happened in the control families but the general tendency has been for the two groups to have more in the moderate group. No further separations have occurred in the Down's group. The initial ill effect on the marriage seems to be a result of the initial emotional trauma but the years of caring for the handicapped child do not seem to be severely detrimental to the relationship between the parents, thus supporting the earlier Oster and van den Tempel findings and the more recent follow-up study by Carr and Hewett (1982).

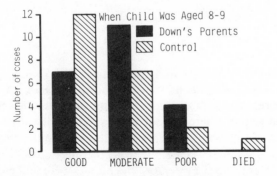

Fig. 9.2   Down's syndrome marriage ratings. ■, Down's parents; □, control

PROFESSIONAL SUPPORT

None of the children in the longitudinal study just described had been enrolled in any specific programme of treatment or early education. All had been to a play group or to the nursery class attached to a special school. Since that time there has been a rapid development of intervention programmes in which parents are taught how to stimulate their handicapped child and how to enhance development in motor, verbal and social spheres (Shearer and Shearer, 1972; Rynders and Horrobin, 1975; Sandow and Clarke, 1978; Cunningham, 1979; Sebba, 1981). A number of longitudinal studies of children who have been enrolled in such programmes are currently being carried out. Not only are the children evaluated at frequent intervals, but in these new studies there are more detailed measures of parent–child interaction and of such variables as the temperament of the child (Berry *et al.*, 1980; Gunn *et al.*, 1981). The effect of such intervention on the later development of children with Down's syndrome has yet to be described. There are major problems, not the least of which being ethical, of conducting comparative studies where one cohort has had some form of intervention programme and another not. There have been some attempts to overcome these difficulties (Connolly, 1978) but in no case is the control group truly comparable. Nevertheless, it appears that children with Down's syndrome are now achieving results on intelligence testing that are higher than those reported earlier as reviewed by Gibson (1978). However, it is still not possible to establish whether this improvement is due to specific intervention programmes, better education provision for the mentally retarded or to the more general improvement in social attitudes to the mentally retarded. Another important question concerns the development of cognitive functioning in Down's syndrome. It will be interesting, and highly relevant to the planning of future services to see if intensive intervention in the early years followed by a suitable education will enable individuals to score mental ages on the tests with evidence of the ability to understand abstract concepts, a level of intellectual functioning which has yet to be described satisfactorily in someone with the Trisomy 21 in all cells.

CONCLUSION

The main value of a follow-up study of this sort is to find some factors that will enable a prediction to be made of the future for the newborn child with a handicap and his family. One such predictor appears to be birth weight, a measure of the general physical well being of the child after the period of interuterine growth. Little can be done to alter or modify the effect of this biological factor. Poor muscle tone may be another measure of the general degree of handicap, as was thought by Penrose and Smith (1966), but early stimulation can improve the tone and power of the children's muscles. Modern child care aids, such as seats which allow babies to look around while at the same time giving maximum support to the back, can to some degree at least compensate for some effects of poor muscle development on cognitive growth. On the other hand, looking at what does not predict later outcome, some of the babies whose health had given risen to much concern in the first year later did very well and, after those early, very anxious months, did not continue to suffer themselves and cause deep distress to their parents. It seems particularly difficult to tell which children would die in the first few years. Although it may be said that very-low-birth-weight babies with Down's syndrome have a greater chance of more severe handicap than more robust babies with the same condition, there is no evidence from this study that the withholding of medical treatment from these babies would ensure that only the brightest and least handicapped would survive. There are compensating factors. Even a child with very low birth weight, much ill health in the neonatal period and severe family difficulties did himself do well when moved to a stimulating environment for part of each week.

The early findings on the marital relationship indicate the extent of the emotional trauma to a couple when an abnormal child is born. However, as the child grows older, there is no evidence that this initial toll of failed marriages will continue relentlessly. Thus the effect on marriages may be considered to be part of the initial grief reaction and not due to the wear and tear of the burden of care. Early support is clearly indicated but removal of the children from the home is not.

Behaviour disorders have already appeared by 8 and 9 years of age. It is the additional handicap of disruptive behaviour accompanying mental retardation that in clinical practice can be seen to produce severe strain on a family, jeopardize the child's place in his family and force admission to a long-stay unit. This longitudinal study must continue to provide some understanding of these disorders before a basis of treatment is developed for those crippling secondary handicaps.

REFERENCES

Berry, P., Gunn, R. and Andrews, R. (1980). Behaviour of Down's syndrome infants in a strange situation, *Am. J. Ment. Defic.* **85**, 213–218.

Brown, G. W. and Rutter, M. (1966). The measurement of family activities and relationships—a methodological study, *Hum. Relat.* **19**, 241–263.

Carr, J. (1975). *Young Children with Down's Syndrome*, Butterworth, London.

Carr, J. and Hewett, S. (1982). Children with Down's syndrome growing up: a preliminary report, *Association for Child Psychology and Psychiatry News*, No. 10.

Centerwall, S. A. and Centerwall, W. R. (1960). A study of children with mongolism reared in the home compared with those reared away from the home, *Pediatrics*, **25**, 678–685.

Chess, S. (1977). Evolution of behaviour disorder in a group of mentally retarded children, *J. Amer. Acad. Child Psychiat.* **16**, 5–13.

Connolly, J. A. (1978). Intelligence levels of Down's syndrome children, *Am. J. Ment. Defic.* **83**, 193–196.

Cornwell, A. C. and Birch, H. G. (1969). Psychosocial and social development in home-reared children with Down's syndrome (mongolism), *Am. J. Ment. Defic.* **77**, 26–32.

Cowie, V. A. (1970). A Study of the early development of mongols, *Inst. Res. Ment. Retard.* Monograph. No. 1. Pergamon, London.

Cunningham, C. C. (1979). Parent counselling in Tredgold's Mental Retardation (Ed. M. Craft), Balliere-Tindale, London.

Dicks-Mireaux, M. J. (1972). Mental development of infants with Down's syndrome, *Am. J. Ment. Defic.* **77**, 26–32.

Gath, A. (1978). *Down's Syndrome and the Family — the Early Years*, Academic Press, London.

Gibson, D. (1978). *Down's Syndrome: The Psychology of Mongolism*, Cambridge University Press, Cambridge.

Gunn, P., Berry, P. and Andrews, R. (1981). The affective response of Down's syndrome infants to a repeated event, *Child Development*, **52**, 745–748.

Hayden, A. H. and Haring, N. G. (1977). The acceleration and maintenance of developmental gains in Down's syndrome school-age children, in *Research to Practice in Mental Retardation*, Vol. 1. *Care and Intervention* (Ed. P. Mittler), University Park Press, Baltimore.

Holt, K. S. (1957). The impact of mentally retarded children on their families, MD Thesis, University of Manchester.

Lambert, N., Windmiller, M. and Cole, L. (1974). A.A.M.D. Adaptive Behaviour Scale. Public School Version, *American Association on Mental Deficiency*, Washington, DC.

Lyle, J. G. (1959). The effects of an institution on the verbal development of imbecile children. I. Verbal intelligence, *J. Ment. Defic. Res.* **3**, 122–128.

Lyle, J. G. (1960). The effects of an institution on the verbal development of imbecile children. II. Speech and language, *J. Ment. Defic. Res.* **4**, 1–13.

Melyn, M. A. and White, D. T. (1973). Mental and developmental milestones of noninstitutionalised Down's syndrome children, *Pediatrics*, **52**, 542–545.

Nihira, K., Foster, R., Shellhaas, M. and Leland, H. (1974). *A.A.M.D. Adaptive Behaviour Scale 1974 Revision*, American Association on Mental Deficiency, Washington, DC.

Oster, J. and van den Tempel, A. (1975). A 21-year psycho-social follow-up of 524 unselected cases of Down's syndrome and their families, *Acta Paediatr. Scand.* **64**, 505–513.

Penrose, L. S. and Smith, G. F. (1966). *Down's Anomoly*, Churchill, London.

Quinton, D., Rutter, M. and Rowlands, O. (1976). An evaluation of an interview assessment of marriage, *Psych. Med.* **6**, 577–586.

Rynders, J. E. and Horrobin, J. M. (1975). Project EDGE: the University of Minnesota's Communication Stimulation Program for Down's syndrome infants, in *Exceptional Infant* 3: *Assessment and Intervention* (Ed. B. Z. Friedlander), Brunner-Mazel, New York.

Sandow, S. and Clarke, A. D. B. (1978). Home intervention with parents of severely subnormal, pre-school children: an interim report, *Child: Care, Health and Development*, **4**, 29–39.

Schonell, F. J. and Watts, B. H. (1957). A first survey on the effects of a subnormal child on the family unit, *Am. J. Ment. Defic.* **61**, 210–219.

Sebba, J. (1981). Intervention for profoundly retarded multiply handicapped children through parent training in a preschool setting and at home, in *Frontiers of Knowledge* in Mental Retardation, Vol. 1. *Social, Educational and Behavioural Aspects* (Ed. P. Mittler), University Park Press, Baltimore.

Shearer, M. S. and Shearer, D. E. (1972). The Portage Project: a model for early childhood education, *Except. Child.* **38**, 210–217.

Siegel, S. (1956). *Nonparametric Statistics for the Behavioural Sciences*, McGraw-Hill, New York.

Stedman, D. J. and Eichorn, D. H. (1964). A comparison of the growth and development of institutionalised and home-reared mongoloids during infancy and childhood, *Am. J. Ment. Defic.* **69**, 391–401.

Tizard, J. and Grad, J. C. (1961). *The Mentally Handicapped and Their Families*, Maudsley Monogrpah, 7, London.

Section IV

Long-term Studies which ask Broader Questions

Longitudinal Studies in Child Psychology and Psychiatry
Edited by A. R. Nicol
© 1985 John Wiley and Sons Ltd.

Chapter 10

Becoming Deprived:
A Cross-Generation Study based on the
Newcastle upon Tyne 1000-Family Survey

F. J. W. Miller, I. Kolvin and H. Fells

This chapter describes the way in which data collected during a longitudinal study of the health of children from 1947 to 1962 has been used from 1979–1981 as the basis of a study of the transmission of deprivation. The design is that of the catch-up longitudinal type (Robins, 1980). The time range of the study is therefore some 35 years covering the birth and childhood, and then the adult and family life, of children born into 847 families living in Newcastle upon Tyne in May and June 1947, and still resident there five years later.

However, this chapter only concerns itself with data from the first nineteen years of the survey. It falls into two parts. First, an account of the origin, purpose and organization of the longitudinal study and the nature of the data obtained and, second, findings concerning the differences between families who moved into deprivation and those did not during a period of economic expansion. In this way it complements the US work (Elder, 1974) which focuses on families catapulted into straightened economic circumstances during the great depression.

ORIGINS OF THE SURVEY

The roots of the Newcastle 1000-Family Study go back to the early 1930s and from them has developed a tradition of local research in child health which has been sustained for fifty years and is characterized by accepting that the origins of health or ill-health are to be found in daily life in home and community rather than in hospital or clinic, and that understanding of those origins is the path to effective prevention or treatment.

Professor J. C. Spence (1933), one of the pioneers of social paediatrics in the UK, had already addressed himself to the study of poverty, sickness and malnutrition in the poorer classes in the city of Newcastle. This early work highlighted the importance of the interaction between malnutrition and infective disease against a background of adverse social conditions, improper and inadequate diet.

In the winter of 1938 Spence's study was repeated with substantially the same results (Brewis *et al.*, 1940). The next 'field' study in 1939 concerned deaths in the first year of life and revealed both the importance of prematurity and infection and the contemporary ignorance of these conditions (Spence and Miller, 1941). Then in 1942 the Nuffield Foundation helped to establish the first whole-time University Chair of Child Health in the country. Spence was appointed but field studies could not be resumed until after 1945 when the question of acute infections in infancy was again taken up.

THE 1000-FAMILY PROSPECTIVE STUDY

Purposes and objectives

The primary question which determined the basic planning of this study followed the 1939 investigation into infant deaths. It was: What is the incidence and what are the types of infective illnesses in children in the first year of life in Newcastle upon Tyne?

If that question could be answered knowledge which would help medical practitioners, doctors and others working in public health, students and their teachers would become available.

Although the survey was designed for one year only, it continued for a second; then until the children were 5 years old and, finally, until most left school aged 15 years. During those fifteen years the purpose of the work changed from a record of illnesses to one of physical growth and social and educational performance and, finally, of entrance to employment or scholastic career. The results were published in three reports between 1954 and 1974, and the final hope was that 'this account of our experience over these 15 years will help readers to understand the interdependence of physical growth, personal development, family function and social environment in determining the character of health and disease in childhood' (Miller *et al.*, 1974).

Organization and methodology

The survey was designed to obtain facts by making an intimate and continuous study of an adequate and representative sample of families in the city. This could be done only through participant observation and the development of a friendly, trusting and lasting relationship with both the families and their general practitioners.

To quote from the introduction to the first report 'surveys and enquiries which make an intrusion into family life demand a justification beyond the mere satisfaction of curiosity. For, indeed, they can be justified only if they are designed to answer questions which are worth answering, which have not been answered before and which cannot be answered in any other way' (Spence *et al.*, 1954). Great care was therefore taken to explain the purpose of the study both to the families, to their doctors and always to remain sensitive to the privilege of access to the homes and scrupulous to avoid anything which might mar the relationship between a family and the family doctor.

The work planned was possible only because a tradition of local study and co-operation already existed between the Medical College and the City Health Committee and a research team could be formed from the existing staffs of the University Department of Child Health and the Maternal and Child Welfare Section of the City Health Department.

The cohort

The cohort to be observed was required to fulfil three conditions.

1 Be a representative sample of the infant population of the city.
2 Be enrolled at birth and as nearly as possible the same age.
3 Be large enough to establish the incidence of all the common types of infective diseases yet of a size which could be visited regularly by a small team of observers.

It was estimated that the size of the cohort required would need to be about 1000 infants and that in the first year each family should have at least eight routine visits at a 6–7 week interval. Provision was also made for 'special request visits'.

About 6000–7000 births were expected in Newcastle during 1947. Therefore one-sixth of that total was chosen. In order that travelling and visiting could be done under the best conditions during a time when each health visitor would be required to meet more than 200 new families, the months of May and June were selected.

This method was known to have some epidemiological disadvantages, but it was necessary to accept what was practical and possible. Enrolment therefore began on 1 May and, by 30 June 1142 infants from 1132 families formed the study group. During the first year only 4 families 'contracted out' and, after removals and deaths, 967 families remained. That number fell by removal from the city to 847 and 750 families at the end of the fifth and fifteenth years.

The observers

Five health visitors (community nurses) were seconded full-time to the survey. They provided to their families the same care and advice as in their usual work and made their usual reports to the Child Welfare Department. The medical staff came from the University Department of Child Health and the health visitors and secretaries from the City Health Department. Everyone helped in the original planning of the study and in its development as the objectives changed and throughout the years worked as a team relying on and understanding each other's rôles and contributions. The secretarial staff was central to all the work of organization and the smooth conduct of the survey, for upon them depended all communications and the maintenance of records.

Visiting and records

Detailed planning began in 1946. The team met regularly and initial records were designed and tested. Since the record was to begin at birth, help was sought from city midwives (50 per cent of infants were expected to be born at home), the matrons of private nursing homes, and the paediatric staffs of the two large maternity hospitals. Contact was made with the health visitors working in the city and also the medical staffs of the children's hospitals. Arrangements were made for the team to be notified when a child from the cohort was admitted to hospital. The survey would not have been possible without the support and acquiescence of the family doctors and they were approached in various ways. The Newcastle branch of the British Medical Association called a meeting of practitioners to explain the origin and purpose of the survey and to ask for help. Immediately afterwards a letter was sent to every family doctor in the city and, after the survey began, two medical members of the team visited doctors in several parts of the town. Initially agreement was sought before a medical member visited a family but soon that became unnecessary.

The identification of the survey families was important and each was supplied with a 'membership' card to show to the family doctor or at the hospital or clinic; they were also given stamped addressed postcards which they could complete by adding their name and address. One of these, dropped in a letter-box, would bring a visit from a member of the team. Soon, however, they were encouraged to report illnesses by telephone or personal calls at the Child Health Department.

It was also necessary to identify correspondence and notes and, after the first few days, a small red 'legal' seal was affixed to each document. This distinctive mark became widely known and soon the children themselves were known as 'Red Spot' babies, a name, a generation later, still warmly remembered by many.

As the work of the first five years proceeded the complexities and uncertainties of family life and the slowness of understanding these stresses became evident. Increasingly the importance of patience as well as observation was appreciated. During those five years, although many of the families were badly housed, the majority enjoyed material standards better than those of twenty years earlier. While there was considerable regard for the health and welfare of children, only too often one or more of the essentials to establish a stable and happy home were missing.

The task of devising a measurement of a family's failure to reach a reasonable standard for the time and place was essential and this is well expressed in the following: 'a satisfactory family is one founded on the marriage of physically and mentally stable parents who live in a harmonious and satisfying relationship with each other and provide a home where the children can find affection, security and responsible care' (Miller *et al.*, 1960). Ultimately the measures used indicated defects or shortfalls from these standards but as far as possible were based on facts and not opinion.

The school years 1952–1962

The five years 1947–1952 were a time of great social change as the country recovered from six years of war and the important early post-war legislation, particularly in relation to health and education, became operative (National Health Service Act, 1946 and the Education Act, 1944). New houses were built, wages increased and living standards, in general, improved. At the same time significant advances, particularly in the treatment of bacterial infections, reduced both morbidity and mortality.

Newcastle shared in these changes as the collection of data proceeded. In 1952 the 847 children remaining in the study began school and until they were age 7 years routine and emergency visiting continued. However, by the end of the sixth year, a change was apparent. Routine visiting was becoming more difficult as more mothers worked outside the home, and it was also evident that the incidence of infective illness was declining and its nature altering. Furthermore, the interests and concerns of parents were also changing. Worry about health was, in most families, beginning to give way to concern about development and, particularly, school or social performance. This increased as the children became older. At this stage the technique of visiting changed. After the children went to school considerable help was given by the Newcastle Education Committee and the individual teachers who had 'Red Spot' children in their classes agreed to notify the survey team whenever a child was absent for more than two days. This brought a special visit to the home.

After the seventh year, therefore, the method of data collection changed. The health-visitor team was reduced from five to one and henceforward each family had only one routine annual visit. But request visits from either doctor or health visitor continued as did visits when children were notified absent from school. The survey team continued to receive or seek notes of hospital attendances or admissions and, later, of school medical records. The routine visit, made by arrangement, was also made the occasion to seek answers to particular questions, e.g. stuttering, enuresis, age of menarche, etc.

Throughout these years there was increasing interest in the concept of 'performance' which, indeed, formed the central theme of the third volume (Miller *et al.*, 1974). Thus, particular studies were mounted in respect of respiratory diseases, of disturbed behaviour, of attitudes to school and attainments therein, weekend work or leisure activities, and of secondary education and the children's hopes and ambitions for the future. Physical growth in height and weight was checked regularly and recorded.

Finally, in 1966 four years after the collection of other systematic data had ceased, data was obtained on the entry of boys to employment and the results of continued education in those who had stayed at school. All these studies could be related to other data and provided facets of 'performance' as described in the third volume (Miller *et al.*, 1974) and all records and data were carefully preserved against the day when they might again be used.

FAMILY SHORTCOMINGS

By 1952, when the children were 5 years of age, the survey team isolated a series of factors which would be simple for students to observe and which would serve as markers or indices of family dysfunction and, therefore, of deprivation, for both the family as a unit and for each child or member. These factors form the basis of the present study. A synopsis of these early reports and the data relating to the school years were presented by Miller *et al.* (1974).

When the 'Red Spot' children were 5 years of age, six main areas of deprivation were delineated. The first five of the six are identifiable at a later point in the life cycle, i.e. when the 'Red Spots' were 10 years of age. The six criteria, their frequencies and subsections are:

A. Family/Marital Disruption (i) Divorce/separation   14.5 per cent
                               (ii) Marital instability
B. Parental illness — Parent incapacitated by illness   12.2 per cent
C. Defective Care of the Child (i)   Personal cleanliness 12.6 per cent
                                 (ii) Domestic cleanliness
                                 (iii) Poor clothing
D. Social Dependence of the Family (i)   Debt   17.5 per cent
                                     (ii) Unemployment
                                     (iii) National Assistance
E. Housing — Overcrowding   18.7 per cent
F. Poor Maternal Capacity (Coping)   15.2 per cent

Each family was given a score of 0 or 1 on each of the above criteria and their scores were added to give a total score of the deprivation. Some families did not show any of the criteria of deprivation while others embraced all six. Conditions in 43 per cent of families fulfilled at least one criterion and 14 per cent at least three criteria. The greater the number of criteria exhibited by a family the greater the degree of deprivation.

All the children with evidence of 'deprivation' at the age of 5 years were identified by their records. Of the 847 families 482 scored 0 (57 per cent), i.e. had no criteria of disadvantage; 365 scored 1 or more (43 per cent); and 116 scored 3 or more (14 per cent).

Further accounts of the method and preliminary findings of the research into deprivation are given elsewhere (Kolvin *et al.*, 1983a,b).

AIMS AND HYPOTHESES

There is a vast literature on deprivation and its consequences, but relatively little about families who were previously reasonably advantaged and then suddenly move into deprivation. In this part of the paper we concern ourselves with three sets of hypotheses in relation to such downward mobility.

1   Ability to identify the factors which precede movement into deprivation. It is hypothesized that these will be primarily social and family circumstances. The presence of such factors may contribute to the vulnerability of such families and therefore are likely to have been present for some time prior to this movement and should be identified over the first five years of the children's lives.
2   In addition to such predictive factors it will be possible to identify other social and family factors associated with deterioration in the status of a family from one of non-deprivation to one of deprivation.
3   Deterioration in family status will be associated with poorer behavioural, cognitive and educational functioning of the children in these families as compared to those who remained without disadvantage.

METHOD

The study group comprises that 10 per cent of 477 families who had been in the 'Red Spot' survey since 1947 and showed no evidence of deprivation in 1952 but displayed such evidence in 1957 when the children were 10 years of age. The sample sizes vary from analysis to analysis but, provided the differences are no more than 1 per cent, we do not comment on such variations.

By the fifteenth year only 423 families remained available for study (an attrition of 11 per cent). Again, we do not comment on variations in sample size from analysis to analysis unless the differences are greater than 1 per cent.

RESULTS

Some data relevant to our hypotheses are presented in Tables 10.1–10.6.

Risk factors

This is an attempt to highlight factors which are predicative of those families who move into disadvantage, that is, while not being rated as deprived when their children were 5 years, were so rated when their children were 10 years. Some hints were available from data gathered during the first year of their children's lives. However, on only a small number of variables were there significant differences although a relatively large pool of variables was studied. Furthermore, none of the differences identified proved substantial (using one-tailed tests, at the first year none of the differences extended beyond the 5 per cent level). Thus, the early data did not provide any major clues as to which families were likely to deteriorate ten years later. The clues obtained related only to social influences such as poor occupational status, a larger family size and families not living in owner-occupier situations (Table 10.1). By the time the children were 5 years old a greater number of risk factors were identifiable (Table 10.2). Again, they were usually social in nature or tended to reflect poor social circumstances. For instance, they primarily related to large family size, poor

Table 10.1 First-year data: Some risk factors

	Not deprived at any time (%) ($n = 430$)	Moving into deprivation 1952–1957 (%) ($n = 46$)	Significance
Social class I + II	16	4	
III	62	60	
IV + V etc.	22	36	$p < 0.05$
House—owner-occupier	19	5	$p < 0.05$
Mean total persons in household	4.5	5.1	$p < 0.05$

Table 10.2 Fifth-year data: Some risk factors

	Not deprived at any time	Moving into deprivation 1952–1957	Significance
Total persons in household (mean)	4.4	4.9	$p < 0.01$
Number of subsequent children (mean)	0.42	0.71	$p < 0.01$
Family size (mean)	2.2	2.8	$p < 0.001$
Poor sleeping arrangements	< 1%	7%	$p < 0.01$
House—owner-occupier*	19%	2%	$p < 0.05$
Mean number of respiratory infections	0.67	1.07	$p < 0.02$
Poor speech at 5 years	9%	30%	$p < 0.001$
Maximum n	430	46	

*Attrition varies from maximum n by 5–10 per cent.

home circumstances (inadequate sleeping arrangements) but also there was an excess of respiratory infections and poor development of speech as compared to the group that remained free of family deprivation.

Defining the differences between groups

Comparison of the groups at the tenth year revealed that disadvantage was compounded of two main circumstances (Table 10.3). First, despite the fact that this was an era of generally improving social and economic circumstances, these families remained static or deteriorated in these respects. Second, there was absence or loss of father.

Table 10.3   Tenth-year: Social data

	Not deprived at any time (%)	Moving into deprivation 1952–1957 (%)	Significance
Loss of father	2	17	$p < 0.01$
Unemployment	0	45	$p < 0.01$
Defective sleeping arrangements	< 0.1	8	$p < 0.01$
Good housing	26	6	$p < 0.05$
Mean total persons in household	4.4	5.2	$p < 0.001$

Subsequent progress of the families

Table 10.4 shows the social and family data at the fifteenth year, that is, five years after the period when a decision was made that the families had deteriorated. The picture had now become much clearer. For instance, a striking feature was the central importance of the father or father substitute: he was frequently absent, often had a job of poor status and was often poorly aspirant in his chosen career. This was compounded by an excess of problems of unemployment, of father being an inadequate provider, participating poorly in domestic tasks, being a poor organizer and was recorded as having a difficult or complex personality. Further, the loss or mere absence of the father is not only a key factor in its own right, but complicates many of the other analyses that relate to the father figure. For instance, in relation to the personality of the father, we had no information on about 30 per cent of the fathers of the families that moved into deprivation but only 10 per cent of the group where there was no deprivation. This meant that there was likely to be an under-representation of fathers with difficult or complex personalities in the former group simply because they were absent. It also meant that both the number of persons in the family and the rate of overcrowding was also under-represented.

Table 10.4 Fifteenth year: Social and family data

	Not deprived at any time	Moved into deprivation 1952–1957	Significance
Father			
Permanently present	85%	66%	$p < 0.01$
Substitute in home	5%	23%	$p < 0.01$
Personality—good	79%*	61%*	$p < 0.01$
Aspirant job status			
(success and promotion)	39%	16%*	$p < 0.01$
More than 6 months			
unemployed in 5 years	5%	20%*	$p < 0.01$
Inadequate provider	8%	34%*	$p < 0.01$
Poorly participates in domestic tasks	7%	21%*	$p < 0.01$
Poor organizer	9%	29%*	$p < 0.01$
Mother			
Poor standard of housekeeping	2%	16%	$p < 0.01$
Poor child/general care	3%	14%	$p < 0.01$
Good premarital employment history	28%	7%	$p < 0.05$
Psychiatric illness	11%	23%	$p < 0.05$
Family			
Activities which include child	70%	44%	$p < 0.01$
Social factors			
Overcrowding	3%	14%	$p < 0.01$
Mean number of persons in home	4.4	5.1	$p < 0.01$
Mean number of younger sibs	0.8	1.3	$p < 0.01$
Housing			
Owner-occupier/Private	29%	5%	$p < 0.01$
Maximum size sample	375	44	

Note: Attrition may vary from maximum *n*.
 Personality of father is based on 336 and 31 families respectively.
*6 per cent or more.

A smaller number of factors related to the mother; particularly poor housekeeping, poorer child and family care, and a higher rate of psychiatric illness. The third series of factors related to housing—those families who moved into deprivation tended to live in houses with a low rateable value, yet they had greater family size, so that there was a larger total number of people in the home and, therefore, they were more overcrowded.

Outcome—intellectual, educational and behavioural

If we look at Table 10.5, which relates to school reports about behaviour and achievement and formal cognitive assessment, we note that although the children of families who moved into deprivation always did worse than those who did not, formal tests seldom gave rise to significant differences from the children

Table 10.5   Last year in primary school (approximately 11 years of age): intellectual, educational and behavioural

	Not deprived at any time	Moved into deprivation 1952–1957	Significance
A. *Cognition*			
Mean IQ (11+ examination)	104.4	103.3	NS
Mean arithmetic	107.6	104.6	NS
English	105.8	103.7	NS
Maximum *n*	367	45	
B. *Achievements* (Teacher reports)			
Reading good	42%	29%	$p < 0.01$
poor	16%	33%	
Craft ability poor*	12%	28%	$p < 0.05$
Maximum *n*	314	42	
C. *Classroom behaviour*			
Good initiative	26%	12%	$p < 0.01$
Good reliability	72%	45%	$p < 0.01$
Poor concentration	20%	40%	$p < 0.01$
Poor persistence	21%	38%	$p < 0.05$
Maximum *n*	316	42	
D. *Other features*			
Never visited the country	6%	23%	$p < 0.05$
Does not read library books	57%	73%	$p < 0.05$
Maximum *n*	361	44	

Note: Data based on *n*.
*Less than 95 per cent at maximum *n*.

from families who were not deprived. The differences that did occur were mainly in relation to poor achievements at reading, craft and general achievements as reported by teachers. Children in the downward mobility group read less in the way of books coming from libraries, were judged to be less persistent in the classroom and had poorer adjustment to new schools. Concentration in class was also poorer and they were generally considered to be less reliable students.

Table 10.6 shows additional information deriving from school. There is a higher rate of poor school attendance. It is also to be noted that teachers thought that those children in families who had moved into deprivation were more likely to become maladjusted and to be more eager to leave school than those from families who did not become deprived. Further, three times more children in families who had not moved into deprivation aspired to skilled employment as compared to those whose families had become deprived.

Finally, there remained the possibility that we are not picking up differences because we had not studied males and females separately. These analyses have

Table 10.6   Outcome of secondary school/early employment: behavioural and cognitive data

	Based on n of	Not deprived	Moved into depri-vation	Significance
A. Behaviour				
School attendance last year less than 90%	360/39	20%	46%	$p<0.01$
Children considered at age 12 years likely to become delinquent or maladjusted (by teachers)	374/43	13%	26%	$p<0.05$
Eager to leave school	304/38	24%	42%	$p<0.05$
Aspiring to skilled employment of those who left school at 15 years	191/29	32%	11%	$p<0.05$
Rated by teachers in top 30				
Good manual dexterity	255/33	35%	14%	$p<0.01$
Good maths test	298/38	31%	14%	$p<0.01$
B. Cognition achievements				
Vocabulary mean	257/38	42.8	39.8	$p<0.02$
Matrices mean	257/38	46.2	43.2	$p<0.02$

been undertaken, but susprisingly, there were few significant differences — no more than would have occurred by chance, and they have been ignored. However, these negative findings are consistent with similar sex specific analyses previously reported in relation to those families who had been disadvantaged and then improved as compared to those who did not (Kolvin et al., 1983b).

DISCUSSION

Much of earlier research has pointed to the importance of the effects of adverse experiences occurring during the preschool years. Subsequent research has pointed to the notion that children remain vulnerable to adverse influences throughout their childhood (Rutter, 1981). This current research afforded an opportunity to study the effects on cognition and behaviour of social and family discontinuities. It was, therefore, possible to study the effects of adverse experiences which impinge on functioning and which reflect maturation at different stages of development. In addition it was possible to ascertain whether the effects were relatively transient, that is occurring prior to adolescence; or more permanent, that is occurring across adolescence (Kagan, 1980, 1981).

The uniqueness of the Newcastle research resides in the fact that it can make contributions to the understanding of the effects of family disadvantage which occurs in the primary-school years on children in families who were not previously disadvantaged. The effects are in terms of cognition and behaviour in the secondary-school years based on longitudinal evidence and some information about entry into employment and the results of continued education of those who remained at school. Elsewhere we have described adverse experiences which created an impact in the earlier or preschool years of life: we have already demonstrated that deprivation in the preschool years has an enduring impact in the school years and also adulthood (Kolvin et la., 1983a,b). This is not to say that all children who experience these circumstances will have a poor outcome, but rather than the risks are substantially greater (Rutter, 1981). Further, the attenuation of the disadvantage may give rise to an attenuation of effect provided the previous adversities were mild for physical development, cognition and behaviour. If the adversities are severe, there is little improvement and even this may soon wash out. Adverse effects are therefore not merely a reflection of the persistence of environmental influences (Rutter, 1983). We now report on the effect of subsequent deprivation, and the current evidence supports the view that adverse experiences in later childhood and adolescence have effects which are not as noxious or enduring as those occurring in earlier childhood. Thus, the earlier childhood experiences appear to be more critical than the later ones. Or, alternatively, children appear more resilient to life stresses and chronic adverse experiences in the second five years of life than they are in the first five years.

The characteristics of families who moved into disadvantage in the years 1952–1957

In studying families who moved into disadvantage, a number of associated factors have been highlighted. First, there are those which provide clues as to which families will move into disadvantage. These are mainly social factors but do not appear sufficient in themselves to give rise to disadvantage at an earlier period in time, but their clustering makes us suspect that they are 'risk' factors which simply make the families more vulnerable to later environmental stress. Examination of the data at the end of this five-year period, that is, when the families have moved into disadvantage, reveals the key factors are evidently unemployment, absence or loss of father and large families associated with overcrowding.

Subsequent circumstances

Five years after moving into disadvantage the picture had become clearer. There was a whole series of unusual or adverse circumstances in relation to fathers and also evidence of deterioration in the care given by mothers to their children. The differences, while significant, were not substantial, but they did provide some indication of the associated mechanisms.

Subsequently, there were few differences of *cognition* between children coming from non-disadvantaged families and children from families that had moved into disadvantage. There were trends but little more than that, despite the large number of cases we were dealing with. This suggests good early foundations are important and subsequent breakdown of caring circumstances are not so damaging to cognitive development. There were, however, some signs of poorer achievements in reading, craft ability, concentration, persistence and so on. In fact, some of the important indicators of poor functioning derive from the school where there were significant judgements about delinquency, eagerness to leave school and poor aspirations of the children coming from families who moved into disadvantage.

To summarize, we identified effects which were behavioural and academic in nature; we have not identified any substantial cognitive effects. It is not clear why there should be this distinction or why disadvantage in the primary-school years had so little impact when it has such a dramatic impact in the preschool years. We can only speculate about possible reasons—the foundation of cognition may have already been laid down in the preschool years and may now be sufficiently robust so as to be able to resist most new adverse influences; or the effects on intelligence may be transient at this stage. However, this does not appear to be the case as they are still present at 15 years. Also there may be some substantial self-correcting mechanisms operative at this time (Hinde, 1982). The first of these alternatives seems to fit the facts best. One other possible hypothesis is that there are age-dependent sensitivities to life stresses (Rutter, 1981)—so that cognition is more sensitive in the pre-school years and achievements and behaviour in the school years—but some would see this merely as a restatement of facts rather than a theory to explain them.

What we have not as yet done is answer questions whether those second-generation children who show immediate reactions to psychosocial stresses continue subsequently to show effects into adulthood. Nor have we so far been able to study some chain effects such as early psychosocial stresses subsequently giving rise to lack of educational qualifications and these in turn to employment difficulties.

There is a vast literature on deprivation and disadvantage and their consequences, but relatively little about families who were previously reasonably advantaged and then suddenly projected into disadvantage as occurred during the great depression. The classic piece of research of families who lived through the Great Depression was that of Elder (1974). He has researched the catastrophe of the Great Depression and his focus has been on families with younger and older children. He looked in particular at the mechanisms by which the effects were mediated; that is, he attempted to understand linkages between the socioeconomic disaster and the subsequent development of those exposed to the disaster. Elder's work encapsulates the best of the sociological approach, as he takes hard data and adds to it information about stability and changes in families and their offspring in relation to the socioeconomic changes in the community and tries to understand the relationships between these changes over a span of time. Elder studied two cohorts—the first was the Oakland group (Elder, 1974) where the children at the time of the depression were in their adolescence and so were capable of understanding the nature of the catastrophe and even make a contribution to the family's attempts to cope with the problems with which they were confronted. However, their study is not really comparable with our study, as their children were at a later stage of development. A greater similarity exists with their second cohort at Berkeley (Elder and Rockwell, 1978) in which the families were exposed to the catastrophe of the depression when their children were in the earlier years of childhood. They addressed themselves to the hypothesis that these children, who were at a more dependent stage of their lives, would suffer more severe and enduring effects. In contrast the Newcastle research is about families that moved into deprivation against the general trend of economic advancement.

The Newcastle research does not have comparable data right up until adulthood—only until school-leaving age and early employment. The Berkeley Study revealed that boys whose families had suffered from the depression and who entered infant school at the time when the depression was still in existence, during these infant-school years appeared to show no effects on psychological stability, social relationships or school achievements. However, in adolescence, the children of those middle- and working-class families who had suffered the full force of the depression had poorer academic aspirations and did more poorly on high-school performance tests than those of families who did not. Elder and Rockwell do not see these as 'sleeper' effects, that is, effects which do not emerge until long after being exposed to an adverse life experience (Bronfenbrenner, 1979 thinks they might be) but rather effects that emerge when the affected children move out of the protected environment of infant schools to the more demanding life situations and achievement expectations of adolescence. Further entry into such secondary settings, such as college or university, will determine the life path of the individual. Those who did not enter college or university tend to start work at an earlier age, undertake manual work and show a pattern of job mobility and in adulthood an excess of health problems. These findings appear to endorse Elder and Rockwell's hypothesis of a greater vulnerability of young children to the stresses of deprivation.

Some of the Newcastle findings covering the secondary-school period, which are described in this report are in accord with the Berkeley study findings.

The picture for the Berkeley girls is rather different—they appeared to do fairly well and appeared more goal-oriented and self-assertive in adolescence. Elder and Rockwell attempt to explain these differences in terms of boys in these deprived families losing respect and affection for their fathers—a type of devaluation—but the girls developed a much stronger tie with their mothers.

The question arises whether in the case of the boys these are persistent or transient effects. The Newcastle research can offer no answer to this question, but the Berkeley study does. First, of those boys who attended university, the previously deprived were more likely than the non-deprived to produce substantial achievements despite previously presenting in adolescence as unambitious, passive and indecisive. The higher achievers from deprived backgrounds moved increasingly to confidence and health. So, for certain of the deprived children, the deprivation proved to be a strengthening and steeling experience. It would, therefore, be unwise to predict a negative developmental trajectory for all the children of the Newcastle families who moved into

Table 10.7   Social class of family of origin and movement into deprivation

	Remained not deprived: Social grouping of family of origin (%)		Moved into deprivation: Social grouping of family of origin (%)	
	Groups 1–3	Groups 4–5	Groups 1–3	Groups 4–5
Characteristics of father: Generation I				
(i) Good personality	82	69	80	20
(ii) Good provider	87	57	64	20
(iii) Poor participation in domestic tasks	4	16	11	39
Characteristics of child aged 15: Generation II				
Classroom behaviour				
(i) Concentration in class good	33	24	31	20
poor	19	25	35	53
(ii) Persistence in class good	20	17	15	13
poor	20	27	31	53
Class achievements				
(i) Reading good	42	38	35	20
poor	13	23	23	53
(ii) Craft good	37	27	35	17
poor	12	15	13	50
Teacher prediction of probability of delinquency and maladjustment at age 12 years	11	20	15	44
Examination successes				
Successfully passed public exams at age 15–16 years	49	24	45	0
Cognition				
(i) Ravens Matrices mean	46.3	45.6	45.7	38.9
(ii) Mill Hill Vocabulary mean	43.7	39.6	40.5	38.7

Note: There are significant social-class effects on 'matrices' for the group that moved into deprivation; for vocabulary for the group that remained not deprived. There is also a significant deterioration effect in the case of the lower social stratum group in the case of matrices and an interaction effect between social class and deterioration on the matrices.

deprivation and appeared to show effects in adolescence. Some may have unexpected successes in later life.

Social class of origin and moving into deprivation

Our data also allowed a study of the importance of the occupational class of origin of those families who moved into deprivation (Table 10.7). The findings presented in this table arouse a number of conclusions. The most important conclusion is that if one's family comes from a lower class of origin and moves into deprivation then the effects appear to be considerable. This is reflected in classroom behaviour and achievements, cognitive ability and exam successes and the teachers' judgements about the probability of delinquency when the children are 12 years old. These effects are apparent whatever the initial social class of the family but to a lesser degree in those coming from higher social strata. It is also evident from the data in the table that there are some social-class effects but it is the interaction of social class and movement into deprivation which constitutes the most damaging experience. This is particularly evident in the case of performance ability as represented by the Raven Matrices. The data in Table 10.7 also suggest that it is not simply a matter of social class which is based on the nature of fathers' employment but rather those additional factors inimicable to family well being which correlate with the social grouping which are most crucial. An example of this is shown by the presence of a series of adverse characteristics of the father which loom very large in the group which comes from a lower social stratum and then moves into deprivation.

While it is true that the size of some of the groups are small, the picture is likely to be reliable.

REFERENCES

Brewis, E. G., Davison, G. and Miller, F. J. W. (1940). *Investigations Into Health and Nutrition of Certain of the Children of Newcastle upon Tyne Between the Ages of One and Five Years (1938–9)*, City and County of Newcastle upon Tyne.

Bronfenbrenner, N. (1979). *The Ecology of Human Development*, Harvard University Press, London.

Elder, G. H. (1974). *Children of the Great Depression*, University of Chicago Press, Chicago.

Elder, G. H. and Rockwell, R. C. (1978). Economic depression and post-war opportunity, in *Research in Community and Mental Health* (Ed. R. A. Simmons), JAI Press, Greenwich, Conn.

Hinde, R. A. (1982). *Ethology*, Fontana, London.

Kagan, J. (1980). Perspectives in continuity, in *Constancy and Change in Human Development* (Eds O. G. Brim and J. Kagan), Harvard University Press, Cambridge, Mass.

Kagan, J. (1981). *The Second Year: The Emergence of Self Awareness*, Harvard University Press, Cambridge, Mass.

Kolvin, I., Miller, F. J. W., Garside, R. F. and Gatzanis, S. R. M. (1983a). One thousand families over three generations: Method and some preliminary findings, in *Families at Risk* (Ed. N. Madge), Heinemann, London.

Kolvin, J., Miller, F. J. W., Garside, R. F., Wolstenholme, F. and Gatzanis, S. R. M. (1983b). A Longitudinal study of deprivation: Life cycle changes in one generation—implications for the next generation, in *Epidemiological Approaches in Child Psychiatry*, II (Eds M. H. Schmidt and H. Remschmidt), G. Thieme Verlag, Stuttgart and New York.

Miller, F. J. W., Court, S. D. M., Walton, W. S. and Knox, E. G. (1960). *Growing up in Newcastle upon Tyne*, Oxford University Press, London.

Miller, F. J. W., Court, S. D. M., Knox, E. G. and Brandon, S. (1974). *The School Years in Newcastle upon Tyne*, Oxford University Press, London.

Robins, L. N. (1980). Longitudinal methods in the study of normal and pathological development, in *Studies of Children* (Ed. F. Earls), Prodist, New York.

Rutter, M. (1981). Stress, coping and development: Some issues and some questions, *J. Child Psychol. Psychiat.* **22**, 323–356.

Rutter, M. (1984). Continuities and discontinuities in socio-emotional development: Empirical and conceptual perspectives, in *Continuities and Discontinuities in Development* (Eds R. Harmon and R. Emde), Plenum, New York (in press).

Spence, J. C. (1933). *Investigations into the Health and Nutrition of Certain of the Children of Newcastle upon Tyne Between the Ages of One and Five years*, Newcastle upon Tyne Health Department.

Spence, J. C. and Miller, F. J. W. (1941). *Infantile Mortality in Newcastle upon Tyne during 1939*, Newcastle upon Tyne Health Department.

Spence, J. C., Walton, W. S., Miller, F. J. W. and Court, S. D. M. (1954). *A Thousand Families in Newcastle upon Tyne*, Oxford University Press, London.

This research was funded by the Economic and Social Research Council. In addition support was provided by the Rowntree Trust, the W. T. Grant Foundation and the City of Newcastle Priority Area Projects.

We would also like to thank Mrs M. Blackburn for administrative help.

Longitudinal Studies in Child Psychology and Psychiatry
Edited by A. R. Nicol
© 1985 John Wiley and Sons Ltd.

Chapter 11

Exploiting Longitudinal Data: Examples from the National Child Development Study

Ken Fogelman

INTRODUCTION

There are now in Britain three national studies, each based on one week's births: in 1946 (National Survey of Health and Development, see, for example, Douglas *et al.*, 1968; Wadsworth, 1979, 1958 (National Child Development Study, Davie *et al.*, 1972; Fogelman, 1976); and 1970 (Child Health and Education in the Seventies, Chamberlain *et al.*, 1975, 1978). Each has taken as its starting point all the babies born in one week in the particular year and has carried out further follow-ups at later ages. The two more recent studies have continued to monitor all the subjects of the original birth population, whereas the 1946 study has been able to include only about one-third of the original sample in its follow-up stages.

Thus each study provides a large sample, ranging from about 5000 to about 15 000, which for almost all purposes can be taken to be representative of the age group concerned. Furthermore, most of the information derived from these studies is not only concerned with simple estimates of incidence and prevalence, but rather with more complex relationships such as those between background and development. It is likely that such relationships are generalizable to a wider age-range, although the exact limits of such generalizations are not clear, and can only be assessed by comparing the findings of successive cohorts.

The main purpose of this chapter is to give an indication of how longitudinal data can and have been used, illustrated by a range of examples drawn from our work on the National Child Development Study (NCDS).

Each of the cohort studies has a number of characteristics which contribute to their special flavour. In addition to the size and representativeness of their samples, none has seen it as appropriate to study the health, or the education, or the social circumstances of their subjects in isolation. Each has adopted a multi-disciplinary approach, as demonstrated by their methods of data collection, the breadth of the data obtained, and the variety of professional backgrounds and interests of those who have worked on them. To an extent

241

this variety of information and approach will be apparent from the examples which I shall give, but this will be incidental to the exploration of what is probably the most important attribute of these studies, their longitudinal nature.

At the time of writing NCDS has just completed the fieldwork for its first adult stage, interviewing some 12 500 people at the age of 23 years. It therefore seems timely now to review the contribution which the study has made to our knowledge of children in their school years.

APPROACHES TO LONGITUDINAL ANALYSIS

For the purposes of this chapter our past longitudinal analyses can, somewhat crudely, be placed into six groups.

1 Change and continuity in characteristics. This is the most simple, essentially descriptive, level of analysis. The general purpose of this approach is to explore the extent to which the characteristics or circumstances of children, in their health, or housing or family circumstances for example, remain stable during their lives.

2 The relationship between early circumstances and later 'outcomes'. In theory both 1 and 2 can be investigated by cross-sectional studies, if retrospective questions on earlier events are included. However, the fallibility of long-term recall is self-evident, whereas longitudinal studies are able to obtain information on the earlier event at or near the time when it occurs.

3 The relationship between changes in circumstances and 'outcomes'. This can be seen as a combination of 1 and 2. Is there an association between a particular change or event and some aspect of a child's development as measured on a later occasion?

4 Changes in relationships. The approach described above will identify relationships, or differences between groups of children defined at one or more points in time, in terms of a developmental characteristic from a single, later occasion. This can be extended to examine whether such relationships change over time. Are, for example, the differences between two groups of children in their development similar at different stages in their lives?

5 Allowing for inputs. The method of analysis here is likely to be essentially as in 4, but the underlying question is somewhat different. Rather than being concerned directly with describing a relationship, and any changes, on two different occasions, it is posisble to ask whether, given an initial relationship, or 'input' — an example would be the intakes of different types of secondary school — is there evidence that subsequent experience (e.g. the type of school attended) changes the relationship (e.g. brings about further differences, not explained by intakes, between children who attended different types of school).

6 The approaches described in 3, 4 and 5 can examine whether a change in

a child's circumstances or experiences relates to a subsequent developmental outcome, and conversely, whether a particular circumstance or experience is related to a change in development. Clearly it is possible to be yet more elaborate and introduce change into both sides of the equation.

Following a general description of the National Child Development Study, I shall attempt to put some flesh on this rather abstract categorization by means of examples from the work which we have carried out in the past few years. In presenting these examples, primarily in order to illustrate the analytical approaches, I shall inevitably not do full justice to the work of my colleagues. Readers who wish to know more about what was done or found for a particular topic will need to refer to the original publication or to Fogelman (1983) where edited versions of many of the original papers are to be found.

NATIONAL CHILD DEVELOPMENT STUDY (1958 COHORT)

The origins of the NCDS can be found in the 1958 Perinatal Mortality Survey, mounted by the National Birthday Trust Fund (Butler and Bonham, 1963). The major purpose of this stage was to identify social and obstetric factors associated with perinatal mortality and handicapping conditions. To this end all the babies born in England, Scotland and Wales in the week 3–9 March, 1958 were studied, by means of a questionnaire completed by the attending midwife, giving details of the pregnancy, labour and birth, and other information from records and an interview with the mother.

The longitudinal element was introduced in 1965, together with the new title, when it became possible for the National Children's Bureau to carry out the first follow-up. Subsequent follow-ups took place when the children were aged 11 and 16 years. In order to maintain the cross-sectional representativeness of the sample at each stage, children born in the same week who had entered the country since the previous stage (i.e. immigrants), were included.

At each of these stages the methods of data collection were basically similar. At each age parents (usually the mother) were interviewed, schools completed questionnaires and each child was medically examined. Schools also administered tests, which varied according to age but always included tests of reading and mathematics attainment. At age 11 years the children completed a small personal questionnaire, and this became a substantial element in the 16-year follow-up.

The examples in the remainder of this chapter are based on the data collected at the above main stages of the study. In addition, however, there has from time to time been the opportunity to collect further data relating to small subgroups, such as those with one parent, and the adopted. Also, since the young people left them, schools have provided us with details of public examination results and, as has been mentioned, a further follow-up at 23 years has taken place.

At all stages the level of participation and co-operation has been gratifyingly high, from the young people themselves and their families, and from the local authority staff and professions who were involved in the organization and administration of our materials. Table 11.1 summarizes the numbers and basic response patterns for the first four stages of the study.

Table 11.1   Numbers and response at each NCDS follow-up

Age (years)	n^* ($= 100\%$)	Some data (%)	Refused (%)	Others without data (%)
Birth	17 733	98.2	—	1.8
7	16 883	91.3	0.5	8.3
11	16 835	90.9	4.9	4.1
16	16 915	87.3	6.7	5.9

*The number from the previous stage, less those who died or emigrated, plus identified immigrants.

Although the response level has been generally high, there has been some reduction. Any reduction introduces the possibility of bias. One advantage of longitudinal studies is that, because children missed at one stage will have data from earlier stages, it is possible to check whether any bias is appearing among those responding. A detailed examination of this question has been reported by Goldstein (1976). In general he found small or non-existent biases in relation to major indices such as social class, region, attainment test scores and measures of physical development. There is, however, evidence of a slight under-representation of some small subgroups of children, who might broadly be termed 'disadvantaged'. For example, 3.4 per cent of the original cohort were born illegitimate, but they compose only 3.2 per cent of those with data at 16 years.

Of course, the above is only a partial story, as it compares those with and without any data at all. Since at each stage there were several methods of obtaining data, it is also quite possible for an individual to have incomplete data at any one stage. In complex analyses drawing upon data from more than one age and several sources the effect is multiplicative, and can lead to a dramatic reduction in the sample available for analysis with complete information on all relevant variables. It is, therefore, vital to investigate response patterns further in the context of each set of analyses in order to check whether any bias is appearing. Fortunately, to date this has not been the case, though we cannot yet know whether this will continue once the 23-year data are added to the picture.

CHANGE AND CONTINUITY

The first set of examples are chosen to illustrate the simplest kind of longitudinal analysis—the description of changes and continuities in children's circumstances or characteristics. Perhaps its most obvious application is in the area of medical conditions.

Among the conditions to which NCDS has paid particular attention are asthma and wheezy bronchitis (Peckham and Butler, 1978). (It must be said that it is often difficult to distinguish precisely between asthma and wheezy bronchitis. Indeed it has been suggested that they constitute part of one disease entity, differing only in degree (Williams and McNicol, 1969).) At the first follow-up just over 3 per cent of children were reported to have had one or more attacks of asthma during their first seven years. At age 11 years, 43 per cent of these children were reported still to be suffering from attacks of asthma, and a further 7 per cent from wheezy bronchitis only. The remaining 50 per cent were reported free from wheezing. On the other hand, 4 per cent of all children were said to have had asthma or wheezy bronchitis for the first time between 7 and 11 years, although of these only 14 per cent were said to have asthma, the remainder wheezy bronchitis alone. None of these figures support the all too common assumption that most children will grow out of their wheeziness at an early stage.

The second example is taken from work on distant-vision screening, by Tibbenham, Peckham and Gardiner (1978). At 7, 11 and 16 years a standard Snellen chart was used, in the course of the medical examination, to test distant visual acuity. For the sake of simplicity Table 11.2 shows the relationship between the findings at 7 and 16 years, although the original paper also incorporated the 11-year data. In this table children have been placed into one of four groups at each age: normal vision (6/6 or better in both eyes); minor defect (6/6, 6/9 or 6/9, 6/9); moderate defect—unilateral or bilateral (6/12 or 6/18 in at least one eye); severe defect—unilateral or bilateral (6/24 or more in at least one eye).

As can be seen there are significant changes of category, both improvement and deterioration (and these are even more marked when the 11-year data are included), some of which may be due to the technical difficulties of vision testing. However, the most important pattern concerns the substantial numbers of

Table 11.2   Distant visual acuity at 7 and 16 years (percentaged)

Vision at 7	Vision at 16				
	Normal	Minor defect	Moderate defect	Severe defect	Total
Normal	81.6	7.2	5.6	5.6	79.6
Minor defect	69.8	12.8	9.3	8.0	12.4
Moderate defect	31.7	14.2	33.1	21.0	5.8
Severe defect	8.9	5.1	24.6	61.3	2.3
Total	75.6	8.2	8.1	8.0	100

children whose vision is normal, or who have only a minor defect, at 7 years, but have acquired a moderate or severe defect by the age of 16 years. Much of this deterioration was probably associated with myopia, although refractive errors and amblzopia are also often first discovered after age 7 years. These results were first published when the role of vision screening was under debate, with some suggestions that regular screening was unnecessary and could be replaced by a single early testing. The results indicate how many children would risk their problem remaining undetected under such a system, since their problems first appear after age 7 years.

A similar question concerning hearing levels during childhood was investigated in a slightly different way (Richardson *et al.*, 1977). In this case the researchers were not so directly concerned with the extent of changes in individual children, but with whether there was evidence of a general increase in hearing impairment as children grew older. Audiometric testing had been carried out at all three ages and for this purpose it was sufficient, and simpler, to compare the straightforward distributions of hearing loss at the three ages (though with such a method it is even more important to check, as they did, that any changes are not the result of response bias).

Figure 11.1 represents median audiometric thresholds at different frequencies at each age. In showing an elevation of thresholds (i.e. diminished hearing acuity) in later adolescence, these findings contradicted those of studies carried out in the 1960s and earlier. On the other hand they are consistent with what others have suggested (e.g. Day, 1970; Lipscomb, 1972) would be the effect of an 'insult' to which young people have been exposing themselves increasingly, namely highly amplified pop music.

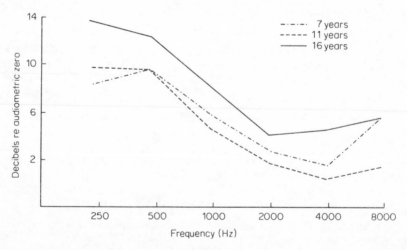

Fig. 11.1   Median audiometric threshold at 3 ages. ·–·–·, 7 years; ------, 11 years; ——— 16 years

Perhaps the most fundamental of all a child's experiences is their family structure, i.e. whether he or she has one parent or two. Frequently the stereotype of a one-parent family is still the illegitimate child brought up alone by the mother. To what extent is this typical? Further, how fully do figures for one age group represent the total situation, or are there large numbers of children who experience being with only one parent for relatively short periods? Figure 11.2 shows that the latter is indeed the case. The figure reveals the substantial amount of change which takes place. Large numbers of children have only one parent for a period which spans one or two follow-ups, and very few children indeed fit the stereotype—just 0.3 per cent of the population.

Another basic and important factor in children's lives is their housing conditions. We know that at any time many children live in unsatisfactory

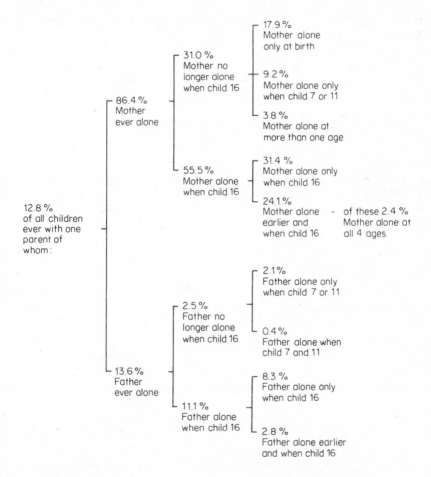

Fig. 11.2 Children in one-parent families at NCDS follow-ups

conditions, in homes which are overcrowded or lack basic amenities, but again a further question is the extent to which this is continuous. Do many families improve their situation as their children grow up, and do others encounter poor conditions for the first time when their children are older?

Table 11.3 (from Essen and Fogelman, 1979) shows the proportions who were in adverse circumstances at each of the three ages. The amenities referred to are: a bathroom, a hot water supply, and an indoor lavatory. Crowding is based on the conventional census definition of more than 1.5 persons per room. Two main patterns emerge from these figures. First, there are considerable changes— about one in five children experience each of these disadvantages at some point, but at most one in twenty-five throughout their childhood. Secondly, children's circumstances generally improve as they get older. For example 15 per cent were crowded at age 7 years, 11 per cent at 11 years, and 7 per cent at 16 years. This is not unexpected in view of what is known about the 'housing cycle' (Donnison, 1967).

Table 11.3   Crowding and amenities at three ages

	Crowding (%)	Sharing or lacking amenities (%)
At all three ages	4	3
At 7 and 11, but not 16 years	4	5
At 11 and 16, but not 7 years	1	1
At 7 and 16, but not 11 years	1	1
At 7 years only	6	8
At 11 years only	2	2
At 16 years only	1	2
Total at 7, 11 or 16 years	19	21

Change in the other direction is relatively infrequent, although it should not be overlooked that even a proportion as small as 1 per cent represents a by no means negligible number of children.

The examples considered so far have been concerned with movement in and out of absolute categories, that is whether or not a child has had a particular condition or experience. It is equally possible to adopt the same approach, but to examine relative positions on a continuous scale, such as an attainment test score. As different tests were used at different ages, it is not appropriate to look directly at changes in raw score, but it is possible to investigate changes in the child's position relative to the scores of other children. For example, in Essen, Fogelman and Ghodsian (1978), we divided scores on the reading and maths tests given at each age into thirds, and then investigated the proportion falling into various categories across ages. Table 11.4 shows the result.

Table 11.4   Percentages of children with each pattern of attainment at 7, 11 and 16 years

	Maths	Reading
Consistently high (top third)	16.5	17.7
Consistently medium (middle third)	7.3	7.1
Consistently low (bottom third)	11.7	17.5
High at 7 to low at 16 years	4.4	3.0
Low at 7 to high at 16 years	3.6	3.5
Less extreme changes	56.6	51.2
Total $n(= 100\%)$	9402	9482

On both tests the majority of children fall into the group comprising those whose attainment changed, but by relatively little (i.e. not by more than from one-third to the adjacent band). The proportion whose attainment is reasonably stable (i.e. in the same third at all three ages) is about half what it would be if attainment at one age predicted accurately attainment at subsequent ages.

The numbers whose attainment changes fairly dramatically are far from trivial. In all, in mathematics about 4.5 per cent and in reading 3 per cent score in the top third at 7 years but are found in the bottom third by 16 years. In both subject areas about 3.5 per cent show an equal amount of change in the opposite direction. It is also the case, as can to some extent be seen in this table, that there is more change between the first two ages, in the primary school years, than between the later ages.

All the examples presented have revealed significant numbers of children who change, in their health, their family background or their attainment levels. In our professional relationships with children it is all too tempting to attach a label of, for example, 'bright' or 'dull' or 'disadvantaged' or 'from a one-parent family' and imagine that we are describing some permanent characteristic. Results such as these demonstrate that our attitudes towards and perceptions of children must incorporate the possibility of change, for the better or worse. Furthermore, policy-makers—not only those at government level but equally, for example, a school which is considering its ability-grouping policy—will need to allow for such change, and for the large numbers of children whose families need temporary help as well as for those with long-term needs.

EARLIER EXPERIENCES AND LATER OUTCOMES

The purpose of the analyses considered so far has been primarily descriptive. No assumptions have been made about causality. In the examples in this section we are certainly concerned with whether some early experience has consequences for later development.

The first such example comes from what is perhaps one of the best known areas of work on the NCDS, the effects of smoking in pregnancy. Early work on the original perinatal data demonstrated that a mother smoking ten or more cigarettes per day during pregnancy increased the foetal plus neonatal mortality rate by 28 per cent and reduced birth weight by an average of 170 g, as compared with non-smokers (Butler and Alberman, 1969). Further analysis indicated that the results were unaffected when statistical allowance was made for possible mediating factors such as maternal age, social class, parity and height. Additionally, it was found that a change in maternal smoking habits during the first four months of pregnancy had the effect of putting the baby into a birth weight or mortality category associated with the new smoking habit. For example, babies of mothers who gave up smoking by the fourth month of pregnancy were no more at risk than those of mothers who had never smoked (Butler et al., 1972).

It was natural that interest should next turn to whether, among the survivors, there was any longer-term association between the child's development and the mother's smoking habit during pregnancy. At the age of 7 and 11 years it was indeed found that there were small but statistically significant differences, again after allowing for other related factors, according to the mother's smoking level during pregnancy, in reading and mathematics attainment and in height (Goldstein, 1971; Butler and Goldstein, 1973).

More recently we have examined the situation once more, at the age of 16 years (Fogelman, 1980). Table 11.5 summarizes the results of analyses of variance. The analyses take into account a number of other factors which also are related to educational attainment and height: child's sex; birthweight; gestation period; father's occupation (social class) at birth; father's occupation at 16 years; birth order; number of younger siblings at 16 years; and mother's age. Also included in the height analyses only were: mother's height; month of measurement; and sexual maturity as indicated by axillary hair growth. Smoking categories relate to the second half of pregnancy and are: none; medium—1–9 per day; heavy—10+ per day.

In this and subsequent tables which report analysis of variance results, the term 'fitted constants' may need some explanation. The technique used produces figures which represent the average differences between the groups under consideration adjusted for the other variables allowed for in the analysis. The fitted constants are not directly interpretable as adjusted means, but the difference between any pair of fitted constants does represent the difference between the adjusted means.

For the height analyses, the fitted constants are in centimetres. Reading and maths scores have been transformed to standard deviation units, that is with a mean 0 and standard deviation 1. Thus, in Table 11.5, the contrast between the average height of the boys of non-smokers and those of heavy smokers is 0.885 cm, after allowing for the other variables in the analysis.

Table 11.5 Smoking in pregnancy and development at 16 years

Mother's smoking during pregnancy	Fitted constants			
	Reading (deviation score)	Maths (deviation score)	Height	
			Boys (cms)	Girls (cms)
None	0.068	0.107	0.484	0.066
Medium (1–9 per day)	– 0.019	– 0.030	– 0.083	0.260
Heavy (over 10 a day)	– 0.049	– 0.077	– 0.401	– 0.326
χ^2	14.54 ($p<0.001$)	34.8 ($p<0.001$)	6.81 ($p<0.05$)	2.14 (NS)

For the reading test the comparable contrast is 0.117 of the population standard deviation.

The differences in average reading and maths test scores are, though highly statistically significant, not very large. The contrast between the non-smokers and the heavy smokers amounts to about one-eighth of the total population standard deviation on the reading test and about one-fifth of a standard deviation on the maths test.

For both attainment tests the differences associated with smoking were approximately equal for the two sexes. For height this was not the case. As can be seen in Table 11.5, for boys there is a contrast of just less than 1 cm, but for girls the difference is smaller and is not statistically significant. At the age of 16 years almost all girls are physically mature and have reached their eventual adult height whereas this is not true for boys. It is therefore possible either that smoking in pregnancy is related to *rate* of growth rather than eventual height, or that real differences exist until the onset of puberty but then disappear in the course of the far greater changes taking place during the pubertal growth-spurt.

The second example of an investigation into the long-term consequences of an earlier experience comes from a very different area, that is the question of the importance of length of schooling. Several earlier studies had demonstrated that autumn-born children do better in school than those born in the summer, but such children typically have spent one term longer in the infants' school, so it was not possible to unravel whether this finding was simply an age-related effect or the result of length of schooling (e.g. Williams, 1964; Thompson, 1971).

The NCDS sample is particularly suited to examine this question. The children were of course all born at the same time of year, and, once those with any formal preschool experience (which was relatively rare at that time) are excluded, they fall fairly neatly into two halves—those who started school in the term before their fifth birthday and those who started a term later.

Once again it is important to take other related factors into account. 'Early' starters are more likely, for example, to come from middle-class families, to be found in Wales, to attend smaller schools and smaller classes, and their general attendance record tends to be better.

Table 11.6 (based on Fogelman and Gorbach, 1978) gives the differences between 'early' and 'late' starters in test scores at age 11 years, adjusted for such related background variables. For this analysis the three test scores (reading, maths and general ability) have been converted to an approximate age-related scale, so that differences are expressed in months. All differences are significant at at least the 5 per cent level.

Table 11.6 Advantages in attainment of early starters over late starters

	Adjusted differences in months
General ability	2.6
Reading	2.3
Mathematics	2.6

CHANGES IN CIRCUMSTANCES AND 'OUTCOMES'

In the previous two sections we have seen how children's experiences and circumstances can change and how a particular experience can relate to subsequent development. The next step is to combine these to ask whether a change, or the particular age at which it happens, is of importance. Is development determined by early experiences or can it be modified by what happens subsequently? Are the experiences of early childhood more important for long-term development than those which occur during adolescence?

Such questions are of interest in relation to two aspects of a child's life which we have already examined descriptively—their housing conditions and whether or not he or she is living in a one-parent family. Children living in poor housing conditions do less well at school (e.g. Davie et al., 1972), as do children in one-parent families (Ferri, 1976) (although in the latter case it appears that this can be explained by other factors; children with one parent do no worse than other children whose families have similar environmental and financial difficulties).

Further analysis has pursued the questions outlined above. In terms of school attainment at 16 years, does the relationship differ according to the age at which the child was in poor housing conditions (Essen, Fogelman and Head, 1978) or lacked a parent (Essen, 1979) Tables 11.7 and 11.8 summarize the main findings of the analyses of variance.

In Table 11.7, the fitted constants for the 16-year test scores are, as before, on a scale with mean 0 and standard deviation 1. Other variables allowed for

Table 11.7   Attainment at 16 years and housing conditions

	Fitted constants	
	Reading	Maths
Crowded (>1.5 persons per room)		
at 7, 11 and 16 years	− 0.171	− 0.142
at 7 and 11 years only	0.065	0.007
at 7 and 16 years only	− 0.253	− 0.201
at 7 years only	0.085	0.040
at 11 and 16 years only	0.070	0.139
at 11 years only	0.047	0.027
at 16 years only	− 0.045	− 0.034
never	0.202	0.164
χ^2	43.7 ($p<0.001$)	30.2 ($p<0.001$)
Sole use of amenities (bathroom, hot water supply and indoor lavatory)		
at 7, 11 and 16 years	0.140	0.138
at 7 and 11 years only	0.041	0.087
at 7 and 16 years only	0.069	0.081
at 7 years only	− 0.004	0.183
at 11 and 16 years only	0.008	− 0.047
at 11 years only	− 0.052	− 0.283
at 16 years only	− 0.009	− 0.023
lacking or sharing amenities at all three ages	− 0.193	− 0.136
χ^2	29.0 ($p<0.001$)	29.0 ($p<0.001$)

in this analysis are: the tenure of the home at each age; social class; family size; sex; region; parents' education; and parental visits to the school. As might be expected, in both subject areas and on both housing measures, the greatest contrast is between those who experienced adverse conditions at all three ages, and those who experienced adverse conditions at all three ages, and those who experienced them at none of the three follow-ups. Comparing the various subgroups who were in poor conditions at only one or two ages, no patterns appear which are consistent across different ages, tests or housing variables. There is some suggestion, looking at those who were in overcrowded homes at one age only, that the more recent the experience the greater the effect on attainment, but the differences are very small.

A similar pattern appears from the analysis of parental situation, though, as had been found in the cross-sectional analyses, the differences in attainment between the single-parent groups and those with two parents do not prove to be statistically significant once other factors are allowed for (these were: sex; social class; family size; number of schools attended; amenities in the house; tenure; whether the home included a room for homework; whether the child had ever been in care; parental aspirations for the child's future education;

Table 11.8   Parental situation and attainment at 16 years

	Fitted constants	
	Maths	Reading
Mother alone at 16 years		
and before 7 years	0.01	0.05
after 7 years only	− 0.04	0.11
Mother not alone at 16 years		
but alone before 7 years	− 0.07	− 0.09
alone at 11 years only	− 0.05	− 0.04
Father ever alone	0.00	0.03
Both parents always	0.15	− 0.06
χ^2	8.7 (NS)	4.2 (NS)

household income; receipt of free school meals; and the reason for the absence of one parent).

These findings are consistent with others from the study, in failing to demonstrate that the experiences of the early years bear a stronger relationship with development by age 16 years than do more recent experiences. Of course 'early' in this context refers to age 7 years rather than the first year or two of life which others might suggest are more crucial. Neither can we rule out the possibility that different findings might appear in more sensitive areas, such as mother–child interaction, not examined in this study. Nevertheless, it is important to be aware that adverse physical or family conditions are likely to be as great in their effects, whatever the age at which the child encounters them.

CHANGES IN RELATIONSHIPS

Among the results from the 7-year stage of the study which received most attention were those which showed the strong association between development and social background, in particular social class and family size. Such findings are now well known and supported by a number of other studies.

Inequalities in attainment between social groups are detectable from the beginning of the school years. But do the differences remain fairly stable, or do schools succeed in reducing inequalities (if indeed that is their aim), or does the gap widen as children grow older?

The simplest way to answer this question is to plot test scores at one age against test scores at a subsequent age for the different social groups. For example, for children of different social class who had the same test score at 7 years, are their average test scores at 11 years the same, or do they differ in some way related to their social class?

Figures 11.3 and 11.4 show the relevant results on the reading tests at 7 and 11 years, for social class and family size respectively (Fogelman and Goldstein,

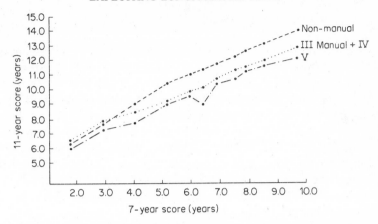

Fig. 11.3   Mean 11-year reading score by 7-year reading score for three social class groups
at 7 years

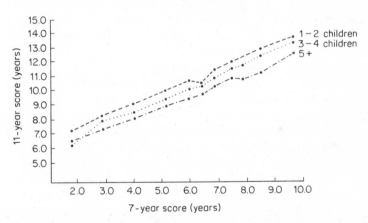

Fig. 11.4   Mean 11-year reading score by 7-year reading Tscore for three numbers of
children in household groups

1976). In each case it can indeed be seen that the groups are separated at age
11 years. Children whose father are in non-manual occupations have, by age
11 years, moved ahead of those children from manual backgrounds who were
reading equally well at 7 years. Similarly, the gap between children from the
largest and the smallest family sizes widens between 7 and 11 years. The same
pattern is found in mathematics attainment, and is confirmed by multivariate
analysis which takes other related background factors into account.

More recently the same investigation has continued to age 16 years, with the
same pattern of results. The gap in attainment between children of different
social backgrounds widens yet further between the ages of 11 and 16 years
(Fogelman *et al.*, 1978).

ALLOWING FOR INPUTS

The above statistical technique has a broader application, which can be labelled 'allowing for inputs'. For example, a cross-sectional study of the effects of ability-grouping policies in schools might relate children's attainment to whether he or she is currently, or recently, in a streamed, setted or mixed-ability class. However, one might properly suspect that any differences found might simply reflect differences in the intake of the different kinds of classes, that there might be pre-existing systematic differences in the attainment of children who are subsequently to experience different systems. Longitudinal studies are well placed to tackle such issues. In examining ability grouping in the secondary school, for example, NCDS has attainment measures not only at 16 years, which can be seen as the outputs of the system, but also at 11 years, i.e. inputs.

The NCDS data provide a broad classification of the ability-grouping policy of each secondary school, whereby each pupil can be placed into one of four main categories, according to the practice with the 12–13-year group of the school (see Tibbenham, Essen and Fogelman, 1978, for an explanation of this choice of measure).

1 Permanent classes formed on the basis of ability. Children take all or most of their lessons with the same class, which contains children of restricted range of ability ('streaming', 'banding').
2 Permanent classes of mixed ability but, for some subjects classes are formed on the basis of ability in that subject ('setting').
3 All classes of mixed ability.
4 Other arrangements.

Simple, raw comparisons between the four groups showed that the highest average test scores at 16 years were obtained by children in mixed-ability schools. However, for the reason given above, multivariate analysis was necessary. It was particularly important to take into account 11-year test scores, and the type of secondary school attended. The greatest proportion of so-called mixed-ability teaching was to be found in grammar schools. Also included in the analyses, as independent variables, were sex, social class, region and the streaming policy of the primary school attended. The results of this analysis are to be found in Fogelman *et al.* (1978) and are summarized in Table 11.9.

On the mathematics test the differences do not reach statistical significance. The differences in reading do just reach significance, but this is largely the result of the contrast between the 'streamed' group and the 'others'. The latter contains a rather meaningless collection of responses which were too unusual, eccentric or vague to be included in one of the three main groups. It also contains relatively few children. Ignoring this group, there is no difference between 'setted' and 'mixed ability' and the contrast between these and the 'streamed' amounts to

Table 11.9   Ability grouping and test score at 16 years

	Fitted constants	
	Reading	Mathematics
Streamed	0.04	0.00
Setted	0.00	0.00
Mixed ability	0.00	−0.06
Other	−0.04	0.05
χ^2	8.9 ($p<0.05$)	3.4 (NS)

only about one-twenty-fifth of a standard deviation. There is, therefore, no evidence in these findings to support a relationship between reading and mathematics attainment and secondary-school ability grouping.

A similar approach has been used to examine a number of other variables related to schooling (Richardson *et al.*, 1983). Table 11.10 presents a selection of these and their relationship with 16-year mathematics test scores — in each case after allowing for mathematics score at 11, social class and type of school.

Table 11.10   School characteristics and 16-year mathematics attainment

	Fitted constants	χ^2
School size		
Under 750	−0.02	
Up to 1250	0.01	1.9 ($p>0.05$)
Over 1251	0.01	
Sex segregation		
Boys in boys schools	0.10	
Girls in girls schools	−0.08	127.5 ($p<0.001$)
Boys in coed schools	0.08	
Girls in coed schools	−0.10	
Pupil-teacher ratio		
−15	0.08	
−16	−0.04	
−17	−0.01	21.3 ($p<0.5$)
−18	−0.03	
>18	0.00	
Present maths-class size		
≤20	−0.13	
−25	−0.03	99.9 ($p<0.001$)
−30	0.06	
31+	0.10	

Our findings are consistent with other studies in showing no relationship between school size and pupils' attainment. Despite commonly held beliefs there is no research evidence to support the idea that pupils of large schools do less well.

The differences associated with the second variable in the table, the sex segregation of the school, are highly statistically significant. However, inspection of the fitted constants makes clear that this is the result not of the contrast between single-sex and co-education schools but of the difference in the average attainment of the two sexes. Boys obtain higher maths test scores on average at this age, and once that is taken into account the results for the two types of school are virtually identical.

The remaining two variables in this table make the distinction between the pupil–teacher ratio of the school, that is the total number of pupils divided by the (full-time equivalent) number of teachers, and the actual class size, in this case as given by the number of pupils in the current mathematics class.

The results for the pupil–teacher ratio variable are not consistent. The highest average test score is found for those in schools with the lowest pupil–teacher ratio, of 15:1 or less, but the next highest is the group with the highest pupil–teacher ratio of greater than 18:1. In any case, even the most extreme contrast is not very large, just exceeding one-tenth of a standard deviation.

Of course pupil–teacher ratio is not a direct measure of class size as it also incorporates senior and pastoral staff who may not teach a full timetable. The final section of Table 11.10 does look directly at the number of pupils in the current mathematics class. There is a clear gradation in the results but, as so often in research on this topic, it is the pupils in the largest classes who have the best average scores, and those in the smallest classes who have the lowest. This runs counter to common sense and every teacher's belief, but is quite consistent with the findings of other studies. One explanation often offered for such results is that, where a school is streamed, higher streams tend to contain more pupils. Although it cannot be ruled out completely this is less likely to be the explanation here as, unlike most other studies, previous attainment has been taken into account. It remains possible that there are other explanations, not involving a direct effect of class size. For example, extra pupils may be allocated to more experienced teachers. Alternatively, it may be that standardized tests are more appropriate to assessing the outcome of a more structured style of teaching which may have to take place in larger classes.

CHANGES IN BACKGROUND AND CHANGES IN OUTCOME

The final example is of the most complex kind of analysis considered here. We have seen how it is possible to relate change in test score, between 7 and 11 years for example, to the social background of the child—social class and family size were the examples taken. This can be extended to examine how changes in test score are related to changes of background during the same period. For example do the socially mobile, those whose fathers change their occupation and thereby move into a different social class category, move ahead of or fall behind those whose social class is unchanged?

The results in Table 11.11 are taken from the analysis already cited (Fogelman and Goldstein, 1976) which investigated test-score change between 7 and 11 years related to social class. The fitted constants in this table compare the reading and maths attainment at 11 years of those whose social class did not change between 7 and 11 years with those experiencing change in various directions. Also allowed for are initial attainment, initial social class, and family size.

Table 11.11   Change in social class and change in attainment between 7 and 11 years

Change in social class		Fitted constants (SD units)	
At 7	At 11	Reading	Mathematics
V	I–IV	0.00	0.00
III manual + IV	Non-manual	0.18	0.22
I–IV	V	−0.21	−0.22
Non-manual	III manual + IV	−0.25	−0.26
χ^2		$(p<0.001)$	$(p<0.001)$

It can be seen that there are relatively large differences associated with the changes in social class. For example, in reading, those whose fathers moved from non-manual to skilled or semi-skilled jobs had an average 11-year score which is one-quarter of a standard deviation behind those who stayed in the non-manual group, for given 7-year score. By contrast, those who moved in the other direction, from the skilled or semi-skilled groups into the non-manual group, also moved about one-fifth of a standard deviation ahead in their reading test score. The mathematics test scores show a very similar pattern.

CONCLUSION

By this rather partial account of a small selection of results from the National Child Development Study, I have attempted to demonstrate some of the kinds of research which are possible, and only possible, with longitudinal data. Of course there are many problematic issues, relating to technicalities of the analyses, consistency of definitions and so on, which I have ignored or glossed over in the limited space available. Nevertheless, I hope that readers unfamiliar with studies of this kind now have some insight into their rich and unique potential.

Some of the analyses discussed may appear complex enough already but yet a further level of elaboration will be possible with the imminent addition of data from the fourth follow-up at age 23 years. Fascinating and important as it is to investigate children's development in terms of, for example, their school attainment or their physical growth during adolescence, there is a sense in which all the results of the study so far are preliminary. They largely depend on assumptions about the relationship between, say, school performance and adult life. With the addition of the 23-year data it becomes possible to explore the association between the various facets of childhood experience and subsequent aspects of their lives in early adulthood: their progress through further and higher education, their careers (and, for many, their experience of unemployment), their personal relationships and family formation. The research team at the National Children's Bureau is now beginning to work with these new data, and results should begin to appear over the next two years.

REFERENCES

Butler, N. R. and Alberman, E. D. (1969). *Perinatal Problems*, Livingstone, London.

Butler, N. R. and Bonham, D. G. (1963). *Perinatal Mortality*, Livingstone, London.

Butler, N. R. and Goldstein, H. (1973). Smoking in pregnancy and subsequent child development, *British Medical Journal*, iv, 573–575.

Butler, N. R., Goldstein, H. and Ross, E. M. (1972). Cigarette smoking in pregnancy: its influence on birthweight and perinatal mortality, *British Medical Journal*, ii, 127–130.

Chamberlain, R., Chamberlain, G., Howlett, B. and Claireaux, A. (1975). *British Births 1970*, Vol. 1, *The First Week of Life*, Heinemann Medical Books.

Chamberlain, G., Philipp, E., Howlett, B. and Masters, K. (1978). *British Births 1970*, Vol. 2, *Obstetric Care*, Heinemann Medical Books.

Davie, R., Butler, N. and Goldstein, H. (1972). *From Birth to Seven*, Longman, London.

Day, F. I. (1970). Auditory fatigue and predicted permanent hearing defects from 'rock-n-roll' music, *New England Journal of Medicine*, 282, 467–470.

Donnison, D. V. (1967). *The Government of Housing*, Penguin, Harmondsworth.

Douglas, J. W. B., Ross, J. M. and Simpson, H. R. (1968). *All Our Future: A Longitudinal Study of Secondary Education*, Peter Davies.

Essen, J. (1979). Living in one-parent families — attainment at school, *Child: Care, Health and Development*, 5, 3, 184–200.

Essen, J. and Fogelman, K. (1979). Childhood housing experiences, *Concern*, 32, 5–10.

Essen, J., Fogelman, K. and Ghodsian, M. (1978). Long-term changes in the school attainment of a national sample of children, *Educational Research*, 20, 2, 143–151.

Essen, J., Fogelman, K. and Head, J. (1978). Childhood housing experiences and school attainment, *Child: Care, Health and Development*, 4, 1, 41–58.

Ferri, E. (1976). *Growing Up in a One-Parent Family*. NFER,

Fogelman, K. (Ed.) (1976). *Britain's Sixteen-Year-Olds*, National Children's Bureau.

Fogelman, K. (1980). Smoking in pregnancy and subsequent development of the child, *Child: Care, Health and Development*, 6, 4, 233–254.

Fogelman, K. (Ed.) (1983). *Growing Up in Great Britain: Papers from the National Child Development Study*, Macmillan, London.

Fogelman, K., Essen, J. and Tibbenham, A. (1978). Ability grouping in secondary schools and attainment, *Educational Studies*, 4, 3, 201–212.

Fogelman, K. and Goldstein, H. (1976). Social factors associated with changes in educational attainment between 7 and 11 years of age, *Educational Studies*, 2, 2, 95–109.

Fogelman, K., Goldstein, H., Essen, J. and Ghodsian, M. (1978). Patterns of Attainment, *Educational Studies*, **4**, 2, 121–130.

Fogelman, K. and Gorbach, P. (1978). Age of starting school and attainment at 11, *Educational Research*, **21**, 1, 65–66.

Goldstein, H. (1971). Factors influencing the height of seven-year-old children, *Human Biology*, **43**, 1, 92–111.

Goldstein, H. (1976). A study of the response rates of sixteen-year-olds in the National Child Development Study, *Britain's Sixteen-Year-Olds* (Ed. K. Fogelman), National Children's Bureau.

Lipscomb, D. M. (1972). The increase in prevalence of high frequency hearing impairment among college students, *Audiology*, **11**, 231–237.

Peckham, C. and Butler, N. (1978). A national study of asthma in childhood, *Journal of Epidemiology and Community Health*, **32**, 2, 79–85.

Richardson, K., Ghodsian, M. and Gorbach, P. (1983). The association between school variables and attainments in a national sample, in *Growing Up in Great Britain: Papers from the National Child Development Study* (Ed. K. Fogelman), Macmillan, London.

Richardson, K., Hutchison, D., Peckham, C. and Tibbenham, A. (1977). Audiometric thresholds of a national sample of British sixteen-year-olds, *Dev. Med. and Child Neurology*, **19**, 6, 797–802.

Thompson, D. (1971). Season of birth and success in secondary schools, *Educational Research*, **14**, 56–60.

Tibbenham, A., Essen, J. and Fogelman, K. (1978). Ability grouping and school characteristics, *British Journal of Educational Studies*, **26**, 1, 8–23.

Tibbenham, A., Peckham, C. and Gardiner, P. (1978). Vision screening in children tested at 7, 11 and 16 years, *British Medical Journal*, **i**, 6123, 1312–1314.

Wadsworth, M. (1979). *Roots of Delinquency: Infancy, Adolescence and Crime*, Martin Robertson, Oxford.

Williams, H. E. and McNicol, K. N. (1969). Prevalence, natural history and relationship of wheezy bronchitis and asthma in children: an epidemiological study, *British Medical Journal*, **4**, 32, 1–35.

Williams, P. (1964). Date of birth, backwardness and educational organisation, *British Journal of Educational Psychology*, **34**, 247–255.

Section V

Treatment and Prevention

Longitudinal Studies in Child Psychology and Psychiatry
Edited by A. R. Nicol
© 1985 John Wiley and Sons Ltd.

Chapter 12

Helping Seriously Disturbed Children

R. M. Wrate, I. Kolvin, R. F. Garside*, F. Wolstenholme,
C. M. Hulbert and I. M. Leitch

INTRODUCTION

Robins (1973) has suggested that in any evaluation of child psychiatry services, two major components merit examination, the first of which is the differential provision and use of such services within the community. The suggestion is that the availability of treatment is frequently decided by social-class factors, but this is more of a problem in the US with its private health-care system than the UK. However, even in the UK, the better educated are more aware of the facilities available and of how to obtain them. It has also been shown that decisions about treatment are influenced not only by the social class and level of intelligence of the patient, but also by the interests and personality of the psychiatrist (Pallis and Staffelmayr, 1973).

Robins' second component is an evelution of the effectiveness of current child-psychiatric services, and this is the main theme of the research described in this chapter. An attempt has been made to compare and contrast the effectiveness of the special services which were available in the north-east of England for children suffering from more serious degrees of psychiatric disorder. For the purpose of this study all children with either psychotic or predominantly organic disorders were excluded, and children were selected aged between 7 years and 12 years 11 months.

Four different categories of placement where children receive special attention for maladjustment or educational backwardness have been used in this study, as follows.

1 Schools geared specifically to maladjusted children—these consisted of residential and day settings.
2 Hospital-based services for maladjusted children—these consisted of outpatient, day or residential services.
3 A comparison group of maladjusted children in special schools for the

*Deceased.

mildly educationally subnormal—again, these were residential and day settings.

4   Finally, a control group of maladjusted children in ordinary schools—either in ordinary classes or in classes specially designed for educationally backward children (remedial classes).

At the beginning of the study the children were diagnosed as suffering from principally either a neurotic or an antisocial disorder. This diagnosis was reviewed annually, and at three defined points during the two years of this trial, the children's behavioural, educational and cognitive development were assessed in various ways.

This research had four main objectives. First, to evaluate the relative improvement within each setting of behavioural, educational, or cognitive development. Second, an attempt was made to identify the types of disorder which responded well in each setting. Third, an attempt to compare the settings was made. As the groups were not directly comparable, a statistical method was used in an attempt to allow for the effect of the nature of the maladjustment, particularly its severity but also its duration and complicating pre-existing family factors. Our objective has been, by use of statistical techniques, to allow for these confounding effects and, hopefully, to permit more valid comparisons to be made between the data. Fourth, the practical utility of current diagnostic systems has been examined with particular reference to outcome.

EFFECTIVENESS OF THERAPY

Earlier reviews of the effectiveness of psychotherapy in seriously maladjusted children came to the conclusion that the results were unimpressive. Such conclusions were based on pooling the results of treatment studies (Levitt, 1957, 1971) or actual systematic clinical study (Shepherd et al., 1971) and both approaches suggested that two-thirds of treated and untreated patients improved markedly so that treatment appeared to make little difference to outcome. However, recent reviews by Kolvin et al. (1981), Rutter (1982) and Kolvin et al. (1984) suggest there is little evidence to support such conclusions. In view of the recency and comprehensiveness of these three latter publications and the detailed literature search of Tramontana (1980), it does not seem sensible to attempt to replicate these in a brief chapter.

HYPOTHESES

The main hypotheses are:

1   These settings differ with respect to improvement in various measures of ability or psychiatric disorder.

2 (a) The responses of children with neurotic disorders differ between each placement, and similarly, (b) the responses of children with conduct disorders differ between each placement.

3 The improvement will be positively or negatively influenced by factors such as sex of child, family size, social factors, parent personality, attitudes and parent–child relationships, and also treatment available.

A subsidiary hypothesis arising from our first two main hypotheses is:

4 Treatment leads to behavioural, temperamental, social, educational and intellectual improvement.

METHOD

Definition of maladjustment

The maladjusted children in this study suffered from disorders which were, in our view, so severe (either in the distress caused to them, their families, or the community, or in the handicap to their inter-personal relationships, behaviour, or education) that they merited intensive treatment. It is in this sense that the term 'maladjustment' is applied throughout this paper, and closely follows that employed by Rutter *et al.* (1970).

The selection of cases

Two distinct samples of maladjusted children were selected for this study. The 'designated' maladjusted sample had been referred for treatment of a psychiatric disorder to a hospital unit or school setting specifically designed to help or treat children with serious degrees of maladjustment. The other sample—the 'screened' maladjusted—consisted of maladjusted children in ordinary or ESN schools in the community who had not been referred for help, but who were identified by means of a two-level screen. The first level consisted of a psychiatric interview. The second level consisted of summed scores from child interview, parent interview, and teacher questionnaires (after appropriate statistical standardization). Thus, the four groups of children studied were as follows.

'Designated' maladjusted

These consist of maladjusted children in, (a) schools for the maladjusted— residential or day settings, and (b) attending hospitals—inpatients or outpatients.

'Screened' maladjusted

(a) Maladjusted children in schools for the educationally subnormal (residential or day), and (b) maladjusted children in ordinary schools (ordinary classes or special).

The children who were receiving help at special schools or hospital units catering for the maladjusted were gathered from ten different educational or hospital establishments. As inclusion in the 'designated' group was the result of a referral for management to one of these types of setting, the group was studied in a similar way to the screened group, so as to permit comparisons. The children in the residential maladjusted schools were educated and also resided in the same setting. The hospital in patients lived in the hospital during the week and returned home at weekends. The hospital out patients attended ordinary schools, lived in their own homes, and attended hospital for therapy. The day-school settings for the maladjusted were more heterogeneous because of the greater degree of variability between establishments. The common factor in this latter subgroup was that the children attended for all or part of their day special schools or units outside ordinary schools which, during the period of the research, catered for maladjusted children who continued to live in their own homes.

By definition, the 'screened' maladjusted group was formed from maladjusted children attending either a residential or day school for the educationally subnormal, and from maladjusted children being educated at an ordinary school, a proportion of whom were receiving special remedial education. To obtain subjects for the educationally subnormal comparison group, the screen assessment described below was applied at three residential and eight day schools for the educationally subnormal. In the initial selection of the 'screened' maladjusted group, a broad match of ordinary schools with the social class distribution of the 'designated' maladjusted group was attempted. After consultation with officials of the Local Education Authority, six ordinary schools were chosen which contained a spread of families throughout the social-class spectrum but with a preponderance falling into the Registrar-General's social classes III and IV.

**The design of the selection screen for
'designated' and 'screened' maladjusted children**

A two-stage selection screen was employed. The first stage consisted of a psychiatric interview of each child of the type devised by Rutter and Graham (1968) and modified by Atkins and Kolvin (1976). Those children considered to be moderately or markedly maladjusted were identified, each child rated for the presence, dubious presence, or absence of specified number of items of behaviour. The second stage of the screen was a teacher questionnaire, designed and fully described by Rutter (1967) and Rutter et al. (1970), and a semi-structured interview with parents to gather information about their children's behaviour (Garside et al., 1973; Kolvin et al., 1975).

Constructing the screen score and group matching

The final screen score was formed from the sum of the scores on the three behavioural scales described above. This technique uses the statistical extreme as an indicator of psychiatric disturbance. No information was available on which to base a differential weighting system, and, therefore, it was decided that the scores on the three components of the screen should be treated as equally important. Consequently, the three scores were simply standardized and summed.

A major concern for the design of the selection screen was that it should identify a maladjusted control group comparable with the 'designated' maladjusted group both in the quantity of symptoms and in the severity of disorders estimated by clinical judgement. The methods used for such selection must give rise to adequate comparability (Shepherd *et al.*, 1966) in order for the findings of the research to be valid (Rutter, 1970). The mean screen scores of the groups were made comparable by simply eliminating the less-severely disturbed until the means of the summed standard scores showed equivalence.

However, despite achieving arithmetical equivalence between the groups, the subjective impression gained from psychiatric interviews, and also from the overall clinical ratings, was that the groups differed in certain quantitative and/or qualitative ways. This is due in part to the methods used, which were essentially symptom counts, and which at times are not adequately sensitive to the severity of an individual symptom. For example, a child with one incapacitating symptom may obtain a low score. Another important matter is the possible bias deriving from the use of psychiatric interview with the child as the initial screen instrument, *as it tends to under-select children with conduct as compared to neurotic disorders* (Rutter and Graham, 1968).

The group-matching techniques were nevertheless retained, as, while less precise than the pairwise matching of individuals, it has the advantage of reducing errors of measurement. Providing initial levels of group maladjustment are much the same, simple comparisons may be made directly between group improvements or reductions in the level of group maladjustment. Where initial levels do differ, such comparisons may be greatly affected by 'regression to the mean' whereby the highest scorers (the most maladjusted) tend to improve more than the lowest scorers (i.e. the least maladjusted) because of statistical effects (Garside, 1956). Some allowance may be made for some of the initial inequalities between groups by using statistical methods, but such statistical control is indirect and involves assumptions which may not be met in practice.

Rates of maladjustment

In the current study, about one-third of the children in the 'screened' maladjusted group attending ordinary schools were found to be as quantitatively disturbed as those in special residential settings for the maladjusted (see Table 12.6).

This finding has important planning and service implications demanding careful thought and sensible interpretation. It should be noted that a randomly drawn school population was not used during this research, but rather schools which were broadly representative of the social class of the 'designated' maladjusted sample; this may explain why the prevalence of maladjustment obtained over this wide age range is rather high.

The prevalence of serious maladjustment in the schools for the educationally subnormal was 38 per cent, which is similar to that found by other authors (Chazan, 1964; Rutter *et al.*, 1970). This high prevalence may, in part, reflect a policy of more readily admitting children with multiple problems (of behaviour, interpersonal relationships, intelligence and educational attainments) rather than on the basis of intelligence and attainments alone. Further, like Chazan and Williams, we found that the rate varied in different schools for the educationally subnormal.

Movement and losses

The original intention had been to gather at least 60 cases in each basic regime. This could have just been managed within the available research resources, and, after allowance for a small rate of attrition, would have sufficed for most statistical investigations. A total population of 275 severely maladjusted children was gathered. Before the initial assessment for research purposes, two families withdrew their children from the research, leaving an effective total of 273. Of these, full parent interview data was obtained on 264. However, even where parent interview data was not obtained, school data was collected.

Between the beginning and end of the study, thirteen children moved to a different type of setting and had been reclassified. The numbers attending each regime had been reduced by attrition and these changes are shown in Table 12.1. The rate of attrition between initial and final assessment was 11 per cent. However, this bare figure poorly represents the true attrition as it simultaneously over, and underestimates the size of, the loss. It ignores the data attrition which one would expect to be caused by difficulty in compiling complete research inventories when there is a high rate of problem families, poor literacy, poor memories, and varying co-operation or availability of the parents. It overestimates the rate in that some parents allowed their children to participate, although they themselves were personally unco-operative. Consequently, information was always sought from the schools and from the children themselves. High attrition rate undoubtedly introduces important biases as the least co-operative and mobile families have often been found to be overloaded with more seriously disturbed children (Robins, 1966; Shepherd *et al.*, 1971). We, therefore, considered it essential to ensure as complete a follow-up data as possible. Reasonably full information was obtained for 264 children, reducing the attrition rate to 4 per cent over the period of study. The different rates of

Table 12.1 Movement of cases during the period of study

'Designated' or 'screened'	Basic regimes	Size of group at initial placement	Change during trial		Size of group at final placement
			In	Out	
'Designated' maladjusted groups	Residential and day schools for the maladjusted*	71	9	5	75
	Hospital patients	72	2	7	67
'Screened' maladjusted groups	Residential and day schools for the educationally subnormal	69	2	1	70
	Ordinary schools*	61	0	0	61
Total population		273	13	13	273

*One maladjusted child from each of these regimes who dropped out before the initial assessment has not been included in this table.

attrition for each group of variables accounts for differences in total numbers in tables presenting the results of subsequent analyses.

Table 12.1 shows the movement between the four regimes during the period of the study. In particular, most movement is observed between groups attending residential schools for the maladjusted, day schools for the maladjusted, and hospital in patient departments (about 10 per cent of cases). Such movement might complicate statistical analyses, but it was found that when these cases were classified according to their initial placement only, measures of change between initial and final assessments did not significantly differ from mean values obtained using alternative forms of classification.

Timing of evaluation

The intermediate follow-up (first follow-up assessment) was at a median interval of fifteen to sixteen months. The final follow-up (second follow-up assessment) was at a median interval of twenty-six to twenty-eight months.

Sex and Age

The mean age of the children in the four regimes lay within a range of one year (10.3, 10.4, 10.9 and 11.1 years), the groups with highest means belonging to the ordinary school and educationally subnormal groups. The sex ratio was just short of two boys to one girl in all the groups except in the case of the schools for maladjusted children where it was five to one.

Follow-up method

We used two methods to compare the effects of the different regimes. The first, a simple clinical method, was to calculate the *outcome* using the formula suggested by Sainsbury (1975) and Kolvin *et al.* (1981) for each child. We calculated the number and percentage who showed good, moderate, and poor outcome for each regime from a clinical assessment of the records at each stage. Significance between groups was tested using the well-established χ^2 test. Outcome is a rather crude way of comparing progress, but has the advantage of presenting data in percentage form and, furthermore, gives added reassurance that the changes had clinical as well as statistical significance. The progress of the children was rated in three ways: in terms of disturbance of emotion (neurotic behaviour), disturbance of conduct (anti-social behaviour), and general disturbance (overall severity). It should be noted that all the children were scored on each of these three ratings of disturbance.

The second, more complex method was to compare regimes by using analyses of covariance. By this method, average *improvement* scores for each regime were compared for every measure separately at each subsequent follow-up.

The special feature of analysis of covariance is that differences between regimes in initial severity and other factors which may affect improvement are taken into account. After carrying out some preliminary analyses, the following factors were taken into account, (a) initial score of the criterion variable, (b) full-scale IQ, (c) index of social risk (representing adverse social factors), (d) index of psychosocial hazard (representing such factors in the child's formative years), (e) index of emotional disorder (representing emotional disorder in the family).

Analysis of covariance compares, for different regimes, the changes that occur in a number of variables after allowance for the effects of modifying factors (covariates). It provides a way of measuring the extent of the mean improvement of each group in each variable in terms of mean change scores. These improvements were made comparable (by dividing by the appropriate standard deviation) and were summed to give an overall improvement score for each regime. This procedure, which gives equal weight to all the variables, was applied to the eighteen variables which conformed to the necessary assumptions underlying analysis of covariance.

Many of the relevant methodological issues are dealt with in greater detail elsewhere, where we report on a parallel study (Kolvin et al., 1981 pp.344–345; see also Chapter 13) in particular the assumptions underlying covariance analysis and also interaction effects.

Comments on the design

The design of this study did not use random allocation of children to relatively homogeneous, specific treatment regimes. Rather it could be described as a 'natural experiment' evaluating the range of services available for seriously maladjusted children in one area of the North of England. As the children were directed on clinical grounds into different regimes, the research lacks the rigorous control of an experimental design. However, this prospective research design often has been usefully employed in behavioural research (Kerlinger, 1969). An important recent study evaluating the specific educational treatment of autistic children is a good example of such a research design (Rutter and Bartak, 1973).

With this 'naturalistic' design, it is essential to seek simple ways of describing the differing treatments and patterns of care provided in different service units, as one wishes to attempt to relate differences in improvement in the children in such service units, not only to the differences in the broad pattern of care, but also to differences in the treatment provided by these units. This design is less than ideal and is likely to yield positive results only if both the patterns of care and the amount and type of treatment vary sufficiently *between* groups and to a greater extent than *within* the groups. These units of service are administratively distinct, and are described in the next section.

BACKGROUNDS OF STUDY CHILDREN AND THEIR SCHOOL TREATMENT SETTING

Family environment and attitude

The study was undertaken in an industrial area in north-east England with a stable population of approximately 800 000 and minimal recent immigration. The general educational provision, supporting educational and health services were of a high standard. As compared with the local population (Neligan *et al.*, 1974), the social class distribution of the families studied showed an excess in the semi-skilled and unskilled categories (20 per cent of local population and 52 per cent of study families).

Parental interviews were undertaken on three occasions and were designed to obtain family, social and behavioural data about the children in the study. The interviews were undertaken by a trained psychiatric social worker, assisted in the early stages by two trained social interviewers. A standardized semi-structured and open-ended technique was used at each of the three interviews, and information gathered on many measures, including parental and early life experiences, family background and other psychological factors. Findings in this section relate to the initial interviews, completed shortly after the child's entry into one of the four regimes.

Social class and employment

In eight families (29 per cent of the study population) there was either no effective breadwinner or he was not gainfully employed or his whereabouts were unknown; and, in a further seven families, the breadwinner had retired; as almost all had been unskilled they had been included in the social class V category. This high proportion of 'out of work' families was nearly five times the regional unemployment rate at that time.

Age and civil status of parents

The average age at initial assessment was 37.4 years for mothers and 40.7 years

Table 12.2 Social class distribution of the families

Social class	Schools for maladjusted	Hospitals	ESN Schools	Ordinary Schools	Total
I + II	2(3)	17(24)	1(1)	6(10)	26(9.5)
III	26(36)	33(46)	19(28)	28(45)	106(38.5)
IV + V unemployed	44(61)	22(30)	49(71)	28(45)	143(52)
Total	72(100)	72(100)	69(100)	62(100)	275(100)

Note: The numbers in brackets are percentages.

for fathers, with no significant differences between groups. Only 68 per cent of the parents in the study were living together, and 12.5 per cent of the children were begin raised in single-parent families.

Family discord

A focused parental interview was undertaken to provide frequency and intensity scores of family discord, and these were summated into a composite score. No significant differences were found between the groups.

Composite scores of adverse experiences

A large quantity of data (thirty-eight measures) on various types of personal, family and environmental adversity was collected. These were combined into conceptually meaningful groups to provide composite scores of adverse experiences. A list of the items which contributed to each composite score is available on request. The composite scores used were as follows.

1   Perinatal (covers six major perinatal difficulties).
2   Physical development (five items of milestone development).
3   Post-natal organic scale (three items covering fits, head injuries etc.).
4   Physical handicap (covers five items, including vision and hearing).
5   Psychological (covers main four life events prior to child's first year, i.e. emotional, financial, and physical illnesses).
6   Psychosocial hazard (six items covering parental separation etc.)
7   Social adversity (six items covering overcrowding and other adverse social experiences).

   In addition, five other composites reflecting family psychiatric disorder were developed—alcoholism and sociopathy (two items); institutionalization (two items); special school or hospitalization (four items); family emotional illness (three items); severe mental illness (three items).
   From examination of Table 12.3, the broad pattern which emerges is that the mean scores of the composites were usually highest (i.e. most adverse) in the groups attending special schools for the maladjusted and educationally subnormal. As it is also the case that the lower occupational strata have the most adverse composite scores, we concluded that these scores broadly reflect social influences.

Maternal factors

Mother's personality

This was measured using the Eysenck personality inventory (Eysenck and Eysenck, 1975). The mean scores of the total sample showed that mothers of

Table 12.3   Comparison of personal, family and environmental adversity in the four groups. Groups ranked according to means of composites

	Schools for maladjusted	Hospitals	ESN schools	Ordinary schools
Scales Related to Birth and Child Development				
a. Perinatal Risk	Intermediate (2.5)	Least Adverse (1)	Most Adverse (4)	Intermediate (2.5)
b. Poor Physical Development	Least Adverse (1)	Intermediate (2)	Most Adverse (4)	Intermediate (3)
c. Post-natal Risk	Most Adverse (4)	Intermediate (2.5)	Intermediate (2.5)	Least Adverse (1)
d. Physical Handicap	Most Adverse (3.5)	Most Adverse (3.5)	Intermediate (2)	Least Adverse (1)
e. Psychological Risk in Neonatal Period	Intermediate (3)	Intermediate (2)	Most Adverse (4)	Least Adverse (1)
Scales Related to Social and Family Factors				
a. Psychosocial Hazard	Most Adverse (4)	Intermediate (2)	Intermediate (3)	Least Adverse (1)
b. Social Adversity	Most Adverse (3.5)	Intermediate (2)	Intermediate (3.5)	Least Adverse (1)
c. Alcoholism and Sociopathy	Most Adverse (4)	Intermediate (2)	Intermediate (3)	Least Adverse (1)
d. Prolonged Institutionalization	Intermediate (3)	Intermediate (2)	Most Adverse (4)	Least Adverse (1)
e. Special School/Hospitalization	Most Adverse (4)	Intermediate (2)	Intermediate (3)	Least Adverse (1)
f. Family Emotional Illness	Least Adverse (1)	Most Adverse (4)	Intermediate (2.5)	Intermediate (2.5)
g. Severe Mental Illness	Most Adverse (4)	Least Adverse (1)	Intermediate (2.5)	Intermediate (2.5)
Total of "Most Adverse"	7	2	5	0
Social Class (Ranked)	3	1 (Best)	4 (Poorest)	2

Note: Ranks 1 = Best : 4 = Poorest or Worst

maladjusted children are significantly more introverted and neurotic than mothers of a random sample of children in Newcastle upon Tyne (Neligan *et al.*, 1976). However, there were no differences between the four groups.

Maternal attitudes

The Maryland self-rating inventory was completed by mothers at the initial interview and provides measures of discipline, indulgence, protection, and rejection (Pumroy, 1966). While the use of questionnaires about parents' attitudes is still the subject of considerable debate, it remains an economic way of obtaining additional information.

Only on the subscales of discipline and indulgence were significant differences between the highest and lowest mean scores of the groups found. There were two broad identifiable patterns: first, parents of maladjusted children in ordinary schools were the most disciplinarian and the least indulgent; second, the parents of children recently admitted into schools for the maladjusted were the least disciplinarian and the most indulgent.

Child-handling techniques

The child-handling techniques customarily used by the parents were assessed by means of the focused maternal interview technique which is described elsewhere (Kolvin *et al.*, 1975) using some of the themes described by Sears *et al.* (1957). Four measures are included—permissiveness, use of negative rewards, use of reasoning, and encouragement of emotive verbalization. Significant differences occurred between the highest and lowest mean scores for two of these. With regard to their use of reasoning and the encouragement of discussion about emotive topics, mothers in the hospital group were most likely to use these techniques while mothers of children in schools for the educationally subnormal were least likely to use them. The lack of any significant differences on the two remaining scales suggests a similarity in handling techniques across the groups.

It is not possible to say whether the parental techniques were influenced by the child's behaviour or vice versa. As maladjusted children in ESN schools received relatively low parental ratings of behaviour difficulties (see later) in comparison with the other groups, it is unlikely that it is the severity of the children's disturbance which determines how the parents respond. Other parent and child factors may be implicated—such as poorer social circumstances and their attendant stresses, and the comparative dullness of the children in these groups.

Family and child sociability

A key function of the family concerns its socialization of the parents and also helping children assimilate and incorporate cultural standards and values.

The Wallin's Neighbourliness Scale (1954) is a simple measure of the number and type of contacts a family employs with its neighbours. It was found that the most socially isolated families were those in the educationally subnormal group and further it is this group who had received least help from professional social workers. It may be their very isolation which places them in a poor position to obtain help from other sources (Bergin, 1966).

The parents' poor social contacts appear to be mirrored by the child's low degree of supervised community contact. The educationally subnormal group again had few extra-familial contacts. Lack of home-based community contacts was also reported by the vast majority of those recently admitted to residential schools for the educationally subnormal and for the maladjusted. This is not surprising as attendance as a residential school is likely to interfere with the maintenance of contacts with home but community isolation may have also predated the admission.

Description of the units of service and treatment received

To minimize selection bias, consecutive children admitted to any of the participating units and who fulfilled the other criteria for the sample were included in the study. As almost without exception every major 'treatment' unit participated, the regimes must be considered broadly representative of services available at that time in the north-east. While it is uncertain that the findings of a local study can be generalized beyond similar communities, the converse is also true—the national picture no more represents local circumstance, than such circumstances represent the national picture. However, provided the local area is carefully described, then comparative local studies may contribute information on critical characteristics, such as family factors and type of behaviour disorder, which continue to be important, irrespective of community differences.

The children selected for inclusion in the study attended one of about fifty different educational or hospital establishments which have been grouped into the four different regimes previously described. In hospitals, educational facilities were available on the premises, while hospital out patients attended their local ordinary schools. Some schools were specifically for the maladjusted and others for the educationally subnormal; for both residential and day provision existed. In ordinary schools, maladjusted children were drawn from both ordinary classes and remedial classes.

Information about the type and amount of treatment received by a child and his family was obtained from a case-note review for each while he attended hospital. For the other children, information was obtained from their schools using a questionnaire covering the following six topics: sessions of individual psychotherapy; group therapy, casework with parents; pharmacotherapy; additional placements before criterion placement; additional placements over the total period of study. All schools replied to the questionnaire, but varied in the amount of information proffered. Staff of schools for the maladjusted appeared to have a comprehensive knowledge of the child's background and of any help given. In contrast, most of the staff of schools for the educationally subnormal and ordinary schools felt that they knew less. Nevertheless, the picture obtained was broadly validated by the parents' account. However, as expected the ordinary schools particularly underestimated the help the child and family had received.

From a simple analysis of additional factual data also available from the schools (pupil:teacher ratios, staff characteristics, psychological and psychiatric resources, community involvement and other factors), it also became evident that there were not only differences between the four types of settings, but also variations within each type of regime.

Length of stay in different settings

The main movement of children over the course of the study occurred between hospital and the maladjusted schools. Inpatients did not usually stay in hospitals for more than six months. About 30 per cent of the total hospital group moved to either residential schools (not necessarily specifically for the maladjusted) or to day units for the maladjusted. Very little exchange took place between residential and day schools for the maladjusted with the majority of children remaining in the same special school throughout the period of study.

For some of the children, however, placement in a residential school for the maladjusted was not necessarily the first nor the final placement. While many returned to ordinary schools, some required further special placement. This pattern of long-term need, perhaps extending into young adulthood, applied to a considerable number of children in residential establishments. As a result of the intractable nature of their disturbance the final placement for some was in a community home or Borstal.

Treatment and management

Table 12.4 shows that the maladjusted children at ordinary schools received little help of any kind, and those at schools for the educationally subnormal barely more. The help given to the hospital group exceeded that given to any group in every category except for treatment prior to the study. The differences are considerable and cover almost every form of help or treatment before or during the course of the study. The group in schools for the maladjusted also received more help, especially in the form of social casework, group therapy, and previous out-patient help, than did the 'screened' maladjusted groups. The principal differences between the maladjusted schools group and the hospital

Table 12.4 'Treatment' and additional resources

	Schools for maladjusted	Hospitals	ESN schools	Ordinary schools
Help prior to study				
(a) Out patient treatment	Much	Some	Little	Very little
(b) In special educational				
unit/setting	Little	Very little	Some	Very little
Help during study				
(a) Individual psychotherapy				
based on more than				
6 sessions	Little	Very much	Little	Very little
(b) Group therapy	Some	Some	Very little	
(c) Social casework	Very much	Very much	Very little	Very little
(d) Pharmacotherapy	Little	Some	Very little	Very little
Further special placement				
during study	Little	Some	Very little	Very little
Social work contact since				
inclusion in study				
More than ten contacts	56	51	18	? very little
Parental dissatisfaction with				
special placement	20%	33%	40%	—

Very little = Under 20 per cent of the sample.
Little   = Between 20 per cent and 40 per cent of the sample.
Some   = Between 40 per cent and 60 per cent of the sample.
Much   = Between 60 per cent and 80 per cent of the sample.
Very much = Over 80 per cent of the sample.

group lies in more individual psychotherapy given to the latter, and more frequent prior treatment given to the former.

The majority of children who attended schools for the maladjusted had previously received from some form of help, (e.g. out-patient or child guidance work, but also for some lengthy periods as a hospital inpatient). Although it was usually children with the more intractable disorders that were transferred to schools for the maladjusted, improvement that may have occurred before their inclusion in a particular criterion group at the beginning of the study should not be ignored. It should be noted, however, that the rate of exclusion from ordinary schools before placement in a residential school for the maladjusted was exceptionally high at 40 per cent. (The next highest — 12 per cent was the group attending a residential school for the educationally subnormal).

Nearly all children who attended the various hospital groups received traditional individual psychotherapy and most parents were counselled by the social worker assigned to the case. Individual psychotherapy was usually brief and was provided weekly or fortnightly and was based upon broad psychodynamic principles and was undertaken either by consultant child psychiatrists or by trainee psychiatrists under consultant supervision. This was supplemented by the milieu therapy which was available daily to all day patients and inpatients. The hospital group more often received psychotropic drugs, probably because of the nature of those disorders displayed by patients in in-patient departments, and the immediate involvement of medically qualified staff. Behaviour therapy principles were well understood by the in-patient teaching and nursing staff, but were not generally employed except occasionally as an adjunct to the therapeutic milieu in specific disorders such as encopresis. In addition to the various daily activities and therapeutic groups in which participation was required, hospital day and in patients also spent at least one session per week in drama therapy.

Thus children in 'designated' residential settings for the maladjusted had very much more therapy of all kinds than did the educationally subnormal group or the ordinary school group.

Remedial education

Information was obtained about the extent, but not the quality, of remedial education. By definition it was readily available in remedial classes and comprised at least a quarter of the school work. About 35 per cent of the children in this group received at least two years full-time teaching in a remedial class. The remainder received remedial teaching for about a quarter of their lessons, for 55 per cent for between one and two years. Additional remedial help was universally available to children in schools for the maladjusted and to those in hospital settings.

Social work contacts

Retrospective information from the schools about the amount and type of counselling that a child and family may have received was supplemented by comparable information obtained from the parents. The comparison between data supplied from these two different sources is discussed below. Reactions and attitudes to help received were also assessed from parents.

Table 12.4 also gives the distribution of social-work sessions since referral. The group from schools for the maladjusted had received the highest average number of sessions of social-work help, followed by the hospital group. The children in schools for the educationally subnormal had fewest contacts with social workers, despite the fact that on nearly all measures of environmental stress or deprivation the educationally subnormal group was found to have an excess over any of the other groups. Comparing parental reports of social-work contact with those obtained from official school records, it is clear that these two sets of accounts coincide remarkably well. The greatest discrepancy occurs in the educationally subnormal group in residential settings, where a higher percentage of parents reported social-work contact that was suggested by school figures. The most likely explanation is that particularly deprived groups were receiving social-work support from several other sources, without the knowledge of the school authorities.

The predominant pattern of social work undertaken tended to involve mothers only. When it did occur, the inclusion of other family members, particularly fathers, was most common where children attended special schools for the maladjusted or were hospital in patients. Although the educationally subnormal group had received some help from social workers, minimal contact existed between parents and school, and this group contained a high proportion of parents who were dissatisfied with the school.

Variations within a regime

It should be noted that the maladjusted schools varied greatly in the amounts and types of treatment they provided, or in the services available to them. Although, in general the availability of help from psychologists and social workers varied considerably, some schools for the maladjusted in particular had a wide repertoire of techniques and professionals at their disposal, and they often employed several in the management of one child. In such a one, a child would typically have received several sessions with a psychiatrist over the course of a year, participated in a daily school group, had some individual counselling sessions at school and, in addition, his parents received frequent therapy (casework) from the social worker attached to the school. Thus, for such a child, the type and amount of treatment received reflected not only the severity of the disorder, but also the local resources available to meet his needs. However, in other schools psychiatric services were virtually non-existent because of their geographical isolation, and liaison with educational and social-service departments was tenuous or difficult to maintain.

Discussion and conclusion

The distribution of adverse parental and family influences amongst the groups closely resembles the pattern of environmental disadvantages previously described. This raises two key issues. First and foremost, there are major differences between the groups with regard to family variables and aspects of the child's wider environment. Second, the harshest conditions are consistently found among the same families, which are those of children in special schools for the maladjusted or for the educationally subnormal. These children, therefore, suffer from multiple social, psychological and frequently severe educational handicaps. One way for making allowance for these differences is by the use of multivariate statistical techniques.

Without the benefit of data from prospective studies, only tentative explanations can be offered as to why the families of children in these long-term placements experience greater parental and environmental adversity. The most plausible explanation is that maladjusted children who, through persistent failure, find their way into a long-term special setting, are those who have been previously or persistently exposed to the most adverse parental and familial influences. For example, the presence of high rates of family discord is a commonly associated feature of children with anti-social problems (Rutter, 1971; see also Chapter 6) and adverse social circumstances and poor family relationships are associated with child psychiatric disorders in general (Rutter and Madge, 1976). Nevertheless, the mechanisms by which psychiatrically disordered children reach such placements are not clearly understood. In any individual case, child behaviour, adverse family relationships, parental attitudes and poor

Table 12.5 Some child behaviour scores—ranked (and some family factors)

	Schools for maladjusted	Hospitals	ESN schools	Ordinary schools	Significance between highest and lowest means
Parent interview					
Neurotic scale	3	4	2	1	$p < 0.01$
Conduct scale	4	3	2	1	$p < 0.01$
Psychosomatic	3	4	1	2	$p < 0.01$
Motor/activity	4	2.5	2.5	1	NS
Global behaviour	3	4	2	1	$p < 0.01$
Temperament					
Activity intensity	4	2	3	1	NS
Mood	2.5	4	2.5	1	$p < 0.01$
Irregularity	4	3	1	2	$p < 0.01$
Teacher scale					
Neurotic subscore	2.5	4	2.5	1	$p < 0.01$
Antisocial subscore	3.5	1.5	3.5	1.5	$p < 0.05$
Total score	3	2	4	1	$p < 0.05$
Psychiatric interview					
Neurotic score[†]	4	3	1	2	$p < 0.01$
Sociability score[*]	3	2	4	1	$p < 0.01$
Motor activity score[*]	4	1	3	2	$p < 0.05$
Inaccessibilty score[†]	3	1.5	4	1.5	$p < 0.01$

Notes: Rank 4 = Highest adverse score or highest deviance
Rank 1 = Lowest adverse score or lowest deviance
Means are presented in rank order for each dimension.
[*]Clinical dimensions
[†] Dimensions derived from factor analysis

discipline combine to produce a complicated picture, and the nature of this combination may be of prime importance in determining the treatment or management plan, including long-term placement. The higher parental discipline and lesser indulgence among the others of maladjusted children in ordinary schools may enable the child to fit into his or her natural environment without resorting to special treatment. A more unlikely explanation for the poor discipline and pattern of indulgence among mothers of special-school children is that parental reactions are secondary to the child's admission to a special school, which the parents see as having low prestige and this generates a sense of guilt or failure which may give rise to over-compensatory permissiveness or indulgence.

The four different regimes clearly differ in the frequency and type of treatment provided, with the two 'screened' maladjusted groups receiving very little help of any kind beyond that generally provided in the educational setting itself. The two 'designated' maladjusted groups differed considerably from one another in the type of treatment received, but within the 'schools for the maladjusted' groups considerable variation existed in frequency of additional treatment. Our overall impression, however, is that the differences in patterns of care and treatment was greater between groups than within any of the four groups (Table 12.5).

FINDINGS ON INITIAL ASSESSMENT

Child behaviour

Parental ratings of behaviour and temperament

The children's current behaviour and temperamental characteristics were assessed, based on focused parental interviews, using a series of reliable five-point unipolar rating scales (Kolvin et al., 1975, Garside et al., 1975). On the basis of this data a broad pattern emerged from the rankings of the mean scores of the groups on the behaviour and temperament dimensions (see Table 12.5). The hospital and the maladjusted school groups had the worse rankings (i.e. most adverse scores). The groups at schools for the educationally subnormal obtained some favourable rankings (i.e. less adverse scores), and the ordinary school group had the most favourable rankings of all.

Teacher ratings

The Rutter Teacher Scale, which has been extensively described in the literature (Rutter et al., 1970), is a short questionnaire of known reliability and validity. Four of the items may be summed to produce a 'neurotic' subscore, and a further six items yield an 'antisocial' subscore. The pattern on the neurotic subscale was similar to that found with the neurotic dimension on the parent-assessed behaviour scale. On the antisocial scale, the pattern differs somewhat from the parental account: the children at special schools (for the educationally subnormal and maladjusted) had high rankings, while the hospital and ordinary-school children had low rankings (i.e. were less deviant).

Some comments need to be made about the different problems which occur when information is obtained from parents and teachers. Apart from some correspondence between the conduct scale and the temperament dimension of 'activity intensity', there is relatively poor agreement between data obtained from parental interview and from teacher ratings of conduct disorder. It may well be attributable to the failure of research workers to find appropriately comparable measures of behaviour, or to the fact that behaviour is situation-specific (Semler, 1960; Kolvin *et al.*, 1977). On the other hand, we did find correspondence between school-reported and parent-reported neurotic behaviour, and this may in part be due to the larger number of scales on the parent inventory related to neurotic behaviour (5) in comparison with antisocial behaviour (2).

Psychiatric interview

The psychiatric interview employed was a semi-structured one (Atkins and Kolvin, 1976), modelled on that originally described by Rutter and Graham (1968). The first part of the interview was designed to set the child at ease and to facilitate the establishment of a relationship between the child and the interviewer. Thereafter, more systematic interviewing included twenty-three specific items, concerning subjects such as anxieties, fears and relationships. In addition, the child was rated on twenty-six features of behaviour or reactions observed by the interviewer. The children attending schools for the educationally subnormal and ordinary schools were interviewed 'blind'; all the children in the specified class, regardless of possible maladjustment, were interviewed. The data was reduced to nine dimensions by summating various items either on the basis of findings from multivariate analyses or because the items appeared to represent a clinical entity. The highest (i.e. worst) overall ranks were obtained by the educationally subnormal and maladjusted school groups. The children in schools for the educationally subnormal had the poorest sociability and also proved particularly inaccessible during interview. Maladjusted children in ordinary schools proved to be the most sociable.

Classification and severity of disorder

When comprehensive information became available from parents, school and interview, the nature and severity of the predominant disorder for each subject was assessed clinically. The distinction of disorders into two broad categories of neurotic and antisocial or conduct disorders is made throughout the literature, whether in clinical studies or in those employing multivariate analysis. Rutter *et al.* (1970) were able to classify 90 per cent of their cases into 'conduct', 'neurotic' and 'mixed conduct' disorders. However, as they found that their 'mixed' group had much in common with their 'pure' conduct disorders, for the purpose of this research it was decided to classify the cases according to one of the two diagnostic groups (neurotic and antisocial, with the mixed included in the latter) or normal variation. Diagnosis was dependent only on the actual presence of symptoms and not on the basis of previous history or causes. The symptoms which suggested a diagnosis of neurotic disorder were anxiety, sensitivity, obsessive-compulsive phenomena, phobias, bodily symptoms, hypochondriasis and hysteria. Conduct disorder was indicated by tantrums, destructiveness, lying, stealing, truanting, abnormal interpersonal relationships and various types of delinquency.

It was possible, without very great difficulty, to classify all cases, and it was not necessary to create an 'other' category. However, probably about 5–10 per cent of the cases could have been classified differently by other research workers applying slightly different criteria. In fact, about two-thirds of the children were classified as suffering from neurotic disorder and the remaining one-third were classified as showing conduct disorder. On forty-one cases a highly satisfactory coefficient of agreement (Kappa; Cohen, 1960) of 0.9 was obtained between the two diagnosticians (IK and RW) for these three unordered categories.

In addition, the cases were rated for severity of disturbance on three separate dimensions: overall disorder, and for severity of *any* conduct or neurotic symptoms, employing four-point scales: 1 = no disorder; 2 = possible disorder; 3 = moderately severe disorder; 4 = markedly severe disorder. Inter-rater reliability on the forty-one cases was as follows: overall clinical severity, $r = 0.67$; conduct dimension, $r = 0.89$; neurotic dimension, $r = 0.58$.

The severe degrees of psychiatric disorders which were encountered in the project is reflected in the figure of 69 per cent of children being rated as showing 'marked' overall severity of disorder. In Table 12.6 the data is arranged to facilitate comparison between the 'screened' and 'designated' groups. Although the 'screened' maladjusted group had arithmetical equivalence to the 'designated' group on the summated screen measures, the two groups differ greatly in relation to the clinically derived measure of severity. Thus arithmetical equivalence of symptoms between the 'screened' and 'designated' groups does not necessarily imply clinical equivalence; the search for arithmetical comparability of symptoms may conceal the variety, complexity and severity of child disturbance. For this reason the variable of overall severity was considered crucial and has been included as a covariate in our measurement of change by analysis of covariance.

Similar differences can be seen for the other clinical dimensions (Table 12.6). For instance, the children in maladjusted school and hospital settings are clinically more severely neurotic and have equal ratings on overall clinical

Table 12.6 Classification and severity (percentage)

Group	Schools for maladjusted (n = 71)	Hospitals (n = 72)	ESN* schools (n = 68)	Ordinary schools (n = 61)	Total (n = 272)
Classification					
Conduct	55	18	46	25	35
Neurotic	45	82	54	75	65
Conduct dimension					
1	14	37	22	47	30
2	17	24	18	23	21
3	14	15	22	15	16
4	55	24	38	15	33
Neurotic dimension					
1	3	0	2	3	2
2	9	5	18	15	11
3	34	24	44	61	40
4	53	71	37	21	47
Overall severity					
1	0	0	0	0	0
2	0	1	0	3	2
3	11	11	38	62	29
4	89	87	62	34	69

1 = Nil;   2 = dubious severity;   3 = moderate severity;   4 = severe.
*One case insufficient information for classification

severity. However, the hospital group has a lesser degree of severity on the conduct dimension, but more on the neurotic dimension than the maladjusted school group. Antisocial behaviour of some severity is a particular characteristic of children in schools for the maladjusted and the educationally subnormal. The information in this table has not, to our knowledge, been studied hitherto, and merits close scrutiny.

The raw data on past duration of disorder is available on request but the essential finding was that children in ordinary schools had the shortest duration of disorder and those in schools for the maladjusted had the longest duration. The importance of duration of disorder is discussed also in Chapter 6 of this volume.

Differences between children suffering from conduct and neurotic disorders

The data so far has been presented in percentages according to the different groups which have been defined for study. It is also of interest that for at least one set of data the children's behaviour is viewed in relation to the diagnostic classification into conduct or neurotic disorder. Consequently, the mean score on each psychiatric interview dimension was calculated separately for the children with conduct and neurotic disorders. (Differences in their family background are presented later.)

It was found that while maladjusted children in ordinary schools, whether suffering from conduct or neurotic disorders, have good sociability, those in schools for the educationally subnormal have poor sociability. As expected, children with conduct disorders had the most adverse mean scores on the antisocial attitudes, acting-out, and motor-activity dimensions, and those with neurotic disorders the most adverse mean scores on the phobic anxiety, interview affect, interview anxiety, and neurotic dimensions, irrespective of regime. Finally, with regard to inaccessibility (poor rapport), the more unfavourable mean scores are held by children with conduct disorders, in particular those in the educationally subnormal group, and least unfavourable in the hospital group.

Physical and neurological functioning

The most striking finding was that only a third of the study population were on or above the median (fiftieth percentile) height for their age, and about 36 per cent were below the lower quartile (twenty-fifth percentile). However, these total figures concealed the wide differences between groups. Poor physical growth was particularly evident in the educationally subnormal group. Similarly, only a third of the study population were on or above the median weight for their age, and 39 per cent were below the lower quartile. These figures broadly resemble those for height and are highly significant. The group with the greatest proportion of underweight children was again the educationally subnormal.

Few children had abnormal neurological signs on examination. Though hard signs were particularly rare, soft signs were more common. A review of the distribution of scores of 'soft' neurological signs led to the decision that an extreme score would be one of 9 or more. Only about one in six children had such a score. An analysis by group indicated that the highest scores occurred in the educationally subnormal group.

To sum up, the educationally subnormal maladjusted group has the highest loadings of adverse social factors, highest mean family size and poorer physical and neurological development than the other groups. It should be noted that poor physical development is commonly found in maladjusted educationally subnormal children (Chazan, 1965) and in ordinary educationally subnormal children (Jones and Murray, 1958). (We were unable to measure the stature of the non-maladjusted children in screened ESN or remedial classes.) The relative absence of children with epilepsy associated with structural brain damage or children with other clear-cut evidence of structural brain damage in this sample is simply because we had decided not to include in the study those children whose major disorder was organic brain disease.

Intellectual and educational functioning

The following measures were employed: Wechsler Intelligence Scale for Children; the Schonell Graded Word Reading Test (Form A) and Spelling Test (Form A); and the Staffordshire Arithmetic Test.

Our study does not have a normal control group, but instead has used a large number of comparison groups. Consequently, the data permit study of:

1 IQ levels and educational attainments of maladjusted children in different settings.
2 Verbal and performance IQ levels and educational attainments in relation to different types of psychiatric disorder.
3 Verbal performance discrepancies in relation to different types of disorder (expressed as differences between the means of verbal and performance IQs for the different groups).

Cognitive development

Table 12.7 shows that the mean intelligence of the maladjusted children was closely tied to the special settings in which they had been placed. Children in schools for the educationally subnormal had mean full-scale IQs more than two standard deviations (30 points) below the Wechsler norm of 100. The mean IQ of all the other groups fell within 1 standard deviation of the norm. Hospital patients had the highest mean IQs. However, the most constant finding for all groups was the discrepancy between the mean verbal and mean performance IQs in favour of the latter. The differences were significant for all groups except the hospital group. The association of social class and intelligence in our groups of maladjusted children is confirmed by the very close correspondence of the ranked order of the mean total IQ for the groups and the social-class rankings.

The next table (Table 12.8) shows the relationships between type of disorder and level of intelligence. Both the mean verbal and performance IQs of children

Table 12.7 Mean IQ and educational attainments (and social class ranked for comparison)

	Schools for maladjusted	Hospitals	ESN schools	Ordinary schools
Mean verbal IQ	92	105	67	92
Mean performance IQ	99	107	73	98
Mean full scale IQ	94	106	67	94
Mean Reading Quotient	75	98	60	85
Verbal IQ – Reading Quotient	17	7	7	7
Social class rankings	3	1	4	2

Table 12.8   Intelligence and type of psychiatric disorder in total sample

Disorder	Number	Verbal IQ		Performance	
		Mean	SD	Mean	SD
Conduct disorder	84	83	18.4	90	19.4
Neurotic disorder	159	91	21.2	95	21.7

with conduct disorders are significantly lower than those of the children with neurotic disorders. The pattern remains broadly the same for the four groups of children we have studied.

As the sample was selected to be representative of certain special settings and not for the maladjusted children generally, the intelligence levels do not reflect the general level intelligence of maladjusted children in the community. Furthermore, the picture in the ordinary school group is especially likely to be an underestimate as there is a degree of overloading with remedial children.

It is tempting to theorize that, in conduct disorder, adverse social influences, truancy (Kolvin and Ounsted, 1968) and the educational failure consequent upon a relatively low IQ (Mangus, 1950; Rutter et al., 1970) interact and thus exacerbate the poor intellectual performance and educational achievements of children with conduct disorders. On the other hand, it may also be the case that delinquency may arise as a maladaptive response to educational failure (Rutter et al., 1970; Sturge, 1982).

Educational attainments

There was retardation in all groups with the exception of maladjusted children in ordinary schools. This is illustrated by considering the discrepancy between verbal IQ and the Reading Quotient which provides a rough indication (Table 12.7) (although the means and the standard deviations of the two tests are not in fact similar). The verbal IQ has been chosen because it is a good predictor of educational achievement. The greatest discrepancies between the means were for the groups in schools for the maladjusted, serving to emphasize the profound need for remedial education among children selected for admission to these schools.

This study cannot answer the question of whether it is severity of maladjustment which determines the severity of educational backwardness, or whether it is those children who are both maladjusted and seriously failing academically who are selected for special placements on a longer basis in schools for the maladjusted. The spelling achievements proved even poorer than the Reading Quotient achievements, but closely parallels the pattern of Reading Quotient already described. Although the reading and spelling deficits of our groups are dramatic enough, the deficits in arithmetic skills for all groups are

Table 12.9 Family differences between conduct-disordered and neurotically-disordered children

	Significance level
1 Social class	*
2 Parent civil state	*
3 Family size	**
'At risk' scores	
4 Perinatal	NS
5 Psychological	NS
6 Physical developmental risk	NS
7 Postnatal risk	NS
8 Psychosocial	**
9 Social	**
10 Physical handicap	*
Family risk scores	
11 Alcoholism/sociopathy	***
12 Prolonged institutionalism (immediate family history)	***
13 Special school/hospital (immediate family history)	*
14 Emotional illness (immediate family history)	NS
15 Severe mental illness (immediate family history)	*
Attitudes and personality	
16 Mother's extroversion	NS
17 Mother's neuroticism	*
18 Discipline (Maryland)	NS
19 Indulgence	NS
20 Protectiveness	NS
21 Rejection	NS
Child-rearing	
22 Total permissiveness	*
23 Negative rewards	*
24 Use of reasoning	*
25 Total family discord	*
Community contact	
26 Neighbourliness	NS

Note: Conduct disorder scores higher on all items.
  *Significant difference ($p < 0.05$)
 **Significant difference ($p < 0.01$)
***Significant difference ($p < 0.001$)
NS not significant

particularly alarming; 97 per cent of the study population obtained an arithmetic quotient of less than 100 (the national average).

Differences between family backgrounds of conduct and neurotic disordered children

Conduct-disordered children are less likely to come from the higher social-class groups, and they are more likely to have experienced the separation or divorce of their parents (23 per cent as opposed to 11 per cent of children with neurotic disorders); conduct-disordered children also come from larger families (in this analysis defined as those with four or more children—68 per cent as opposed to 44 per cent). Seven indices of adverse family experience (the 'at risk' variables) were considered; on three of these, significant differences were found, and on the remaining four, the trend was for the conduct group to experience higher levels of adversity (Table 12.9).

Of the five global scores of family psychiatric disorder, four produced significantly higher scores for the conduct-disordered group. The children of these families were more familiar with the problems of alcoholism and sociopathy (46 per cent versus 17 per cent of the neurotic disordered); institutional experience (22 per cent versus 8 per cent); periods of care in special schools or psychiatric hospitals (24 per cent versus 13 per cent), and intra-family mental illness of a severe nature (16 per cent versus 8 per cent). The conduct and neurotic groups did not differ on the criterion of family history of 'emotional illness'. The various personality and attitudinal measures revealed only one significant difference between the groups. The mothers of conduct-disordered children obtained higher scores on the neurotic dimension of the EPI than mothers of neurotically disordered children.

Three child-handling variables showed a significant difference between the groups. The parents of conduct-disordered children were more permissive, used negative rewards more often (i.e. physical punishment, deprivation of privileges, and isolation), and were less likely to reason with their children. The total family discord score reflects the degree of interpersonal conflict within a family. This discord score was significantly higher in the conduct-disordered group.

Some idea of the extent to which families related to the wider community was available from the 'neighbourliness' rating. On this index the families of conduct- and neurotically disordered children did not differ significantly, although the families of conduct-disordered children tended to have fewer community and neighbourhood contacts.

FOLLOW-UP FINDINGS

Outcome (Table 12.10)

A steady reduction in symptomatology was usually noted in all four groups over the two years of the study. This was reflected in the very much smaller percentage

Table 12.10 Outcome in percentages

	(A) Schools for mal-adjusted	(B) Hospitals	(C) ESN schools	(D) Ordinary schools	Significance $p<0.05$	$p<0.01$
Overall severity						
After 1 year						
Good	8	13	17	43	(B)>(A)	(B)>(C)
Moderate	31	49	22	11		
Poor	61	38	61	46	(D)>(C)	(D)>(A),(B)
After 2½ years						
Good	20	37	16	43		
Moderate	40	46	26	13		(D)>(A),(C)
Poor	40	17	57	43		(B)>(A),(C),(D)
Antisocial behaviour						
After 1 year						
Good	11	34	17	36	(B)>(C)	(B)>(A)
Moderate	37	35	36	41		
Poor	52	31	46	23		(D)>(A),(C)
After 2½ years						
Good	18	51	21	47		(B)>(A),(C)
Moderate	37	31	31	26		
Poor	45	18	48	25		(D)>(A),(C)
Neurotic behaviour						
After 1 year						
Good	25	32	41	49		(B)>(C)
Moderate	31	41	16	16	(D)>(A)	
Poor	45	28	44	35		
$n=$	(65)	(68)	(69)	(61)		
After 2½ years						
Good	42	51	41	60	(B)>(A) ⎱ Almost i.e.	
Moderate	29	37	24	11	(D)>(C) ⎰ $p<0.1$	
Poor	29	12	35	28	(D)>(A)	(B)>(C)
$n=$	(65)	(65)	(68)	(60)		

of cases showing moderate or marked degrees of disturbance at the final assessment than at the initial assessment; and the very much greater percentage of the cases showing nil or 'dubious' severity at the end of the program compared with the beginning of the programme. This steady decrease in severity proved less marked at the intermediate follow-up than at the final assessment. However, such raw percentages merely describe clinical status, or how well the patients were at follow-up and therefore this data has not been presented. They do not take into consideration what we have previously defined as outcome, that is, how well the patients are at follow-up in relation to their status at the onset. The outcome findings are presented in percentage form as good moderate or poor in Table 12.10. In the analyses simple comparisons have been undertaken of each groups with every other group using a χ^2 technique.

Overall severity

Overall severity was a measure based on clinical judgement, taking all information into consideration. After one year both the ordinary school group and the hospital group have the most satisfactory outcome. The two special-school groups have poor outcome in more than 60 per cent of the cases. After 2½ years the percentage with good outcome is only high in the hospital group and the ordinary school group. Furthermore, all groups excepting the hospital group have a high percentage of the cases showing poor outcome. At this point in time the hospital group have significantly better outcome than the other three groups and the ordinary school group do better than the maladjusted school and the ESN school groups.

Antisocial behaviour

The hospital and the ordinary-school groups show very similar patterns of good outcome—each of them doing significantly better than the maladjusted school group and the ESN school group. After 2½ years the pattern remains remarkably similar. Again, there is not very much change in the case of the ESN school and the maladjusted school groups.

Neurotic behaviour

Satisfactory outcome is achieved by the hospital group after one year. After 2½ years the hospital group again has the highest percentage of cases with a satisfactory outcome, but this only proves significant in comparison with the ESN school group. On the other hand, the ordinary-school groups do particularly well in relation to good outcome, but this is counterbalanced by poor outcome in some 28 per cent of the cases—and they only do significantly better than the maladjusted school group.

Improvement

Our data has well demonstrated the great variability of behaviour and emotions of children according to their type, severity and their location. This merely underlines the difficulty of achieving comparability of type of disorders and of severity of disorder in any controlled study. It also reinforces the view that simple analyses of follow-up data of maladjustment provide simple and crude answers. In theory to obtain more precise answers and a more sophisticated level of understanding only multivariate analyses begin to meet the requirements. In practice, the findings using such multivariate techniques proved broadly similar to the outcome findings.

Of the twenty-eight possible variables that were gathered, only the following eighteen proved to be suitable for this type of analysis, that is, met the theoretical assumptions underlying the statistical analysis (covariance) and also had complete data: teacher questionnaire, 3 variables; cognitive data, 1 variable; parent interview—behaviour data, 3 variables; parent interview—temperament data, 3 variables; psychiatric interview, 4 variables; global assessment, 4 variables. We excluded certain data related to cognitive functioning and personality because relevant information was not available at the first follow-up.

The adjusted difference between initial and follow-up scores for the four groups at first and second follow-ups are presented in Figure 12.1a and b. These figures are based on the data described above. The change scores were made comparable by statistical means and were therefore capable of direct arithmetical summation. The strength of this summarizing analysis is that it summates data from diverse sources—classroom questionnaire, parent interview, psychiatric assessment of the child, and, finally, a clinical assessment of severity of disturbance. The latter assessments are by far the most sensitive and valid indices of change in maladjustment as they are not solely symptom counts. The total count on the Rutter Teacher Scale may, in a sense, be considered duplicative but it too contains data not included in the Rutter Neurotic and Rutter Antisocial subscores. On the other hand, we considered that these two latter scores merited representation in their own right. However, whether parts of the data are omitted or included, the broad pattern tends to remain the same.

The importance of multiple criteria

It is worthwhile commenting on the variability in the improvement of the various groups in relation to different facets of child behaviour over the study periods. Some broad patterns are discernible over the *first year* of the study and these are best commented on as average improvement over all groups at the *first follow-up*. Over this period of the study there were only moderate levels of improvement in behaviour as perceived by school staff and at psychiatric interview. On the other hand, the level of improvement in behaviour based on parental reports was quite considerable but not surprisingly there were only a few changes in temperament. Finally, there was little improvement in reading over this period. The variability observed from base to first follow-up is again observed in the base to *second follow-up*. On this occasion deterioration of behaviour, as described by the teachers, was noted. However, ratings of behaviour based on interview of parents showed continuing improvement. Again, for measures based on psychiatric interview, there was reasonably consistent improvement over the second year. These findings are of crucial importance in that they demonstrate the necessity of gathering data from a variety of sources when attempting to measure change. Furthermore, they underline the fact that one source of evidence may suggest that there has been improvement at a particular time, whereas another source may suggest that there has been no improvement, or even deterioration, and this situation may be reversed later. Therefore, when measuring change in children, *it is only sensible to draw data from multiple sources because one source is likely to provide only a partial picture of the changes that are occurring.*

Between group differences in improvement (Figures 12.1a and b)

Analysis of improvement was undertaken year by year with the following results. The maladjusted children in ordinary schools did well in the first year, doing

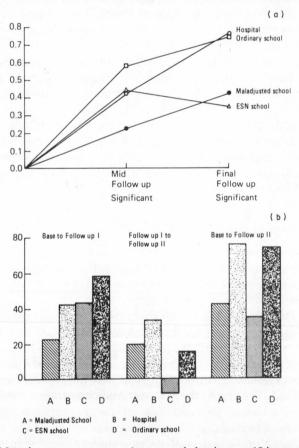

Fig. 12.1 (a) Mean improvement scores (aggregate behaviour on 18 items at start, midline and final follow-up). □, ordinary school; O, hospital; △, ESN school; ●, maladjusted school. (b) Histograms of improvement by groups. A maladjusted school; B, hospital; C, ESN school; D, ordinary school

significantly better than those in maladjusted schools ($p < 0.01$). The hospital group and the educationally subnormal school group also did significantly better than the maladjusted-school group ($p < 0.05$). At the second follow-up, maladjusted children in ordinary schools and in hospitals improved significantly more than both the ESN- and maladjusted-school groups ($p < 0.01$).

To determine how the children faced during their second year in the study, improvement over the first follow-up period was subtracted from improvement over the second follow-up period (see Figure 12.1b). The picture that emerged was that maladjusted children in ordinary schools do well in the first year, but only moderately in the second; maladjusted children in schools for the educationally subnormal do moderately well in the first year but poorly in the second; the hospital patient group do consistently well in both years; and, finally, the group of children in schools specifically for the maladjusted did only moderately well in the first year but did comparatively well in the second year. It can be seen that the changes from the base to the second follow-up are compounded of changes occurring over the two previous years, and that the rates for these changes vary considerably from group to group and from year to year.

Differences between groups according to type of disorder
(Figures 12.2a, b and c)

For *conduct-disordered children*, at the first follow-up the children in ordinary schools do best. Improvement in the ordinary school is significantly greater than in the other three groups and the educationally subnormal group is better than hospital and maladjusted school groups. At the final follow-up, the superiority of improvement in the ordinary-school group persists in relation to the other three groups, and the hospital group shows significantly more improvement than the maladjusted and ESN school groups. In the case of *neurotic disorders*, the pattern is different; the maladjusted school groups shows the least improvement compared with each of the other groups at the first follow-up. At the final follow-up, the hospital settings have the greatest improvement closely followed by ordinary schools—this improvement proved significantly better than the ESN school group.

Further, when we compared the effects of different management settings on children with *conduct disorders* we found that the group at schools for the maladjusted did very poorly the first year and comparatively well the second.

The hospital group did poorly the first year but were the most improved group during the second year. The educationally subnormal group did well during the first year but very poorly the following year. The group in ordinary schools were the most-improved group during the first and were the second-best group during the second year. Comparing the effects of these different management settings on children with *neurotic disorders*, we found that those groups at

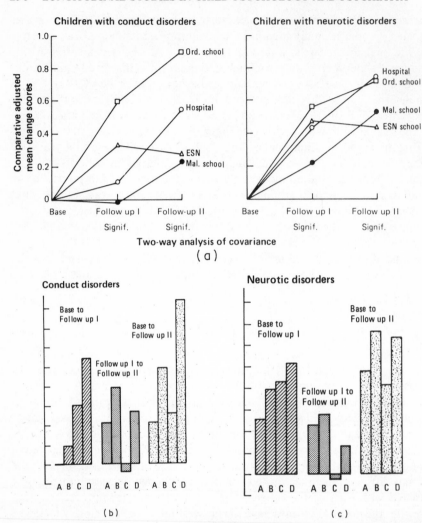

Fig. 12.2   (a) Improvement by diagnosis in four management groups over 2 years. □, ordinary school; O, hospital; Δ, ESN school; ●, maladjusted school. (b) Histogram of improvement (conduct disorders). (c) Histogram of improvement (neurotic disorders). A, maladjusted school; B, hospital; C, ESN school; D, ordinary school

schools for the maladjusted showed an approximately equal amount of improvement over the first and second years. The hospital group did well over the first year and were the most improved group over the second year. The educationally subnormal group did well over the first year but very poorly indeed over the second year. The neurotic children in ordinary schools were the most improved over the first year but improved only moderately over the second year.

Interaction between factors

A further statistical technique was used which allowed us to study the interaction of several factors, for example, diagnosis (whether the children fell into conduct or neurotic categories) and sex (male and female). From this analysis, three conclusions can be drawn—first, whether one classification has an independent effect, such as males do better than females; second, whether another also has an independent effect, such as children with conduct disorders do better than those with neurotic disorders; and, third, whether the classifications interact with each other—in other words, whether for example, boys with conduct disorders do better than girls with neurotic disorders. These are complex analyses and the findings are only given in brief.

The principal findings were that on one-third of the eighteen measures of behaviour and cognition studied, children with neurotic disorders showed significantly more improvement than children with conduct disorders. However, a notable but surprising finding was that there was greater improvement by children with conduct disorders in ordinary schools than by children with neurotic disorders in other settings. Finally, no interaction was detected between sex (male or female) and treatment settings (maladjusted schools, hospitals, ESN schools and ordinary schools).

Predicting improvement

We used multiple regression analysis to identify factors which were important in predicting improvement. We studied a number of factors covering: adverse early life experiences; social factors or influences; psychiatric or emotional disorder in parents; parental attitudes and family patterns of child-rearing; parental discord; maternal personality; children's age, sex and ordinal position.

A number of significant predictions were identified which appear sensible and meaningful on the basis of clinical experience. The most common predictor of slow improvement proved to be evidence of a poor or adverse social environment. Another set of common predictors of poor improvement were poor mother–child or father–child relationships. Less frequent but equally important were parental management techniques—poor improvement was predicted by lack of evidence of willingness to reason with the child and lack of a reasonable degree of firmness and discipline. Other less frequent parental predictors included a family history of serious mental illness; poor identification with the wider community standards; family stresses in the children's early years of life; and introversion of mothers.

Changes in classification

An important question which has so far received little attention is whether there is a change of diagnosis over the course of time, that is, whether there is a syndrome shift. Workers from the Isle of Wight Study (Graham and Rutter, 1973) in their follow-up in adolescents deny that such a shift occurs. A comparison of the baseline and follow-up diagnoses (Table 12.11) shows that a syndrome shift *did* occur during our study which was highly significant in the 'screened' group, that is, maladjusted children in ordinary and educationally subnormal schools, but this shift is not significant in the 'designated' groups. The shift comprised an increase in the percentage of cases diagnosed as having conduct disorders, so that by the final follow-up more than half of the children in the 'screened' group were diagnosed as having conduct disorders. This shift may have been due to the downward social-class gradient of our sample, with the associated heavier loadings of adverse social factors; such factors are more likely to promote conduct disorders.

Table 12.11   Syndrome shift in percentages

| Diagnosis | At base | At final follow-up | Final follow-up | |
			Deemed	Screened
Conduct	35	48	42	58
Neurotic	65	46	53	41
Other	0	6	5	1

CONCLUSIONS

Introduction

In this study we have surveyed and compared the progress of groups of maladjusted children in different management settings. Previously, the fate of children with psychiatric disorders in such settings has been largely a matter for speculation. Our study has shown that children with psychiatric disorders improve whether or not they are given specific help. Although this is not a new finding (Robins, 1970; Shepherd *et al.*, 1971; Robins, 1973; Kolvin *et al.*, 1981), we did find differences in the extent of improvement in relation to different types of disorder and different management settings.

The outcome of maladjustment within these settings was studied both irrespective of, and also according to, the type of disorders from which the children were suffering. We must stress that the nature of the groups included made it impossible to allocate maladjusted children to the very different settings we studied on a random basis, although such a random allocation (Kolvin *et al.*, 1981) would have been desirable on scientific grounds.

A number of important questions remain. How comparable are the groups studied? What is the explanation for the different rates of improvement of the different groups over the two years of the study? Why did the educationally subnormal children do so poorly at the final assessment? Why did the neurotic children in hospitals do so well at the final assessment compared with those in other special settings? Why did children with conduct disorders in ordinary schools do so well at the final assessment? What are the explanations for the differences in outcome for children with conduct and neurotic disorders? What part does treatment play? These and similar questions are discussed below.

Comparability of maladjustment of the groups studied

Like Shepherd *et al.* (1971), we used a quantitative and additive approach to symptomatology in order to achieve comparability between the groups. Our information was obtained from three different sources—parents, teachers and psychiatric interview and we confirmed the findings both of Rutter *et al.* (1970) and of Shepherd *et al.* (1971), that there was only a limited overlap in the disorders reported by each of these three sources. Although we assembled study groups which were quantitatively equivalent according to our screen measures, on clinical grounds the severity of psychiatric disturbance was found to be much more marked in the groups of children in hospitals and in schools for the maladjusted. In addition to clinical severity, we also found other quantitative differences between the various groups, in particular the poorer socialization and much more adverse home and family circumstances of those attending hospital and in special schools.

Effectiveness of treatment

The question of effectiveness of treatment is bound up with the question of comparability of the groups, and the latter has to be viewed in terms of type and severity of the maladjustment and social and family factors. There are indubitably differences between the groups in relation to all these factors and these are not only quantitative but qualitative as well. For instance, children in ordinary schools have the least in the way of *conduct problems* and their disorders are *least severe*. In the appendix we argue that we have tried to make allowance for such differences and conclude that while the findings of ordinary schools seeming to cope well with the maladjusted children in their care are not invalidated, the extent of improvement or change *may have been over-estimated*. This brings us to the subject of outcome.

Though crude, the technique of measuring outcome has the merit of being based on clinical measures of severity as rated by the clinician. And the clinician is likely to take into consideration qualitative behavioural factors in making such ratings. This will be discussed in greater detail elsewhere, where it is argued that with the type of design we are confronted with in this research, outcome scores more fairly reflect change, particularly in a clinical sense and, further, are less liable to inexplicable distortion which may occur with complex statistical analyses (Kolvin *et al.*, 1984). It is interesting to note that good plus moderate overall outcome is only achieved by 56 per cent of the ordinary school group and 83 per cent of the hospital group. Though we do not have sufficient cases to provide an estimate of a base rate of spontaneous improvement, it is evident that this is less than the traditional 66 per cent suggested by Levitt (1957, 1963, 1971) and Shepherd *et al.* (1971). Further, as already intimated, this ordinary-school group was significantly less maladjusted and had less in the way of cases of severe conduct disorders.

A word needs to be said about spontaneous recovery as reflected by the measure of outcome. First, the antisocial behaviour of maladjusted children who remain in ordinary schools is quantitatively the least severe of all the groups studied and it is also likely to be the least complex. It needs to be noted that antisocial behaviour tends to be intransigent to treatment (Kolvin *et al.*, 1981; Robins, 1970). Second, there were numerous in-depth cognitive and personality assessments of the children and interviews with their families, and there is evidence from the literature that such contact with cases has a therapeutic impact. Third, there were regular requests for information from the schools to whom it must have been obvious that we were enquiring about vulnerable children. In these circumstances, it is inconceivable that no informal help was made available to these children. We must, therefore, conclude that these were less than ideal controls which were likely to give at least some overestimation of spontaneous recovery.

Our improvement and outcome data also suggests that antisocial behaviour is an important prognostic factor—those groups with the most severe degrees of antisocial behaviour at the baseline assessment have the poorest outcome. This suggests that one cannot allow for such differences adequately by statistical means but only by random allocation. Severity of neurotic behaviour does not appear to have similar prognostic characteristics. As we consider outcome is a better measure of change in relation to our research design (see Appendix), it is worthwhile commenting on outcome of the conduct and neurotic categories separately. For conduct disorders good outcome is rare, except in the ordinary school group, and poor outcome is common: however, in the neurotic group poor outcome is only a phenomenon of the educationally subnormal and ordinary school groups.

Table 12.12   Comparative outcome of conduct and neurotic disorders in percentages (moderate outcome excluded)

	Conduct category		Neurotic category	
	Good	Poor	Good	Poor
Schools for maladjusted	14	53	26	20
Hospitals	15	23	42	15
ESN Schools	6	58	24	57
Ordinary schools	28	43	48	43

We present the bare percentage outcome at the second follow-up in Table 12.12. Our outcome findings are closer to those of the well-controlled and systematic study of Miller *et al.*, 1972, who evaluated the treatment of phobic children and report that 73 per cent of the treated group were successful as opposed to only 34 per cent of the untreated group (a difference of 39 per cent). In our neurotic group treated in hospitals 85 per cent were successful (that is, had good and moderate outcome) as against 57 per cent of those in ordinary schools (a difference of 28 per cent).

Differing outcomes in different management/treatment programmes

The outcome for untreated maladjusted children in ordinary schools was relatively good, especially for children with conduct disorders and this was particularly evident when allowance was made for the different initial levels of severity of the criterion variables. As this group had received little in the way of specific psychotherapy, the difference must have been attributable to some other factors such as the major differences between the groups in family socio-economic circumstances and other adverse emotional and psychological influences. When allowance was made for such factors by analysis of covariance, the magnitude of differences of improvement between groups was reduced and the children with neurotic disorders in ordinary schools were then found to do as well as those in hospital settings. Some of our findings resemble those of Shepherd *et al.* (1971). Their sample, like ours, had a heavy loading of working-class families and only a few upper-class families. Furthermore, they found that social factors were important in predicting improvement, as we found in our regression analysis.

Other adverse environmental experiences, either of a social or psychological nature, occur comparatively infrequently in the families of maladjusted children in ordinary schools (Table 12.3). This not only suggests that a favourable environment is associated with better outcome, but also that there may be crucial environmental factors which, if present to any great extent, may bring about the exclusion of the child from ordinary-school settings; even if these factors are present only to a slight degree, they have predictive importance. This suggestion is supported by previous findings that marital discord (Wolff, 1961) and adverse social and intrafamilial emotional factors (Sundby and Kreyberg, 1968) are predictive of poor outcome. Although we have allowed for some such factors in our more complex analyses (covariance), children with conduct disorders in ordinary schools still show remarkable improvement and those with neurotic disorders also show excellent improvement (Figure 12.2 b and c). However, there are questions about whether such statistical techniques can adjust sufficiently for such adverse social and family experiences (Campbell and Erlebacher, 1975) and further whether indices of adversity used for these purposes are sufficiently sensitive. Like Campbell and Erlebacher, we suggest that covariance does not adjust sufficiently for the fundamentally different adverse environmental experiences of controls selected from a superior population and further, our control findings using covariance are likely to constitute *an over-estimate but are not invalidated* (see Statistical Appendix). Again like Campbell and Erlebacher, we can propose that the only valid way to answer such questions is by longitudinal studies of children with maladjustment who have high and low levels of social and psychological disturbance in their family and who have been randomly allocated to different treatment settings (Kolvin *et al.*, 1981).

Maladjusted children in ordinary schools

Another finding of interest is that the mothers of maladjusted children in ordinary schools are comparatively more firm (disciplinarian and less indulgent). This suggests that such child-rearing factors, together with positive social factors, are predictive of improvement.

As far as factors intrinsic to the children are concerned, the maladjusted children in ordinary schools also have higher mean intelligence scores than those in educationally subnormal schools which suggests that higher levels of intelligence are associated with greater improvement. In a comparative sense, the better improvement of maladjusted children in ordinary schools is less evident when they have neurotic disorders rather than conduct disorders.

We have also demonstrated that the main improvement of maladjusted children in ordinary schools occurred during the first year. Over the second year the extent of the improvement was less than that achieved by the hospital groups and, indeed, as far as neurotic disorders are concerned, was even less than that of the groups in schools for the maladjusted.

Hospital groups

The children in the hospital groups were similar to the children in the ordinary school groups both with regard to cognitive levels and in the comparatively enlightened maternal approach to child rearing. While the neurotic children in the hospital group had very high initial levels of disturbance, assessed overall, they responded comparatively well to treatment (Figure 12.2a). However, the pattern of improvement differed between conduct and neurotic disorders— conduct-disordered children showed little improvement over the first year and their main improvement was over the second year, while neurotically disordered children showed a major improvement over the first year but less, although still considerable, improvement over the second year. The main differences in management as compared with the two special school groups (maladjusted and educationally subnormal) is that the children in the hospital groups were given more treatment of all kinds, had fewer adverse temperamental characteristics and had a higher mean level of intelligence. All these factors suggest that:

1   All else being equal, children with neurotic disorders respond better to intensive and concentrated psychotherapeutic help, such as is provided in hospitals, than to the help available in any other special setting that we have studied. On the other hand, children with conduct disorders respond best to management in ordinary schools. Further, despite the qualitative differences which lead children to receive hospital treatment, such children with neurotic disorders do as well as those children whose behaviour is not severe enough to cause them to be extracted from ordinary schools (see Figure 12.2a).

2   Despite severity of disturbance, maladjusted children with higher IQs appear to have a better prognosis than those with lower IQs. This proved more true for those with neurotic disorders. It could be concluded that the IQ of the children is of considerable prognostic importance. However, the question arises of how *independent* is the effect of IQ as a predictor of outcome. We have some evidence on this theme from our analysis of covariance where IQ was used as a covariate and where it proved to have little *independent* effect. This does not mean IQ is unrelated to outcome but, rather, that its effects were absorbed by other covariates, such as measures of social factors.

3   It is evident that the majority of the children in the hospital group spend most, if not all, of the second year in ordinary schools. Hence, most of the improvement of children with conduct disorders from hospital settings over this period could possibly be attributable to the effects of attendance in ordinary schools after initial treatment. This suggests that the social modelling obtained in ordinary schools may be crucial in encouraging improvement in maladjustment, whether caused by conduct or neurotic disorder.

Schools for the maladjusted

The groups in schools for the maladjusted differed from the hospital group in having more adverse intra-familial, social and psychological experiences, less intensive treatment, lower mean IQs and more negative temperamental characteristics. Nevertheless, the initial level of clinical disturbance was substantially the same for both groups. On most factors, other than initial level of clinical disturbance, children in maladjusted schools are worse than children in hospital settings, and so it is probably this clustering and interaction of adverse factors within the child and environment that determine this group's relatively poor outcome over the two-year follow-up. However, while this group improved comparatively little over the first year (especially those children with conduct disorders), children with either type of disorder did relatively well over the second year. This supports the argument that the response to help of children in such schools occurs only with time and the delay in response is due to the intractability of their disorders.

Educationally subnormal

Sundby and Kreyberg (1968) have shown that poor IQ is an important prognostic factor of adverse outcome. Naturally, our educationally subnormal group had the poorest mean IQs and almost always had the poorest outcome (Figure 12.2a, b and c). One of the clearest findings of the study is that maladjusted children in schools for the educationally subnormal do not flourish beyond their first year of admission. This is likely to represent the maximum repsonse to a helpful educational environment without specific psychotherapeutic intervention.

This appears true of educationally subnormal children both with neurotic and with conduct disorders (Figures 12.2 b and c). The educationally subnormal groups differ from the ordinary school groups in having an abundance of family and environmental problems, and also a poorer mean IQ. It is not possible to determine with any certainty which of these two factors was most instrumental in determining poor outcome. Similarly such factors were also noted in schools for the maladjusted. Another possibility is that the poorest eventual outcome of educationally subnormal children with neurotic and conduct disorders was attributable to the smaller amount of help they received. The precise answer cannot be determined, as those who started with least intelligence and had the worst family experiences also received least help and improved least.

Overall findings

Our overall findings suggest that maladjustment, whether of conduct or neurotic variety, is often better contained, *wherever possible*, in ordinary schools in ordinary classes, rather than in special schools. The finding has support from the work of Roe (1965), Lunzer (1960) and Shepherd *et al.* (1971). For instance, Roe demonstrated that tutorial classes (special classes in ordinary schools) were associated with significant improvement; the improvement in children in residential schools for the maladjusted proved to be non-significant, and the children in day schools for the maladjusted not only did more poorly but, indeed, showed overall deterioration. However, Roe's findings have to be viewed with caution as her's was a one-year follow-up only and our research has shown differing rates of improvement from year to year for the different groups of maladjusted chidlren. Indeed, our findings do not support Rutter's (1970) contention that two years is too long for a follow-up study. We have demonstrated clear trends towards improvement year by year, but especially in the second year, and it was only with a stage-by-stage analysis that a clear picture emerged of the differences between settings.

These findings and conclusions should not be interpreted as belittling the value of special-school settings, because there are frequently certain qualitative differences, both in personality and behaviour of maladjusted children, and in their home environments, which preclude ordinary schools from managing them. Further, we must add the caution that the good effects of ordinary schools, as found using covariance analysis, are likely to have been over-estimated (but not invalidated) by those very qualitative differences. Inevitably, therefore, some such children will need to be catered for in special settings which are necessarily schools for the maladjusted. Our own interpretation of our findings would be that perhaps more maladjusted children than at present could be better catered for in the ordinary stream of education.

Educational themes

For administrative reasons, it was not possible to obtain data on IQ at the intermediate follow-up, and therefore IQ was not included in our final analysis. However, as far as improvement in reading ability is concerned, the children at schools for the educationally subnormal again showed the least improvement of any of the groups, on both first and second follow-ups, irrespective of how we reorganized our data. This probably reflects both the multiplicity of handicaps of children in this setting and the frequent lack of appropriate educational and other facilities. The admission procedures, facilities and curricula provided for maladjusted children in educationally subnormal settings should therefore be re-examined.

Finally, it is also important to note that no difference could be found between specific maladjustment settings and ordinary schools with regard to broad cognitive improvement.

Some questions and implications

What is the best way to help educationally subnormal children who are maladjusted? The clearest finding of our study is that maladjusted children in schools for the educationally subnormal do not flourish beyond the first year in that setting. We have speculated that this could be attributable to factors within the child, within the school, within the family or within all of these. We have argued that poorer outcome is likely to be caused by a combination of a multiplicity of handicaps in the child, of adverse life experiences, of the scarcity of psychological help available to educationally subnormal children, and of the poor contact between families and the school.

The staff in schools for the educationally subnormal maintain that a number of children with very complex disorders are often diverted to schools for the educationally subnormal — not so much for their serious educational problems, but rather because of their adverse home and social circumstances and complicating maladjustment. Our findings corroborate this claim. For instance, the children identified as maladjusted by the first stage of screening in schools for the educationally subnormal proved to have high mean combined standard scores of maladjustment almost equivalent to those found in schools for the maladjusted and much higher than those found in remedial classes in ordinary schools. In view of the weight of evidence that children with neurotic disorders do well in hospital settings, there is a good case for screening children going into educationally subnormal settings for neurotic disorder, and for giving them more appropriate therapy. Some of them may have to be diverted to child guidance or hospital settings or, with appropriate support, could be maintained in special classes in ordinary schools. Some could be diverted to those schools for the maladjusted which are prepared to cater for children over a wide range of intelligence. However, if the bulk of these children are to be maintained in schools for the educationally subnormal, more resources are needed, such as: more staff training in developing special skills to deal with maladjustment; the possibility of special units or adjustment classes within schools for the educationally subnormal (an adjustment class would be a special class catering more specifically for maladjusted children); seeking ways of increasing contact with families and of helping them with the social and psychological problems. This is likely to include the presence of a social worker on the school staff; and a redesigned curriculum to meet the needs of these children.

Where should children with conduct disorders be managed? The subject of conduct disorders is very complex. The evidence is that, initially, neither hospitals nor schools for the maladjusted cope with such children appreciably better than do schools for the educationally subnormal. Ordinary schools appear to have the best results in this respect. We suspect that there are important quantitative differences (in terms of severity) and qualitative differences in conduct disorders retained in ordinary schools and those diverted to special settings. Nevertheless, with our more refined analyses, taking a variety of environmental influences into account, children with conduct disorders in the in patient and out patient hospital settings show greater improvement eventually than do those in the other two special settings. Furthermore, the progress of those in schools for the maladjusted takes place only over the second year, while the progress of those in schools for the educationally subnormal comes to a halt at the end of the first year. While some of the children with conduct disorders currently in schools for the educationally subnormal could possibly be maintained, at least for a while in remedial units of ordinary schools, we believe that careful consideration would have to be given to qualitative factors in the children or their families which might hinder the success of such a venture.

In general, this study illustrates that children with neurotic disorders show greater clinical improvement than those with conduct disorders. This general conclusion is confirmed by analysis of covariance, with the one exception that children with conduct disorders who are in ordinary schools do better than those in any other setting. The ordinary-school group contained children both in remedial classes and ordinary classes. Although we have not analysed those separately in relation to diagnosis, the implication is that children with conduct disorders do at least as well in remedial classes in ordinary schools as they do in schools for the maladjusted. This is consistent with the previously noted comment often reported by teachers of remedial classes, that both antisocial and neurotic behaviour of children with educational problems frequently subside spontaneously soon after admission to a remedial class. It is not clear how remedial classes achieve this without specifically focusing on maladjustment. It may be because the child is taken out of a crisis situation in which their behaviour had become maladaptively interlocked with staff-management procedures, or it may be because such classes have some features in common with schools for the maladjusted—for example, the smaller size of the class and the possibility of tailoring management and curriculum to the individual child. In addition, in a remedial class it is more possible to keep in touch with ordinary society so that the child is provided with normal models, normal conditioning and the greater expectation of comforting behaviour than is usually the case in schools for the maladjusted. Further, maladjustment in educationally subnormal children may also be helped by attention being directed to their educational deficiencies.

Apart from remedial classes, there are the maladjusted children in ordinary classes in ordinary schools. Our evidence suggests that such children with conduct disorders do very well compared with children in any other setting (after allowance for quantitative differences). This suggests that certain children with conduct disorders might well be retained in ordinary schools, but we must again emphasize that there may be important quantitative and qualitative factors which preclude certain children with conduct disorders being maintained in ordinary schools with any reasonable degree of ease.

Where should children with neurotic disorders be managed? Our data shows that children with neurotic disorders in the long term fare best in hospital settings and worst in settings for the educationally subnormal. Children with neurotic disorders (like those with conduct disorders) show greater improvement in ordinary schools than those in schools for the maladjusted. This again suggests that some of these children should be retained in ordinary schools.

Recommendations

There seems to be a strong case for trying to retain more maladjusted children in ordinary schools. Additionally, it seems reasonable to expand the provision of remedial or adjustment classes in such schools. Such views are strengthened by three considerations—first, the greater ease with which children can be reintroduced into ordinary classes as opposed to when they return from a special school; second, the comparative ease with which special classes could be organized in ordinary schools; and, third, the reduction in cost compared to running a school for the maladjusted. Of course, such a proposal is not a panacea. Nevertheless, it broadly coincides with the recommendation in section 10 of the Education Act, 1976—that no child with special needs should unnecessarily be separated from its home.

Taking fuller consideration of the quantitative and qualitative differences puts these proposals into better perspective; we calculate that about 30 per cent of maladjusted children in ordinary schools (including remedial classes) are rated as showing marked severity of disturbance whereas the corresponding figures at 60 per cent in schools for the educationally subnormal and almost 90 per cent in hospitals or schools for the maladjusted. These percentages show that the disorders are quantitatively more severe in the special settings. We have already suggested that children in special settings have disorders which are also more complex and qualitatively different. It may be precisely these qualitative differences that originally led to the extraction or exclusion of some of these children from the ordinary stream of education. This is likely to be true for some proportion of the children placed both in special educational and in hospital settings, and this proportion must be assessed, if possible, if not precisely, then by an informed guess.

It may be argued that qualitative differences apply mainly to children with marked severity of disorder, and then only to that percentage difference representing the excess of such children in a special setting over those in ordinary schools. Crude estimates of the percentage of children with qualitatively different disorders in various settings would appear to be about 55 per cent of those in schools for the maladjusted and in hospital settings; and 30 per cent of those in settings for the educationally subnormal. In other words, it is suggested that as many as half of those children in schools for the maladjusted could be contained in ordinary schools.

Some guidance as to which children with conduct disorders could be retained in the ordinary stream of education is available from our multivariate studies and is entirely in accord with clinical expectation. Our results have shown that ordinary schools may well be able to manage more maladjusted children with conduct disorders particularly those whose differences from the norm are mainly quantitative. Hence, only those children who are quantitatively different and incapable of being maintained in ordinary schools should be considered as candidates for special schools. The qualitative differences may be related to very adverse home background, reflected by factors such as an accumulation of negative social influences, disturbance of family relationships, less in the way of direction and firm management by the parents, and a family which has less in the way of identification with wider community standards.

Similar considerations apply to children with neurotic disorders. Again, we suggest that as many as a half of children with neurotic disorders in schools for the maladjusted could be contained in ordinary schools, provided that there were appropriate facilities.

These suggestions do not imply either a reduction in the number of special schools or an expansion of these services; rather, that the places available, which are currently thought to be insufficient, could be used more selectively. More selective use of these settings would entail their organization to contain a higher percentage of children with more complex conduct disorders; staff might rightly argue that this would radically change the character of their schools. An expansion of services would also be necessary for large senior schools, to deal with this problem. It would be naive to offer these as firm recommendations but we advance them rather as proposals for exploration by the educational authorities. Indeed, not all ordinary schools would favour trying to retain and cope with seriously maladjusted children. Some children may be regarded as so disruptive that the staff would not be able to continue to teach, and other children would therefore suffer.

Why are schools for maladjusted children apparently comparatively unsuccessful? We attempted to make allowance for some qualitative factors by incorporating related quantitative variables in the analysis of covariance. The argument has been that those children whose behaviour is both quantitatively and qualitatively different find their way into schools for the maladjusted and hospital settings. While there are no quantitative differences in severity between those in schools for the maladjusted and those in hospitals there are certainly qualitative differences for which one cannot make full allowance with statistical techniques. Perhaps the most important of these differences is that some of the children in schools for the maladjusted are those who have previously failed to respond to the psychological help provided by hospital in patient and out patient services (including child-guidance services). With the importance of social and family influences to which our work has pointed, most of which take their toll before the child ever gets to school, it is not unexpected that treatment in schools for the maladjusted, which provide help mainly at a very much later stage of development of the child and against very adverse family and social backgrounds, has little power to counteract rapidly such crucial influences. It is, therefore, not surprising that our analyses have demonstrated that there is no improvement in conduct disorders until the second year. Further, the improvement curves associated with school settings for the maladjusted, are almost linear (Figures 12.1 and 12.2) suggesting that such improvement will continue. If we had not studied the children year by year, we would not have become aware of this cumulative impact and would have been more pessimistic about the overall outcome of treatment in such special schools. However, major questions remain; in particular, how long should maladjusted children be maintained in special schools, and when should they be reintroduced into their ordinary schools? Our findings suggest that early reintroduction for some would be beneficial. However, the decision for each individual would depend on many factors—the child's initial diagnosis and subsequent improvement, the family background, the resources available in the ordinary school, and last but not least, cost effectiveness of the special placement.

Finally, in view of the adverse social and family environment, we recommend that trained social workers should invariably be attached to schools for the maladjusted.

A major consequence of such proposals would be the expansion of special provisions within the ordinary schools. There are also sound economic reasons for supporting such a policy—for instance, it is becoming prohibitively expensive to maintain maladjusted children in special schools. Hence, rather than increasing the number of places in special schools, we are suggesting that funds be allocated to the provision of specially trained staff and appropriate facilities in ordinary schools. Certain disturbed children are manageable only in small groups, which implies more classrooms and staff. However, as Anderson (1976) points out, these are not the only alternatives. We should regard this additional help in ordinary schools as a range of continuum of services as follows: an ordinary class with no special additional help; an ordinary class with ancillary help provided (Hulbert et al., 1977); an ordinary class but with part-time withdrawal of children for specific help or access to a teacher with specific skills; a special class for selected activities only; and, finally, a special class for most activities. Furthermore, the number of children managed by such staff are likely to be increased over the school year as children who are responding to help can more easily be returned to ordinary classes. If these staff are engaged in teaching, supporting social workers and/or school counsellors may be needed to help both in the school and to liaise with the families (Harvey et al., 1977). Such resources will be especially useful with the current expansion of foster placements for disturbed or deprived children.

The above proposals sound rather familiar—while they derive from research, they appear to support the imaginative policy of greater integration of children with special needs including disturbed children into ordinary schools—where possible—as recommended by the Warnock Report (1978). This chapter, therefore, appears at a time of change in the practice of special education in the UK with a coming together of ideas deriving from committee conclusions and research findings. For instance, funds are currently being allocated in the UK for the implementation of the Warnock Report proposals and similar changes are under way in the US (Strain and Kerr, 1981).

Educational administrators, whether national or regional, will want to judge whether they are using their available funds effectively and wisely, and may wish to make decisions based on informed educational opinion (including research findings) whether to develop a policy of supporting more special schooling for psychologically handicapped children rather than more special schools (Anderson, 1976).

STATISTICAL APPENDIX

Statistical measures of improvement — covariance analysis

Corrections between the groups — quantitative differences

There are well-established techniques for making allowance for initial quantitative differences between the groups. In the present study, mean improvement scores of various measures of maladjustment of the different groups of children were adjusted by analysis of covariance. This adjustment is necessary because of the effect that factors, such as initial severity of maladjustment and social factors, have upon measures of improvement of maladjustment. The effect of using analysis of covariance is therefore, to arrive at approximately the same results as would have been obtained had all the groups of children in question been matched with respect to the distorting factors or influences. It will be remembered that corrections were made to allow for such initial differences between groups and for this purpose we used five variables (covariates). However, we found the variable which dominated all others, on average by a factor of 10, was the *initial level of severity* of disturbance.

Our research design can be described as a *quasi-experimental* one. In such a situation we have to deal with a number of allied methodological objections. *First*, analysis of covariance involves the assumption that within-group regression slopes are the same for all the groups. We have dealt with this by using only those variables for which this assumption is justified. *Second*, it is well known that analysis of covariance, based as it is on observational (fallible) data, leads to undercorrection because it does not take errors of measurement into account (Snedecor and Cochran, 1967). This qualification applies to our analysis, as indeed it must to most studies in the behavioural sciences. It will be seen in our findings that the use of covariance has resulted in the improvement in ordinary schools and hospitals being increased; had errors of measurement been taken into account, then these increases may have been greater. We hope that this particular difficulty was met by the majority of our variables being sufficiently reliable to make the disturbing effects of errors of measurement small. As there may be other important influences other than initial level of disturbance which may affect the results, we have been careful to allow for as many of these as possible.

Corrections between the groups — qualitative differences

Finally, there are qualitative differences between the groups which have to be taken into account. Our results suggest that maladjusted children in ordinary schools do significantly better than those at schools for the educationally subnormal or maladjusted. However, it must be remembered that, while there is arithmetical equivalence between groups in terms of screen measures used, in terms of clinical severity of disorder there is not necessarily equivalence. It could well be that in certain cases a comparison has been made between, on the one hand, children with crippling neurotic disorders with circumscribed symptomatology or with intractable conduct disorders which cannot be coped with in an ordinary school setting, and, on the other hand, children with neurotic disorders or conduct disorders with relatively widespread but not severe symptomatology who can remain in ordinary schools, but who nevertheless have equal symptom counts. Although we recognize that it is not possible to make complete allowance for qualitative differences by the use of covariance, in this study we have attempted to take account of such qualitative differences of child behaviour by using quantitative variables related to them as covariates.

The most serious objection to analysis of covariance is advanced by Campbell and Erlebacher (1975) who contend that it does not correct sufficiently for the adverse environmental experiences of fundamentally different groups of children, because the adjusted changes are insufficient 'to overcome the inevitable regression artefacts coming from the fact that controls were selected from a superior population'. The one group of children in our study who might be considered to be relatively favoured were the children in ordinary schools and while the important practical finding that these schools coped well with the maladjusted children in their care is not invalidated, the *extent* of improvement or change may have been overestimated. Elsewhere, Kolvin *et al.* (1984) we point out that this overestimation is likely to be a reality and determined by the excess of children with conduct disorders (and their complexity and severity) in these special school settings.

We do allow that there may be *qualitative differences* between the populations over and above those which we have attempted to allow for by analysis of covariance and, consequently, differences in improvement must not necessarily be equated with differences in effectiveness between settings. Some authorities suggest that a more appropriate statistical procedure in the case of a quasi-experimental design is analysis of variance (Nunnally, 1964 — considering differences between pre-test and post-test measures as constituting a within-subject factor in repeated measurement analysis of variance). However, since analysis of variance involves similar assumptions to those described above in relation to covariance (and these are not mentioned by Nunnally), and also does not provide adjusted mean scores, we considered it less suitable for our purposes.

Clinical measures of outcome

This follows Sainsbury (1975) as modified in Newcastle (Kolvin *et al.*, 1981). Sainsbury pointed out that the problems associated with outcome 'stems from the situation, often crucial in clinical studies, in which patients at the top (or bottom) of the scale have no room to improve (or worsen)'. He suggested a formula to solve the problem and it simplifies to the following:

$$O = 3M_2 - M_1$$

where O = outcome; M_1 = initial score; M_2 = final score.

In 'measuring' outcome by Sainsbury's method, the initial score is not merely subtracted from the final score, but a differential weighting of three to one is introduced. Therefore, using this measure of outcome is much the same as carrying out an analysis of covariance when the regression coefficient of final upon initial score is one-third (Kolvin *et al.*, 1981).

In using this method the children's behaviour was rated by a child psychiatrist on three occasions: at base, at midline assessment and at final follow-up. No attempt was made to assess improvement, which is a more difficult task but rather each child was merely rated on a four-point scale of (a) no disturbance, (b) slightly disturbed, (c) moderately disturbed and (d) markedly disturbed. The range of outcome scores was divided into three categories corresponding to good, moderate and poor outcome (Kolvin *et al.*, 1981).

Elsewhere we argue that our measure of outcome, though crude, may be less subject to the distortions that occur through attempts at correction for differences between groups, particularly when the differences are qualitative as in a quasi-experimental design (Kolvin *et al.*, 1984). In particular, it is less liable to overestimates of outcome in the case of superior populations.

ACKNOWLEDGMENT

One of us (IK) would like to acknowledge the support of the DES.

REFERENCES

Anderson, E. M. (1976). Annotation: Special schools or special schooling for the handicapped child? The debate in perspective, *J. Child Psychol. and Psychiat.* **17**, 151–156.

Atkins, M. and Kolvin, I. (1976). *Born Too Soon or Born Too Small* (Eds G. A. Neligan, I. Kolvin, D. McI. Scott and R. F. Garside), Clinics in Developmental Medicine No. 61, Heinemann Medical Books, SIMP, London.

Bergin, A. E. (1966). Some implications of psychotherapy research for therapeutic practice, *J. Abnormal Psychol.* **71**, 235–246.

Campbell, D. T. and Erlebacher, A. (1975). How regression artifacts in quasi-experimental evaluations can mistakenly make compensatory education look harmful, in *Handbook of Evaluation Research*, Vol. 1 (Eds E. L. Struening and M. Guttentag), Sage, London.

Chazan, M. (1964). The incidence and nature of maladjustment among children in schools for the educationally subnormal, *Brit. J. Educ. Psychol.*, **34**, 292–304.

Chazan, M. (1965). Factors associated with maladjustment in educationally subnormal children, *Brit. J. Educ. Psychol.*, **35**, 277–285.

Cohen, J. (1960). A coefficient of agreement for nominal scales, *Educational and Psychological Measurement*, **20**, 37–46.

Eysenck, S. B. G. and Eysenck, H. J. (1975). *Manual of the Eysenck Personality Inventory*, Hodder and Stoughton, London.

Garside, R. F. (1956). The regression of gains upon initial scores, *Psychometrika*, **21**, 67–77.

Garside, R. F., Hulbert, C. M., Kolvin, I., van der Spuy, H. I. J., Wolstenholme, F. and Wrate, R. M. (1973). Evaluation of psychiatric services for children in England and Wales, in *Roots of Evaluation* (Eds J. K. Wing and H. Hafner), Oxford University Press for Nuffield Provincial Hospitals Trust, Oxford.

Garside, R. F., Birch, H., Scott, D. McI., Chambers, S., Kolvin, I., Tweddle, E. G. and Barber, L. M. (1975). Dimensions of temperament in infant school children, *J. Child Psychol. Psychiat.* **16**, 219–231.

Graham, P. and Rutter, M. (1973). Psychiatric disorder in the young adolescent: a follow-up study, *Proc. Roy. Soc. Med.* **66**, 1226–1229.

Harvey, L., Kolvin, I., McLaren, M., Nicol, A. R. and Wolstenholme, F. (1977). Introducing a school social worker into schools, *Brit. J. Guid. and Counsel.* **5**, 26–40.

Hulbert, C. M., Wolstenholme, F. and Kolvin, I. (1977). A teacher-aide programme in action, Part II, *Special Education: Forward Trends*, **4**, 27–31.

Jones, A. P. and Murray, W. (1958). The heights and weights of educationally subnormal children, *Lancet*, **i**, 905.

Kerlinger, F. N. (1969). *Foundations of Behavioural Research—Educational and Psychological Inquiry*, Holt, Rinehart and Winston, New York.

Kolvin, I. and Ounsted, C. (1968). Survey of boys on psychiatric remand, *Medicine, Science and the Law*, **8**, 88–95.

Kolvin, I., Wolff, S., Barber, L. M., Tweddle, E. G., Garside, R. F., Scott, D. McI. and Chambers, S. (1975). Dimensions of behaviour in infant school children, *Brit. J. Psychiat.* **126**, 114–126.

Kolvin, I., Garside, R. F., Nicol, A. R., Leitch, I. M. and Macmillan, A. (1977). Screening school children for high risk of emotional and educational disorder, *Brit. J. Psychiat.* **131**, 192–206.

Kolvin, I., Garside, R. F., Nicol, A . R., Macmillan, A., Wolstenholme, F. and Leitch, I. M. (1981). *Help Starts Here: The Maladjusted Child in the Ordinary School*, Tavistock Publications, London.

Kolvin, I., Wrate, R. M. and Nicol, A. R. (1984). Treatment is effective, for presentation.

Levitt, E. E. (1957). The results of psychotherapy with children: An evaluation, *J. Consult. Psychol.* **21**, 189–196.

Levitt, E. E. (1963). Psychotherapy with children: A further evaluation. *Behav. Res. Ther.* **60**, 326–329.

Levitt, E. E. (1971). Research on psychotherapy with children, in *Handbook of Psychotherapy and Behaviour Change* (Eds S. L. Garfield and A. E. Bergin), Wiley, London.

Lunzer, E. A. (1960). Aggressive and withdrawing children in a normal school, *Brit. J. Educ. Psychol.*, **30**, 119–123.

Mangus, A. J. (1950). Effects of mental and educational retardation on personality development of children, *Amer. J. Ment. Defic.* **55**, 208–212.

Miller, L. C., Barrett, C. L., Hampe, E. and Noble, H. (1972). Comparison of reciprocal inhibition, psychotherapy and waiting list controls for phobic children, *J. Abnorm. Psychol.* **79**, 269–279.

Neligan, G. A., Prudham, D. and Steiner, H. (1974). *The Formative Years: Birth, Family and Development in Newcastle upon Tyne*, Oxford University Press for the Nuffield Provincial Hospitals Trust, Oxford.

Neligan, G. A., Kolvin, I., Scott, D. McI. and Garside, R. F. (Eds) (1976). *Born Too Soon or Born Too Small*, Clinics in Developmental Medicine No. 61. Heinemann Medical Books, London.

Nunally, J. (1964). *Educational Measurement and Evaluation*, McGraw-Hill, New York.

Pallis, D. J. and Staffelmayr, B. E. (1973). Social attitudes and treatment orientation among psychiatrists, *Brit. J. Med. Psychol.* **46**, 75–81.

Pumroy, D. K. (1966). Maryland parent attitude survey: A research instrument with social desirability controlled, *J. Psychol.* **64**, 73–78.

Robins, L. N. (1966). *Deviant Children Grown Up*, Williams and Wilkins, Baltimore.

Robins, L. N. (1970). Follow-up studies investigating childhood disorders, in *Psychiatric Epidemiology* (Eds E. Hare and J. K. King), Oxford University Press, London.

Robins, L. N. (1973). Evaluation of psychiatric services for children in the United States, in *Roots of Evaluation* (Eds J. K. Wing and H. Hafner). Oxford University Press, Oxford.

Roe, M. C. (1965). *Survey into Progress of Maladjusted Pupils*, ILEA, London.

Rutter, M. (1967). A children's behaviour questionnaire for completion by teachers: preliminary findings, *J. Child Psychol. Psychiat.* **8**, 1–11.

Rutter, M., Tizard, J. and Whitmore, K. (1970). *Education, Health and Behaviour*, Longman, London.

Rutter, M. (1970). Follow-up studies investigating childhood disorders — Discussion, in *Psychiatric Epidemiology* (Eds E. Hare and J. Wing), Oxford University Press for Nuffield Provincial Hospitals Trust, Oxford.

Rutter, M. (1971). Parent–child separation: Psychological effects on the children, *J. Child Psychol. Psychiat.* **12**, 233–260.

Rutter, M. (1982). Psychological therapies in child psychiatry: Issues and prospects, *Psychological Medicine*, **12**, 723–740.

Rutter, M. and Bartak, L. (1973). Special education treatment of autistic children: A comparative study. II. Follow-up findings and implications for services, *J. Child Psychol. Psychiat.* **14**, 241–270.

Rutter, M. and Graham, P. (1968). The reliability and validity of the psychiatric assessment of the child. I. Interview with the child, *Brit. J. Psychiat.* **114**, 563–579.

Rutter, M. and Madge, N. (1976). *Cycles of Disadvantage: A review of Research*, Heinemann Educational, London.

Rutter, M., Tizard, J. and Whitmore, K. (1970). *Education, Health and Behaviour*, Longman, London.

Sainsbury, P. (1975). Evaluation of community mental health programmes, in *Handbook of Evaluation Research*, Vol. 2 (Eds M. Guttentag and E. L. Struening), Sage, California.

Sears, R. R., Maccoby, E. E. and Levin, H. (1957). *Patterns of Child-Rearing*. Harper and Row, New York.

Semler, I. J. (1960). Relationship among several members of pupil adjustment, *J. Educ. Psychol.* **51**, 60–68.

Shepherd, M., Oppenheim, A. and Mitchell, S. (1966). Childhood behaviour disorders and the child guidance clinic: An epidemiological study, *J. Child Psychol. Psychiat.* **7**, 39–52.

Shepherd, M., Oppenheim, B. and Mitchell, S. (1971). *Childhood Behaviour and Mental Health*, University of London Press, London.

Snedecor, G. W. and Cochran, W. G. (1967). *Statistical Methods* (6th edn), Iowa State University Press, Ames, Iowa.

Sturge, C. (1982). Reading retardation and anti-social behaviour. *J. Child Psychol. & Psychiat.*, **23**, 21–32.

Strain, P. S. and Kerr, M. M. (1981). *Mainstreaming of Children in Schools*, Academic Press, New York.

Sundby, H. S. and Kreyberg, P. C. (1968). *Prognosis in Child Psychiatry*, Williams and Wilkins, Baltimore.

Tramontana, M. G. (1980). Critical review of research on psychotherapy outcome with adolescents, 1967–1977, *Psychol. Bulletin*, **88**(2), 429–450.

Wallin, P. (1954). A Guttman scale for measuring women's neighbourliness, *Amer. J. Sociol.* **59**, 243–246.

Warnock Report (1978). *Special Educational Needs. Report of the Committee of Enquiry into the Educational Needs of Children and Young People*, HMSO, London.

Wolff, S. (1961). Symptomatology and outcome of pre-school children with behaviour disorders attending a child guidance clinic, *J. Child Psychol. Psychiat.* **2**, 269–276.

Longitudinal Studies in Child Psychology and Psychiatry
Edited by A. R. Nicol
© 1985 John Wiley and Sons Ltd.

Chapter 13

What Sort of Therapy Should Be Given For What Sort of Problem?

A. R. Nicol, A. Macmillan, I. Kolvin and F. Wolstenholme

A most notable development in clinical child psychiatry over the last fifteen years or so has been the development of a wide variety of approaches to treatment. From our modern armamentarium of behaviour modification; dynamic therapy, both individual and group; family therapy; drug, educational and social therapies; we look back with some scorn at the so-called 'traditional child guidance approach'. This term is associated with the idea of a team of psychiatrist, psychologist and social worker who work together in fixed roles on all cases; prolonged psychoanalytically based treatment with other approaches considered as inferior and makeshift; long waiting lists and an ivory-tower image. The new techniques, while promising and exciting, have their problems too. All too easily, they can develop into a succession of fads and fashions. Power struggles can develop between rival factions and self-appointed 'gurus'.

How can child psychiatry benefit fully from the wealth of enthusiasm that the new ideas bring yet avoid imposing fads and fashions on the children and their families? The answer must lie in objective evaluation and comparison of the different types of therapy. Are the different approaches as different as they at first seem? If so, what type of treatment works for what type of disorder? Do the characteristics of the therapist and his personal style make a difference? These sort of questions are vital to the development of psychotherapy yet are very hard to answer. It is very difficult to carry out effective research in psychotherapy while keeping the therapy that is being investigated in its natural state. For some purposes, laboratory studies of therapy have been very illuminating, using social situations that bear some resemblance to therapy. However, firm answers are only likely to come from studying therapy itself in its natural setting—or as near to it as one can get.

Within the field of naturalistic research into psychotherapy the most widely held view is that evaluation should be carried out on tightly circumscribed diagnostic groups. In this way, the effects of specific types of therapy on specific problems can be investigated. The disadvantage with this approach, especially in child psychiatry, is that a great deal of common morbidity does not fall into neat, well-defined categories. Also, such strictly circumscribed disorders are comparatively rare so that studies have to be carried out on small samples. For the investigation of the full range of disorders, to detect long-term outcomes and, equally important, to search for generalization of effects, large-scale longitudinal studies are essential. These need to use a spread of outcome measures which sample different types of behaviour and, if possible, in different situations.

Before turning to the practicals, it is necessary to pause for a moment to consider the rather special place of theory in psychotherapy research. It could be said that such theory has two overlapping and intertwinning functions. The first of these is the straightforward need to have theories which generate testable hypotheses about how therapy works. This starts from the reasonable basis that therapy interaction and the changes that hopefully arise from it are understandable in the same way as other psychological events. Goldstein and Simonson (1971), for example, indicate some of the ways in which psychotherapy is understandable in terms of social psychological principles. The second use of theory has more to do with the 'schools' of psychotherapy—psychoanalysis, behaviour therapy and so on. Each of these are serious attempts to elucidate the mysteries of human emotions and motivation (although some other contenders can hardly be described as such). However, they also serve an essential function as the therapists guide and friend in the difficult task of practical therapy. Very often, theories of therapy assume the shape of ideologies and firmly held belief systems which fire their proponents with enthusiasm and *esprit de corps*.

Since, for the most part, psychotherapists have nailed their colours to one or other theoretical mast, it is not surprising that much psychotherapy research has been in the form of comparisons of one type of therapy with another—for example behaviour therapy with dynamic therapy. The difficulty with this approach is that the theoretical or ideological underpinning of a particular therapist's work may be a rather poor guide to the quality of the interaction he or she established in the therapy setting. For example, in the excellent comparative study of Sloane *et al.* (1975) the behaviour therapists were rated as having higher accurate empathy than the short-term analytically oriented therapists, although this is a quality generally associated with insight therapies! Other studies have contrasted different forms of delivery of therapy, for example individual contrasted with group therapy. In both cases, it is of course possible to see the comparison as a contest between different therapies. However, a more constructive approach is to see such work as hopefully enabling us to focus down on those common factors which really constitute the active ingredients of therapy. Equally important is the task of identifying which type of therapy is best for which type of problem.

In this chapter, we will present some results from a school based comparative study of three types of intervention that we have carried out in the north of England.

These are: parent counselling–teacher consultation, behaviour modification and Axlinian group therapy. The aim of this presentation will be to compare the results of the three approaches and see if we can add to the debate on the crucial ingredients of therapy. We will describe the process of therapy and then examine the outcomes once therapy is complete. We will be looking to see if this longitudinal study gives us any insights into the effectiveness of therapies in relieving problems and into the way the therapists work.

THE PROJECT

Our project is of special interest in this context because we compared different types of therapies using a wide range of measures from various different sources and over long time spans. We compared the effects of three different types of intervention with a no-treatment control group and with each other. The children that took part in the project were 322 children in six schools, all 11 years of age at the beginning of the project who had been identified as maladjusted by a multiple criterion screening technique. To screen the children, data were collected through a teacher behaviour scale (Rutter, 1967), a self-report scale of neuroticism (Eysenck, 1965) and a sociometry measure of isolation and rejection by peers (MacMillan et al., 1978). This screen was applied to all children in two consecutive year cohorts of the six schools. Cut-off scores were then applied to identify those children who scored highly on one or a combination of the scales. Details can be found in the definitive account of the project (Kolvin et al., 1981).

The children selected by the screen were included in the study. A battery of further assessments was then carried out. This included a further self-report scale: the Barker Lunn Scale (Barker Lunn, 1969). Other tests used were the Devereux Elementary School Behaviour Rating Scale (Spivack and Swift, 1967) and parent reports of the childrens behaviour by questionnaire (Rutter et al., 1970) and interview (Kolvin et al., 1975) and of the children's temperament (Garside et al., 1975). Verbal and non-verbal ability tests were also administered (The NFER Scales see Kolvin et al., 1981). Background demographic data was also collected.

Following assessment, cases were randomly allocated to treatment groups by school class. The three treatments, parent counselling–teacher consultation, group therapy, and behaviour modification, together with a no-treatment control group were introduced into each of the six schools that the children attended. Thus the effects of school differences were controlled for. Following treatment, three follow-ups were carried out using all the measures of functioning at school, from parents, peers and self that have been described above.

The three interventions were seen as differing from each other along two different dimensions: degree of directness in the approach to the child and emphasis on behavioural versus 'insight' approaches. Parent counselling–teacher consultation was carried out by trained social workers. It was an 'indirect' approach in that there was no direct contact with the child, the work of the social worker being entirely with the parent and teacher. The first task was to establish a foothold in the school so as to become, to all intents and purposes, a school social worker. At the same time the social worker made home visits to assess, and then provide help, for any family difficulties. There were up to ten visits to the families, most receiving four to six calls in all. The social worker was also in a position to perform a linking function between home and school. The programme took place over a year. The parent counselling–teacher consultation regime was the only one under discussion here where there was regular contact with the parent. This gave us the opportunity to get a 'consumer response' measure at the end of treatment from the mothers. A total of eighty families were involved in this regime.

The other two therapies, group therapy, involving 60 children, and behaviour modification, involving 68 children, were particularly suitable for comparison. Both took place within the school and during the school day. They were both short-term treatments taking place over six months within a single academic year and, as mentioned above, within the same six schools. At this point the similarities end. There was every opportunity for the two treatments to develop along their own lines. Behaviour modification was the less-direct approach in that teachers were trained to undertake the therapy. It was directed by a psychologist and psychiatrist who developed a training programme for thirty-nine teachers who had regular contact with the seventy-two target children. All teachers were given an introductory training manual. This was followed by a series of 3-hourly seminars. Time sampling and behaviour analysis were carried out for each of the children and treatment plans were then developed, individually tailored to the childrens problems. The directors remained closely involved as consultants throughout the project.

The group therapy was carried out by the same social workers who had previously received special training in school social work in the parent counselling–teacher consultation regime who had had additional training in group therapy techniques. The seventy-three children were taken in seventeen single-sex groups of four to five children per group. Each group ran for ten sessions. There was extensive and continuous supervision of the therapist's work by a psychiatrist and a psychotherapist. Details of the project together with extensive reports of both the therapy processes and outcomes can be found in Kolvin *et al.* (1981).

In this chapter we will concentrate on the aspects of the research which may throw light on the practical question of choice of therapy. All three therapy conditions were compared with controls at three time points: End of treatment, eighteen months (midline follow-up) and three years (final follow-up) after the baseline measures. Analysis was carried out by calculating change scores between the various follow-up points for each subject. The treatment groups were then compared on the change measures. Because social and ability factors are known to be strong prognostic indicators of childhood disorders these were taken into account in the statistical analysis which was by analysis of covariance. Initial score on any baseline measure will inevitably influence the size of the change score for statistical reasons (regression) so initial levels were allowed for in the analysis as well. The techniques were similar to that used in Chapter 12 in this volume. Significant differences quoted here are the results of pair-wise comparisons (Winer, 1971).

FOLLOW-UP FINDINGS

Many of the positive findings in the study were in the form of composite scores of the many different individual measures listed above. Since in this chapter we are trying to disentangle the specific contribution of the three approaches, we will focus mainly on those changes that showed up on individual scores. We will touch on some of the composite scores when we come to examine change over time.

There were rather few changes as a result of parent–teacher counselling when compared with the control group. The only two changes on single scores were in a Devereux measure at eighteen-month follow-up of 'importance of doing well' and three-year follow-up measure of child withdrawal based on parent interview. There were no changes on composite scores. In the individual questionnaire to parents which asked a series of questions specific to that regime (and therefore not suitable as a comparative measure) there were a number of positive responses which to some extent put a question mark against the unimpressive findings of the objective measures. For example, 68 per cent of the mothers agreed that it helped to have someone to talk to. We will return to this theme in the discussion.

The behaviour modification and group therapy regimes are, as mentioned above, particularly suitable for comparison so it is convenient to present the results side by side.

First, two self-reports measures were administered, the Junior Eysenck Personality Inventory (Eysenck, 1965) and the Barker Lunn School Attitude Scale (Barker Lunn, 1969). It was only in these two scales (and the ability scales) that the children were directly approached and the results used in our analysis of outcome measures. The Junior Eysenck Personality Inventory is an attempt to detect in a child and adolescent population the basic dimensions of personality that have arisen out of factor studies of self-report personality questionnaires. It consists of an extroversion scale, a neuroticism scale and a lie scale. The Barker Lunn scale was developed for a study to investigate the effect of ability streaming in British junior schools, the scales being derived originally from statements made by children during group discussions. Ten subscales were developed on the basis of homogeneity of structure and internal consistency. In our analyses (Kolvin *et al.*, 1981, Appendix 2) we found that the scales fell into two groups on the basis of the patterns of intercorrelation between individual scales. The first group consisted of seven scales which concerned attitudes to school and work. Attitude to school, interest in school work, importance of doing well, attitude to class, 'other' image of class, conforming versus non-conforming and relationship with teacher. The second group comprised three scales which reflected attitudes to the self in the school context. There were anxiety about school work, social adjustment and self-image in terms of school work. It is these latter scales which seem particularly relevant to the assessment of emotional state.

Table 13.1   Significant improvements over control group in behaviour modification and group-therapy regimes: Self assessments

	Improvement over controls		
	Behaviour modification only	Both treatments	Group therapy only
Immediate post treatment	Nil	Barker Lunn: attitude to school	Nil
Base to midline follow-up	Nil	Barker Lunn: anxiety about school work JEPI: neuroticism	Barker Lunn: poor social adjustment
Base to final follow-up	JEPI: intro-version	Nil	Nil

The comparative changes in the various self assessments at the follow-ups are shown in Table 13.1. It can be seen that significant improvements in anxiety-based measures seem to have occurred as a result of *both* treatments at midline follow up, this result having disappeared by final follow-up. At immediate post treatment there was a similar common improvement in attitude to school but the anxiety measures fell just short of significant improvement on our more rigorous test of pairwise comparisons. Two scores which had more to do with individual social adjustment (Barker Lunn Social Adjustment and JEPI Introversion) showed separate changes for the two treatments.

Having examined the available self-report measures we will now turn to direct assessments such as attainments tests and reports of significant others in the child's environment such as teachers, peer or parents. In our study, all these sources of data were used.

Peer choice and attitudes towards the study children were measured by a sociometric technique (Macmillan *et al.*, 1978). As can be seen, there were significant improvements over controls on measures of isolation, but these occurred at different time points in the two treatments.

As for teachers observations, these were measured by the Rutter 'B' Teacher Behaviour Scale (Rutter, 1967) and the Devereux Elementary School Behaviour Rating Scale (Spivack and Swift, 1967). These scales again revealed similar patterns of change for the two treatments except that there was a significant improvement in anti-social behaviour at final follow-up in group therapy and at end of treatment behaviour modification showed gains in the Devereux Subscore 'Creative Initiative'.

A variety of parent reports were made on the children. These included a behaviour interview (Kolvin *et al.*, 1975) a temperament interview (Garside *et al.*, 1975) and the Rutter 'A' scale (Rutter *et al.*, 1970). There was less similarity in the changes on these home measures than on the other measures reported above. There is little to show for either intervention immediately post treatment largely because only the more superficial questionnaire measure was given at this time. The behaviour modification showed some early deterioration on the Rutter 'A' scale. By final follow up, the behaviour modification showed

Table 13.2 Significant improvements over control group in behaviour modification and group therapy regimes: assessment by others

	Improvement over controls		
	Behaviour modification only	Both treatments	Group therapy only
Immediate post treatment	Devereux teacher report of: lack of initiative Peer report of: isolation	Devereux teacher report of: need for closeness	
Base to midline follow-up	Rutter 'A' parent questionnaire: deterioration of antisocial behaviour	Academic attainment: (a) verbal (b) non-verbal	Parent interview: psychosomatic symptoms
Base to final follow-up	Parent interview of: antisocial behaviour	Rutter 'B' teacher report of: neurotic behaviour	Rutter 'B' teacher report of: anti-social behaviour Peer report of: isolation

improvement in antisocial behaviour. The only significant unitary change on parent report for group therapy was psychosomatic symptomatology at midline follow-up.

We regard the reports of parents as particularly significant for two reasons. First, parents are in a position to observe their children at closer quarters than other observers. Second, their reports reflect behaviour in a setting quite independent from that where the treatment occurred. The positive findings thus reflect a possible generalization of the treatment effect.

Finally, group measures of attainment were made at each follow-up point. The only significant improvements over the controls occurred at midline follow-up where again both behaviour modification and group therapy showed the same favourable changes.

Treatment effectiveness with different types of problem

It has long been recognized that blanket terms such as 'behaviour problem' or 'maladjusted' are inadequate descriptions of children's disorders. Of the many different types of problems (see, for example Rutter and Hersov, 1976) the vast majority of the disturbed children in ordinary schools have either neurotic disorders or conduct disorders. Neurotic disorders are characterized by an excess of depression, anxiety, phobias, obsessional symptoms whereas conduct disorders are characterized by persistent antisocial behaviour such as stealing, lying, truancy, aggressiveness and so on. It is now well established that the different types of disorder have other distinguishing features apart from manifest behaviour. Conduct disorders, for example, are more clearly associated with family discord (see Chapter 15 this volume) and also carry a worse prognosis (Robins, 1966).

In our study, a psychiatric assessment of the type of disorder was made on each child from examination of all the available data and interview schedules. At follow-up, those with conduct disorders were compared with those with neurotic disorders. When this comparison was made for the total sample, irrespective of treatment, it was found that, as expected, the neurotic youngsters showed more improvement than those with conduct disorders.

We then focused more closely on the effects of different treatments on conduct and neurotic disorders to see if there were any differences in effectiveness on these different types of problem. In fact we found no differential effectiveness at all—the results seemed exactly the same for neurotic and conduct disorders.

A second way to examine differences in effectiveness between treatments was to derive statistical summaries of the various questionnaire scores rather than make a clinical rating based on a human judgement about each case. A principal component factor analysis of all the individual results except the Devereux teacher scale and the Barker Lunn self-report scale contrasted, as expected, neurotic and antisocial behaviour. Aggregate measures derived from the addition of standard scores of nine neurotic items and five antisocial items were then examined to see if there were any differences between the different treatments. Again no difference between the effectiveness of different treatments on different measures was found.

The overall magnitude of change

So much for the separate areas of functioning that showed change, but what about the magnitude of the changes? Our findings on this question were quite extensive but they can be summarized by examining the change scores for an aggregate measure of the fourteen items of disturbance which made up the neurotic and antisocial aggregate measure mentioned above.

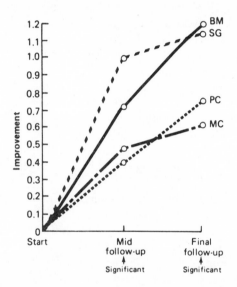

Fig. 13.1 Improvement on overall maladjustment

It can be seen that on an aggregate of these fourteen measures, there is a rapid improvement, particularly in group therapy, in the period up to the midline measure. In the period between eighteen months and final three-year follow-up the improvement clearly is not only maintained but, in the behaviour modification group, it continues to increase. This progressive improvement over the control long after active treatment has finished was a phenomenon we observed quite frequently in the various follow-ups we carried out, particularly in the behaviour modification regime but also group therapy on some measures.

To summarize, the above results are some of those from our research which are relevant to the question of which type of therapy is best for which type of problem. We will now turn to some of the lessons that may be learned from them, in particular the difficult process of translating the findings into practical lessons.

DISCUSSION

Let us consider first of all the apparent lack of effectiveness of the parent counselling–teacher consultation regime. The casework in this regime was designed to be in the task-centred casework tradition (Reid and Epstein, 1972). This comprised a preliminary assessment in order to delineate problem areas followed by the setting up, with the client, of tasks which would form the content of the treatment sessions. There have been quite a lot of descriptive accounts of the application of task-centred casework in different settings (Reid and Epstein, 1972; Reid, 1979) and to our knowledge, three evaluative studies. The original evaluation of Reid and Shyne (1969) compared task-centred with traditional casework and found that, despite its short time span it was more effective, both in measures of overall problems and in various specific areas such as spouse and parent–child relationship, emotional climate of the home and parents perception of self. The authors note that their method was less effective with child-related than with marital problems. It would be foolish to draw conclusions about our study from one as diverse in context as the Reid and Shyne study, especially as our focus was clearly on the school and parent–child relationships, however, the possibility remains that more family-centred measures may have revealed changes which did not generalize to effect the behaviour of the child.

The original Reid and Shyne study was carried out in a social work agency in the US, Reid has carried out a more recent study (Reid, 1979) in which the clients comprised a deprived inner-city population. In this study, change was measured along problem dimensions which were designed individually for each case. There was a control group which received supportive attention and, in a later phase, was given the task-centred approach so that cross-over effects could be looked for. The results suggested that the task-centred treatment did bring about specific changes, but no information is given as to the areas of functioning where the changes occurred. We are not able, therefore, to evaluate whether the results were truly different from ours or whether the content areas which were included in the evaluation accounted for the differences from our study. The Reid study did also include some major design problems, for example at some points in follow-up the change ratings were made by the therapists themselves—a highly contaminated measure.

A third study of task-centred casework is the British study of Gibbons *et al.* (1978) where a task-centred approach was used with self-poisoning patients. Measures of mental state and of social functioning were made. It was in the latter that the changes were found. This again raises the possibility that a spread of measures focused more on the recipient of the casework rather than on the child, as in our study, might have yielded different results. There is clearly a need for further independent evaluation on this interesting and widely applicable form of intervention. We will return to the teacher component of the parent–teacher counselling in a moment.

We turn next to the two most successful treatments, the behaviour-modification and group-therapy regimes. The striking finding here is not only that the two approaches were successful but that the good results seemed to come in remarkably similar content areas. In fact, rather surprisingly, this result is in line with many other results of comparative studies in both the child (Miller et al., 1972) and adult literature (Luborsky et al., 1975; Bergin and Lambert, 1978).

At midline, eighteen-month follow-up it was the anxiety measures that showed the most consistent changes together with the measures of academic performance. It is worth mentioning that the anxiety measures also showed significant differences at the immediate post treatment stage with the parent–teacher counselling coming out particularly poorly. Changes on the more stringent pair-wise comparison tests were non-significant. These observations bring us to consider a traditional classification of outcome in the healing professions which is into the relief of discomfort on the one hand, and the improvement of function on the other. These two aspects of improvement do not always run together, improved function is often only achieved at the expense of some discomfort — as with the improvement of function in a joint with exercise following immobilization for a fracture.

Frank (1973) in his discussion of the effectiveness of the psychotherapies, highlights the relevance of this distinction between discomfort and function. There is considerable evidence that a wide range of inert placebos act as a source of increased hope and comfort, and in this the psychotherapies are no exception. Frank postulates that the improvement in self-report mood and anxiety scales, often found following psychotherapy, is in fact equivalent to a placebo effect. Such effects, as was found in the work of Frank and his colleagues, can be surprisingly long lasting and, according to their evidence, could well persist up to the eighteen-month follow-up. Whether this is such a plausible explanation in young adolescence where so many changes occur so rapidly, is of course debateable. Another interpretation would be that the children are, in fact, making their own sense of the therapy experience and one which may not respect the distinction between the different types of therapy.

The remarkable eighteen-month improvement in school-attainment measures in another area where there is similarity in the improvement shown by the two regimes. This is less easy to explain since the approach to the children in work-related areas seems on the face of it to have been so different. It may be linked to the findings concerning the levels of anxiety, for example the lower manifest anxiety of the treated children may have allowed them to offer a better performance at school or at least in the immediate test situation. There are in fact other studies which suggest that there may be benefits of counselling in terms of the children's academic progress (see Kolvin *et al.*, 1981, Chapter 8, for review). The mixed bag of studies available, while suggesting that there may be overall benefits of therapy, gives no indication of superiority of a particular type of therapy. Clearly, from our results, it will be important to include both a longitudinal element in any further studies in this area and also to consider ways in which the improvements might be maintained over long time periods.

The reports made by others: peers, teachers and parents might be considered to reflect objective performance more than discomfort as distinguished by Frank (1973). In fact, the changes are both much more diverse and also appear later. These facts are consistent with the operation of both a generalization effect and the results, possibly, of more specific effects of the different therapy regimes. When we come to the details of what type of therapy seems most effective for what type of change, it is again somewhat paradoxical that the more antisocial trends in school behaviour seem to have responded to the more permissive group therapy rather than the more directive behaviour modification regime. Review of the results of the statistical analyses confirms these different results of treatment can only be considered as suggestive, since there are no significant interactions of therapy with broad types of behaviour.

Before commenting generally on the importance of longitudinal studies in therapy research, let us return to the parent counselling–teacher consultation regime to consider its school component more specifically. The point here is that the other two regimes which turned out to be effective, both involved trained staff in direct contact with the child. The training did, of course, differ quite a lot, and in the case of behaviour modification was limited to in-service training of interested teaching staff. Macmillan (1984) has specified the emphasis in the behaviour modification intervention which may have contributed to its superiority over teacher consultation. These include specifying clear and discernible features of the child's behaviour on which the teacher can focus; developing successive objectives as the treatment proceeds; stressing the link between behaviour and consequences and finally a stress on the teacher increasing rates of positive responses and encouragement.

Let us finish by looking at the conclusions that can be drawn from the data we have presented and examine how the nature of these conclusions is influenced by the particular methodology used.

The first conclusion is that there is a marked difference in the effectiveness of parent counselling–teacher consultation on the one hand and behaviour modification and group therapy on the other. Within the area of outcome measures employed in this study this distinction is quite clear but there remains the possibility that for parent–teacher counselling, there could be undetected changes. The alternative possibility is that, while task-centred casework is a useful technique, the approach used in this particular study failed to engage the families adequately.

The second conclusion is that there are similarities in outcome between the behaviour-modification and group-therapy regimes. Here again methodological considerations are central to the interpretation of outcome. In this broad-based study an important strategy has been to group together discrete items of behaviour into the global groupings of conduct and neurotic disorders and we have referred to this above. In addition, another grouping has been necessary and that is of the presumed 'active ingredients' of therapy into packages — for example behaviour analysis and reward system into the behaviour modification package or the provision of group interpretations of emphatic reflection of feeling into the group-therapy package.

We might postulate, therefore, that for each child in therapy, there is a specific change which constitutes an individual response of that child's disorder to the particular therapy and a non-specific change which is shown by all children. These latter changes may be related to the children's assessment of the therapy experience which may not emphasize distinctions in technique in the same way as we as research workers did. Our results constitute a summation of these numerous individual responses. Thus, elements that are common to all the children's responses will be amplified while specific responses will be submerged. It is perhaps not surprising, therefore that the 'non-specific' improvements are clearer and easier to interpret while the 'specific' improvements are rather patchy and inconsistent. What strategies might be used to explore the specific as well as the non-specific responses? This is easy with more discrete disorders such as monosymptomatic phobias. Unfortunately, the bulk of disorders which present in the school situation are not so easily classified. Some studies with adults using more specific therapies for more specific diagnostic entities have been able to identify and compare the specific and non-specific components of therapy. This is easier in the case of behaviour therapy (Paul, 1966, 1967; Gelder et al., 1973) than with dynamic therapies.

The third conclusion is that the approach by the teachers in this behaviour modification regime was more effective than that in the parent counselling–teacher consultation regime. We have already discussed reasons why this might be.

A fourth conclusion is that there is a progressive improvement over time. This most important finding has been commented on previously (Wright et al., 1976) but could in fact only have been demonstrated fully in a research of the scale of our project with its wide spread of measures and long-term follow-ups. Not only was there a progressive improvement over time for the two most effective therapies but there was a progressive generalization from self-report measures to those which constitute external reports of the child's performance. Wahler et al. (1979), in discussing the dearth of evidence concerning generalization effects in child-behaviour therapy calls for more studies which adopt an 'inductive approach' with a sampling of a wide range of behaviours in different settings. This is precisely the contribution that our study has been able to make and it does, in fact, provide a wealth of information on the generalization to home and school functioning.

Studies of adult psychotherapy have not typically shown the progressive improvement that was shown in our study but rather an initial improvement followed by a catch up by the control group in longer-term follow-ups. A similar picture emerged from the treatment study of phobia of Hampe and his colleagues (Hampe *et al.*, 1973). There are several reasons why our results may have differed from those of other studies. For example, in many of these studies it is likely that control groups received treatment from other agencies so that they may have caught up with the treatment group rather than the treatment groups deteriorating. Alternatively, the effect may have been due to the great maturational powers of the young, which makes them able to capitalize on the initial advantages of therapy. A third possibility is that the community basis of our study was all important. For example, it may be that the treatment of children in an environment where they will spend many subsequent years sets off chains of events in the environment which operate through positive feedback loops to maintain adaptive behaviour.

It is clear that the weight of our evidence is against the idea that schools can only be places to gain academic knowledge. It does seem that if sufficient expertise and careful supervision are brought to bear different techniques derived from psychotherapy practice could add a new dimension of emotional learning to the curriculum, and this is badly needed. The children need to be engaged directly in this enterprise. Exactly which of the multiplicity of techniques is used seems less important but more focused evaluation on individual disorders may reveal distinctions which could give more guidance on this question. The application of these brief techniques need not be prohibitively expensive, and choice between the two most effective approaches is likely to be influenced by local circumstances such as the skills available in any particular locality and the preferences of decision-makers.

REFERENCES

Barker Lunn, J. C. (1969). The development of scales to measure junior school children's attitudes, *Brit. J. Educ. Psychol.* **39**, 64–71.

Bergin, A. E. and Lambert, M. J. (1978). The evaluation of therapeutic outcomes, in *Handbook of Psychotherapy and Behaviour Change* (2nd edn) (Eds S. L. Garfield and A. E. Bergin), Wiley, New York.

Eysenck, S. B. G. (1965). *Manual of the Junior Eysenck Personality Inventory*, University of London Press, London.

Frank, J. D. (1973). *Persuasion and Healing: A Comparative Study of Psychotherapy*, (revised edition) John Hopkins University Press, Baltimore.

Garside, R. F., Birch, H., Scott, D. McI., Chambers, S., Kolvin, I., Tweddle, E. G. and Barber, L. M. (1975). Dimenions of temperament in infant school children, *J. Child Psychol. Psychiat.* **16**, 219–231.

Gelder, M. G., Bancroft, J. H. J., Gath, D. H., Johnston, D. W., Mathews, A. M. and Shaw, P. M. (1973). Specific and non-specific factors in behaviour therapy, *Brit. J. Psychiat.* **123**, 445.

Gibbons, J. S., Butler, J., Urwin, P. and Gibbons, J. L. (1978). Evaluation of a social worker service for self poisoning patients. *Brit. J. Psychiat.* **133**, 111–118.

Goldstein, A. P. and Simonson, N. R. (1971). Social psychological approaches to psychotherapy research, in *Handbook of Psychotherapy and Behaviour Change* (Eds A. E. Bergin and S. L. Garfield), Wiley, New York.

Hampe, E., Noble, H., Miller, L. C. and Barrett, C. L. (1973). Phobic children one and two years post treatment, *J. Abnorm. Psychol.* **82**, 446–453.

Kolvin, I., Garside, R. F., Nicol, A. R., Macmillan, A., Wolstenholme, F., Leitch, I. M. (1981). *Help Starts Here*, Tavistock, London.

Kolvin, I., Wolff, S., Barber, L. M., Tweddle, E. G., Garside, R. F., Scott, D. McI. and Chambers, S. (1975). Dimensions of behaviour in infant school children, *Brit. J. Psychiat.* **126**, 114–126.

Luborsky, L., Singer, B. and Luborsky, L. (1975). Comparative studies of psychotherapy, *Arch. Gen. Psychiat.* **32**, 995–1008.

Macmillan, A. (1984). Unpublished PhD Thesis, University of Newcastle.

Macmillan, A., Walker, L., Garside, R. F., Kolvin, I., Leitch, I. M. and Nicol, A. R. (1978). The development and application of sociometric techniques for the identification of isolated and rejected children, *Journal of Assn. of Workers for Maladjusted Children*, **6**, 58–74.

Miller, L. C., Barrett, C. L., Hampe, E. and Noble, H. (1972). Comparison reciprocal inhibition, psychotherapy and waiting list control for phobic children, *J. Abnorm. Psychol.* **79**, 269–279.

Paul, G. L. (1966). *Insight vs. Desensitization in Psychotherapy*, Stanford University Press, Stanford.

Paul, G. L. (1967). Insight vs. desensitization in psychotherapy two years after termination, *J. Consult Psychol.* **31**, 333–348.

Reid, W. J. (1979). *The Task Centred System*, Columbia University Press, New York.

Reid, W. J. and Epstein, L. (1972). *Task Centred Casework*, Columbia University Press, New York.

Reid, W. J. and Shyne, A. W. (1969). *Brief and Extended Casework*, Columbia University Press, New York.

Robins, L. N. (1966). *Deviant Children Grown Up*, Williams and Wilkins, Baltimore.

Rutter, M. and Hersov, L. (1976). *Child Psychiatry: Modern Approaches*, Blackwell, Oxford.

Rutter, M. (1967). A children's behaviour questionnaire for completion by teachers: preliminary findings, *Journal of Child Psychology and Psychiatry*, **8**, 1–11.

Rutter, M., Tizard, J. and Whitmore, K. (1970). *Education, Health and Behaviour*, Longman, London.

Sloane, R. B., Staples, F. R., Cristol, A. H., Yorkston, N. J. and Whipple, K. (1975). *Psychotherapy vs. Behaviour Therapy*, Harvard University Press, Cambridge Mass.

Spivack, G. and Swift, M. (1967). *Devereux Elementary School Behaviour Rating Manual Devon Pa*, The Devereux Foundation.

Wahler, R. G., Berland, R. M. and Coe, T. D. (1979). Generalization processes in child behaviour change, in *Advances in Clinical Child Psychology*, Vol. 2 (Eds B. D. Lahey and A. E. Kazdin), Plenum Press, New York.

Winer, B. J. (1971). *Statistical Principles in Experimental Design* (2nd edn). McGraw Hill, New York.

Wright, D. M., Moelis, I. and Pollack, L. J. (1976). The outcome of individual psychotherapy: increments at follow up, *J. Child Psychol and Psychiat.* **17**, 275–285.

Longitudinal Studies in Child Psychology and Psychiatry
Edited by A. R. Nicol
© 1985 John Wiley and Sons Ltd.

Chapter 14

Stress and Protective Factors in Children's Lives

E. E. Werner

In this chapter I will highlight some of the lessons we learned from a longitudinal study of a multi-racial cohort of 698 children, born on the island of Kauai whom we followed until the end of the second decade of their lives. My objectives are:

1 To provide a longitudinal perspective on the children's capacity to cope with perinatal stress, poverty and serious disruptions of the family unit.
2 To examine sex differences in vulnerability and resistance to biological and psychosocial stress.
3 To identify protective factors within the children and their caregiving environment that discriminated between resilient youngsters and peers who developed serious learning and/or behaviour problems in the first and second decades of life.

I will conclude with a discussion of the implications of our findings within the framework of a transactional model of human development.

METHODOLOGY

Kauai, with some 32 000 inhabitants, lies at the north-west end of the main chain of the Hawaiian islands. Settled between the eighth and thirteenth century AD by voyagers from the Society Islands and Tahiti, the island was first visited by Europeans in 1778 when Captain Cook landed on its shores. In the nineteenth and twentieth century, Kauai encountered successive waves of immigrants from south-east Asia and Europe, many of whom intermarried with the local Hawaiians. The majority of children in this birth cohort are of Oriental or Polynesian descent. Most of the fathers worked as semi- or unskilled labourers on the island's sugar plantations; most of the mothers did not graduate from high school (see Table 14.1).

The study began with an assessment of the reproductive histories and the physical and emotional status of the mothers in each trimester of pregnancy,

Table 14.1 Distribution of 1955 birth cohort by ethnicity and socioeconomic status (Kauai Longitudinal Study)

Ethnic group	n	Percentage in each SES category		
		Upper (1, 2)	Middle (3)	Lower (4, 5)
Japanese	217	14.3	54.4	31.3
Part- and full-Hawaiian	147	2.0	31.3	66.7
Filipino	115	2.6	15.7	81.7
Other ethnic mixtures	105	5.7	26.7	67.6
Portuguese	42	7.1	33.3	59.5
Anglo-Caucasians (Haole)	17	76.5	23.5	0

from the fourth week of gestation to delivery. It continued with an evaluation of the cumulative effects of perinatal stress and quality of caretaking environment on the physical, cognitive and social development of the offspring in the post-partum period, and at ages 1, 2, 10 and 18 years. In addition, we monitored the records of educational, health and social agencies for two decades. Attrition rates remained relatively low. Ninety-six per cent of the 1955 birth cohort participated in the two-year follow-up, 90 per cent in the ten-year follow-up and 88 per cent in the eighteen-year follow-up. For two subgroups, the offspring of psychotic parents, and the teenage mothers, we now have data that extend into their twenty-fifth year of life. (Details of our methodology and data base can be found in three books: *The Children of Kauai* (Werner *et al.*, 1971); *Kauai's Children Come of Age* (Werner and Smith, 1977); and *Vulnerable, but Invincible* (Werner and Smith, 1982).)

While the focus of this report is on young people who were vulnerable, we could not help but be deeply impressed by the resiliency of most children and their capacity for positive change and personal growth. This is especially remarkable since our study took place during a period of unprecedented social change that included Statehood for the former territory of Hawaii, the arrival of many newcomers from the US mainland and the after-effects of two prolonged wars in south-east Asia (in Korea and Vietnam).

RESULTS

Our study was conducted on an island with educational, medical, and public-health facilities that compared favourably with most communities of similar size on the US mainland. Yet the magnitude of the casualties among the children and youth in this cohort was impressive.

The casualties of pregnancy and the first decade of life

Deleterious biological effects resulting in reproductive casualties exerted their peak influence in the very early weeks of pregnancy, when 90 per cent of the fetal losses in our study occurred. Of pregnancies reaching 4-weeks gestation, an estimated 237 per 1000 ended in loss of the conceptus. The rate of loss formed a decreasing curve from a high of 108 per 1000 women in the 4–7 week period to a low of 3 in 32–35 weeks of gestation.

In contrast, neonatal and infant mortality rates were very low on Kauai, reflecting a minimum number of unfavourable influences in the first weeks of postnatal life. There were only 13.8 deaths under 28 days per 1000 liveborn and all were attributed to pre- and perinatal causes.

At birth, 9 per cent of the cohort had some congenital defects, of which 3.7 per cent were serious enough to require long-term, specialized care for either severe physical handicaps and/or severe mental retardation. Eight per cent of the liveborn weighed below 2500 g.

By age 2 years, paediatricians found 14 per cent of the children to be below normal in physical development. This included children with congenital defects of the central nervous, musculo-skeletal, and cardiovascular systems, and children born prematurely.

Sixteen per cent of the children in the cohort were considered to be below normal in intellectual development, and 12 per cent were rated below normal in social development by the psychologists. Judgments were based on results of the Cattell and Vineland tests and behaviour observations during the developmental examinations.

Had the two-year follow-up been restricted to paediatric examinations, only 46 per cent of all below-normal children would have been detected. Had the follow-up study been limited to psychological examinations, a little over two-thirds (70 per cent) would have been pinpointed. This finding highlights the need for the use of multiple criteria and interdisciplinary cooperation in the assessment of young children.

At age 10 years, an interdisciplinary panel consisting of a paediatrician, a psychologist, and a public-health nurse reviewed each child's record to isolate any evidence of significant physical, learning, or behaviour problems and to identify any need for medical treatment, remedial education, or mental health care. The following groups of children were identified:

1 For moderate to marked physical handicaps (congenital and acquired defects of the central nervous system, vision, or hearing, heart anomalies, and orthopaedic problems) 7 per cent were in need of continuous medical care.
2 Long-term (more than 6 months) remedial education in such basic skills as reading, spelling, grammar, arithmetic, were required by 14 per cent.

3 Special classes for the mentally retarded were needed by 3 per cent.

4 Three per cent were in need of placement in classes for the learning disabled. These were children of normal intelligence with serious reading and perceptual-motor or attention problems.

5 Long-term (more than 6 months) mental health services were needed by 4 per cent. Four out of five in this group of children were 'acting out'; the others were diagnosed as having childhood neuroses or as schizoid or sociopathic personalities.

6 Short-term (less than 6 months) mental-health services were needed by 10 per cent. The overwhelming majority in this group were shy or anxious children who lacked self-confidence and had developed chronic nervous habits to deal with their insecurities.

By age 10 years more than twice as many children in this cohort needed remedial services for either learning or behaviour problems than were in need of medical care for physical handicaps.

The casualties of the second decade of life

By age 18 years, 15 per cent of the cohort had a record of serious delinquencies documented in the files of the Police Department and the Family Court. Among the delinquents were youths who were, or had been involved in, larceny, burglary, malicious injury, assault and battery, sexual misconduct (including rape); possession, sale, and abuse of hard drugs; and in repeated acts of truancy, running away from home, curfew violations, and unlawful hunting.

Mental-health problems by age 18 years were found among approximately 10 per cent of the cohort. These were documented in the Mental Health Register, the records of the Department of Health's Division of Mental Health, and other Social Service records. They included youths who had made one or more suicide attempts; youths who had been sent to the Hawaii State Mental Hospital or local hospitals for mental-health reasons; youths treated as out patients of the Kauai Community Health Center; and youths who, on the basis of our eighteen-year interviews, were judged to have serious conflicts and high anxiety that led to maladaptive behaviour. The majority of such troubled youth had a record of multiple problems.

Conclusions

Approximately one out of every three children in this birth cohort had some learning or behaviour problems during the first decade of life, and approximately one out of every five youths had records of serious delinquencies or mental-health problems in the second decade. Some were exposed to major perinatal insults that prevented normal development; many more lived in chronic poverty or in a persistently disorganized family environment. Frequently *biological* and *psychosocial* risk factors interacted and exposed these children and youths to cumulative stresses too difficult to cope with unaided.

The joint influences of reproductive risk and the quality of the caregiving environment

For 56 per cent of the children in this cohort, the prenatal and perinatal periods were free from complications. Thirty-one per cent suffered complications of only a mild nature; for 10 per cent, complications of moderate severity were present; and for 3 per cent they were considered severe. Of the infants who died before the two-year follow-up, more than three-quarters were from the very small group with severe perinatal complications. Among the surviving children, only 2 per cent had severe complications.

During the developmental examinations at 20 months, we found a *direct* relationship between severity of perinatal stress and the proportion of children considered to be below normal in physical, intellectual or social development. This trend was especially pronounced among children who had experienced moderate or severe perinatal stress. In the latter group were children with major congenital defects, who required long-term medical care (see Table 14.2).

By age 10 years, differences between children exposed to various degrees of perinatal complications and those born without perinatal stress were less pronounced than at 20 months and centred on a small group of survivors of moderate and severe perinatal stress. The greatest effect of perinatal complications was found in the proportion of children with physical handicaps related to central nervous system (CNS) impairment, children requiring placement in special institutions or classes for the mentally retarded (MR) or learning disabled (LD), and children in need of long-term mental health (LMH) services of more than six months duration.

By age 18 years, four of five survivors of the small group who had suffered severe perinatal stress had persistent and serious physical, learning, or mental-health problems. The rate of mental retardation in this group was ten times, the rate of serious mental health problems was five times, and the rate of serious physical handicaps was more than twice that found in the total cohort. Among the survivors of moderate perinatal stress, the rate of serious mental-health problems was three times, and the rate of mental retardation and of teenage pregnancies was twice that of their peers in the 1955 cohort.

At each of the follow-up stages, however, we found significant interaction effects between characteristics of the caretaking environment and degrees of perinatal stress that produced the largest deficits for the most disadvantaged children (see Table 14.3).

As early as 20 months, these effects were seen in several ways. First, children growing up in middle-class homes who had experienced the *most severe* perinatal

Table 14.2   Two, ten- and eighteen-year outcomes by severity of perinatal stress: 1955 birth cohort (Kauai Longitudinal Study)

	Total cohort (%) ($n = 698$)		Moderate perinatal stress (%) ($n = 69$)		Severe perinatal stress (%) ($n = 14$)
Criteria at age 2 years					
Pediatrician's rating of physical health status below normal	14.2		23.1		35.7
Psychologist's rating of intellectual development below normal	13.5		21.5		28.6
Cattell IQ > 1 SD below mean	9.6		15.4		21.4
Criteria at age 10 years					
Physical handicap (moderate-marked)	6.0		7.0		22.2
PMA IQ > 1 SD below mean	10.7		9.9		30.6
In MR class or institution	2.3		3.5		16.7
Criteria at age 18 years					
Physical handicap (moderate-marked)	6.0		6.0		14.5
Mental retardation	3.0		6.0		29.0
Serious mental health problem	3.0		9.0		14.5
Delinquency record	15.0		17.0		21.5
Teenage pregnancy	6.0	(F)	14.0	(F)	—
Proportion of children and youth with some problem at 2, 10 or 18 years	33.0		36.0		79.0

complications had mean scores on the Cattell Infant Scale almost comparable to children with *no* perinatal stress who were living in poor homes. Second, the most developmentally retarded children (in physical as well as intellectual status) were those who had experienced *both* the most severe perinatal complications *and* who were also living in the poorest homes. Third, SES differences provided for a *greater* difference in mean Cattell scores for children who had experienced severe perinatal stress than did perinatal complications for children living in a favourable environment.

Although the correlation between SES and family stability ratings was low, the difference in mean Cattell scores at 20 months between children who had experienced *severe* perinatal stress, but who were growing up in a *stable* family environment, and those with *serious* perinatal stress who were living in an *unstable* caretaking environment was nearly as dramatic as that found for differences between children from middle-class and poor homes. Unstable caretaking environments also produced a significant increase in the proportion of children in poor health at 20 months, especially among those who had

Table 14.3 Proportion of children with physical health problems, mean Cattell IQ at 2 years and mean PMA IQ at 10 years by socioeconomic status and degree of perinatal stress: 1955 birth cohort (Kauai Longitudinal Study)

Variable	Severity of perinatal complications			
	None (%) (n = 388)	Mild (%) (n = 222)	Moderate (%) (n = 69)	Severe (%) (n = 14)
Physical health status at 2 years (below normal)				
(Very) high SES	7.5	16.7	16.7	50.0
Middle SES	10.9	15.9	22.0	22.2
(Very) low SES	12.2	13.8	21.4	66.7
Cattell IQ at 2 years	Mean score (and standard deviation)			
(Very) high SES	102 (12)	100 (11)	104 (20)	95 (13)
Middle SES	100 (12)	100 (11)	98 (14)	91 (8)
(Very) low SES	98 (11)	96 (12)	93 (12)	61 (37)
PMA IQ at 10 years	Mean score (and standard deviation)			
(Very) high SES	112 (11)	113 (12)	114 (11)	110 (11)
Middle SES	108 (12)	106 (13)	105 (12)	101 (13)
(Very) low SES	99 (11)	100 (11)	99 (12)	94 (14)

undergone severe perinatal stress, in spite of the availability of prepaid and easily accessible health-care services provided by the plantations.

The impact of the caretaking environment appeared even more powerful at age 10 years. First, children *with* and *without* severe perinatal stress who had grown up in middle-class homes *both* achieved mean PMA IQ scores well above the average. Second, PMA IQ scores were seriously depressed in children from *low* SES homes, particularly if they had experienced *severe* perinatal stress. Third, the family's socioeconomic status showed significant associations with the rate of serious learning and behaviour problems. *By age 18 years, ten times as many youth with serious coping problems were living in poverty as had survived serious perinatal stress.*

Conclusions

Perinatal complications were consistently related to later impaired physical and psychological development *only* when combined with persistently poor environmental circumstances (e.g. chronic poverty, family instability, or maternal mental-health problems). Children who were raised in more affluent homes, with an intact family and a well-educated mother, showed few, if any, negative effects from reproductive stress, unless there was severe CNS impairment.

The bidirectionality of child–caretaker effect

Although most of the children and youths with serious and persistent learning and behaviour problems in this community were *poor*, it needs to be kept in perspective that *poverty alone* was not a sufficient condition for the development of maladaptation.

In *both* poor and middle-class homes, infants with 'difficult' temperaments who interacted with distressed caretakers in a disorganized, unstable family, had a greater chance of developing serious and persistent learning and behaviour problems than infants perceived as rewarding by their caretakers and who grew up in stable, supportive homes. Let us briefly illustrate this bidirectionality of child–caretaker effects by a comparison of the records of children with learning disabilities and long-term mental-health problems.

Sixty per cent of the LMH children and 30 per cent of the LD children had records of moderate perinatal stress, low birthweight, congenital defects, or CNS dysfunctions. Controls of the same age and sex, from the same SES and ethnic background, did not display these factors to a significant extent.

More frequently noted among the LMH and LD children than among the controls were infant temperamental traits that appeared distressing and non-rewarding to the caretakers and that may have contributed to initial difficulties in attachment and bonding. These disturbed child–caretaker transaction patterns were observed in the postpartum period and during home visits at year 1 by public-health nurses and were noted independently by psychologists and paediatricians during the developmental examinations at 20 months.

By the tenth year, public-health nurses, social workers, and teachers who were unaware of the earlier child–caregiver transactions noted a pronounced lack of emotional support in the homes of most of the children whose problems persisted throughout adolescence.

The prognosis for childhood learning disabilities and mental health problems

Among children in need of placement in a *learning disability class* by age 10 years, serious problems persisted throughout adolescence. Agency records of *four out of five* indicated continued academic underachievement, confounded by absenteeism, truancy, a high incidence of repetitive, impulsive acting-out behaviour that led to problems with the police for the boys and sexual misconduct for the girls, and other mental-health problems less often attended to. Rates of contact with community agencies were nine times as high as that for control-group youths matched by age, sex, socioeconomic status, and ethnicity.

Group tests at age 18 years showed continued perceptual-motor problems for most, as well as deficiencies in verbal skills and serious underachievement in reading and writing. Self-reports revealed a pervasive lack of self-assurance and interpersonal competency, and a general inadequacy in utilizing their intellectual resources. High 'external' scores on the Nowicki Locus of Control Scale were indicative of the youths' feeling that their actions were not under their control. Only *one out of four* in this group was rated improved by age 18, the lowest proportion among all the groups of youth at risk.

Among children considered in need of *long-term mental health services* at age 10 years more than three out of four had contacts with a variety of community agencies during adolescence, the majority as consequences of persistent, serious behaviour problems. Rates of contact were six times as high as that for controls matched by age, sex, socioeconomic status, and ethnicity.

Psychosomatic and psychotic symptoms, sexual misconduct or problems with sexual identity, assault and battery, theft and burglary, drinking and drug abuse, and continued poor academic performance, coupled with absenteeism and truancy, left these youths few constructive options for the future as they reached young adulthood. Only *one out of three* in this group was judged to have improved by age 18 years.

The prognosis was much more favourable for the children who, at age 10 years, had been considered in need of *mental health services of less than 6 months duration*. In the absence of early biological stress and early family instability, the majority of childhood behaviour problems in this group appeared to be temporary, though at the time painful reactions to stressful life events.

Six out of ten children in this group were rated improved by age 18 years. With few exceptions the improved cases had been troubled by a lack of self-confidence, anxiety and/or chronic nervous habits in childhood.

Conclusions

The majority of problems identified in middle childhood had improved spontaneously by the time the cohort reached age 18 years, although positive changes in behaviour were noted more often for middle-class than lower-class children. Children with learning and/or behaviour problems that *persisted* into late adolescence had higher rates of moderate to severe perinatal stress, low birthweight, and 'chronic conditions leading to minimal brain dysfunctions' noted by paediatricians in infancy *and* tended to live more often in chronic poverty or amidst parental psychopathology than children whose problems were transient. They also tended to elicit more negative responses from their caretakers.

Sex differences in vulnerability and resistance to stress

Sex differences in susceptibility to both biological and psychosocial stress were noted, making boys more vulnerable in childhood and girls more vulnerable in adolescence.

At birth, and throughout the first decade of life more boys than girls were exposed to serious physical defects of illnesses requiring medical care, and more boys than girls had serious learning and behaviour problems, necessitating remedial services or special-class placements.

Boys who were at high risk because of constitutional factors (moderate to severe perinatal stress; congenital defects) were more vulnerable amidst a disordered caretaking environment than girls with the same predisposing conditions. There were significant sex differences in the effects of poverty, family instability, and lack of educational stimulation in the home, which led to a higher rate of childhood problems (i.e. need for long-term remedial education, need for long-term mental-health services, repeated serious delinquencies) for high-risk boys than for high-risk girls.

Nearly three times as many boys than girls had records of serious delinquencies by age 18 years, but the sex ratio of other disordered behaviour shifted from a majority of boys in childhood to a majority of girls in late adolescence. By age 18 years more than twice as many girls as boys had developed serious mental-health problems.

More boys than girls with serious learning and/or behaviour problems in childhood had *improved* by age 18 years, and *new* problems in the second decade appeared more frequently among the girls than the boys.

Related to this trend was the cumulative number of stressful life events experienced by each sex that led to disruptions in their family unit. Boys with serious coping problems had experienced more adversities than girls *in childhood* (such as departure of older sibs, sporadic maternal employment, marital discord, maternal mental-health problems, father absence, divorce and remarriage of mother). Girls with serious coping problems reported more stressful life events in adolescence (such as problems in their relationships with their parents, parental divorce or chronic conflict that led to temporary separation of one parent from the family, and maternal mental-health problems). Among girls with serious mental-health problems by age 18 years, a high proportion became pregnant, married during their teens and reported marital stress of their own. Among *both* sexes significantly more such stressful life events were reported in childhood *and* adolescence for lower-class than middle- and upper-class children.

Conclusions

Sex differences in susceptibility to biological and psychosocial stress changed *with time*, and with the different cognitive and social demands of childhood and adolescence. Overall, however, more females than males in this birth cohort appeared to be able to cope successfully, in spite of reproductive risks, chronic poverty, or family distress.

Key predictors of serious coping problems

About a dozen variables were among the key predictors of serious coping problems in our study. Among the variables that characterized the *caregiving environment* were a low level of maternal education; a low standard of living, especially at birth, but also at ages 2 and 10 years; and a low rating of family stability between birth and age 2 years. Among the *biological* variables were moderate to severe perinatal stress, the presence of a congenital defect at birth, and of a moderate to marked physical handicap at age 10 years. Among the *behavioural* variables were maternal ratings of very-low or very-high infant activity level at year 1, a Cattell IQ score below 80 at age 2 years, a PMA IQ score below 90 at age 10 years, and a recognized need for placement in a class for the learning disabled or for six months or more of mental health services by age 10 years.

Singly or in combination these variables appeared in our multiple-regression equations as key predictors of serious learning and behaviour problems, with the predictive power increasing steadily from birth to age 2 years, from ages 2–10 years, and from ages 10 to 18 years. Predictions for children from poor homes could be made with greater certainty than for children from middle-class homes, reflecting a greater likelihood of some *continuous* malfunction of the child–caretaker/environment interaction across time for the children of poverty than for the children of affluence.

The presence of *four or more* of these predictors in the records of the children by age 2 years appeared to be a realistic dividing line between most children in this cohort who developed serious learning and/or behaviour problems by age 10 or 18 years, and most of the boys and girls who were able to cope successfully with the developmental tasks of childhood and adolescence. We chose this cut-off point to select the resilient children.

Characteristics of stress resistant children and youth

A number of constitutional, ecological and interpersonal variables discriminated, over time, between high-risk children, born and reared in chronic poverty, who appeared to be stress resistant and peers of the same age, sex and low SES who developed serious coping problems in childhood and/or adolescence. All of the resilient youths (thirty males; forty-two females), about 10 per cent of the total cohort, 'worked well, loved well and expected well' when we last interviewed them at age 18 years. None had developed any serious learning or behaviour problems or sought or received any mental-health services during the first two decades of life.

Key factors in the caregiving environment that appeared to contribute to their stress resistance in the midst of chronic poverty were: the age of the opposite-sex parent (younger mothers for resilient M, older fathers for resilient F); the

Summary Table 14.4   Significant discriminators between high-risk resilient M and F and children and youth with serious coping problems at 10 and 18 years (low SES homes)

High-risk M			High Risk F	
at 10 years	at 18 years		at 10 years	at 18 years
×	×	Birthorder	×	×
		Infant perceived as 'cuddly', 'affectionate'		
×	×	(year 1)		
		Infant perceived as 'good-natured', 'even-		
×	×	tempered' (year 1)		
		Infant has (sleeping, feeding) habits		
		distressing to mother (year 1)		×
		Mother's way of coping with infant (year 1)		
	×	Ratio of positive/negative interactions		
		Attention given to infant (year 1)	×	×
		Prolonged separation of infant from mother		
×	×	(year 1)	×	×
	×	Prolonged disruption of family life (year 1)		
		Father absent from household since birth	×	
		Serious or repeated illnesses of child (birth-		
×	×	year 2)	×	×
×	×	Physical status of child (20 months exam)	×	
		Behaviour patterns of child (during 20 months		
×		exam) Ratio of positive/negative interactions	×	
×		Social orientation of child (20 months)	×	×
×	×	Autonomy of child (20 months)		
		Information processing skills of child		
		(20 months)	×	
	×	Self-help skills (SQ) of child (20 months)	×	×
		Parent–child interaction (during 20 months		
×	×	exam) Ratio of positive/negative interactions	×	×
×		Conflicts between parents (birth–year 2)	×	×
	×	Total cumulative life stresses (birth–year 2)	×	×
		Serious or repeated illnesses of child (years		
×	×	2–10)	×	×
	×	Emotional support in home (years 2–10)		
	×	Parents' illnesses (years 2–10)		
	×	Father died or permanently absent (year 2–10)	×	
		Father absent temporarily (years 2–10)	×	×
		Mother works long term (>1 year) outside		
	×	of home (years 2–10)		
×	×	Death of sibling (years 2–10)		
×	×	Older sibling left home (years 2–10)		
×	×	Conflict between family members (years 2–10)	×	×
		Total cumulative life stresses (years 2–10)	×	
×	×	N of children in household (by year 10)		×
		N of additional adults in household (besides		
		parents) (by year 10)		×

(continued)

Summary Table 14.4 — *continued*

High-risk M			High Risk F	
at 10 years	at 18 years		at 10 years	at 18 years
×	×	Bender-Gestalt error (<4) score of child (year 10)	×	×
	×	Problems in family relationships (years 10–18)		×
		Problems in relationship with mother (years 10–18)		×
		Problems in relationship with father (years 10–18)		×
		Self-concept (year 18)		×
	×	Total cumulative life stresses (years 10–18)		×
×	×	Age of opposite-sex parent	×	×
×		Evidence of low mental functioning in parents (parental IQ in school records)		×
		Evidence of parental mental-health problems during offspring's infancy	×	
		Evidence of parental mental-health problems during offspring's childhood		×
		Evidence of parental mental-health problems during adolescence		×

number of children in the family (four or less); the spacing between the index child and next-born sibling (more than two years); alternate caretakers available to the mother within the household (father, grandparents, older siblings); the workload of the mother (including steady employment outside of the household); the amount of attention given to the child by the primary caretaker(s) in infancy; the availability of a sibling as caretaker or confidante in childhood; structure and rules in the household in adolescence; and the presence of an informal multigenerational network of kin and friends, including neighbours, teachers and ministers, who were supportive and available for counsel in times of crises.

Although they had been exposed to higher-than-average rates of perinatal stress and low birthweight, the resilient children among the poor had fewer serious or repeated illnesses in the first two decades of life. Their mothers perceived them to be very active and socially responsive when they were infants, and independent observers noted their pronounced autonomy and positive social orientation when they were toddlers. Developmental exams in the second year of life showed advanced self-help skills and adequate sensori-motor and language development for most. In middle childhood these children possessed adequate problem-solving and communication skills and their perceptual-motor development was age appropriate. Throughout childhood and adolescence their activities and interests were less sex-typed than those of their peers. In late adolescence the resilient youth had a more internal locus of control, a more positive self-concept and a more nurturant, responsible and achievement-oriented attitude toward life than peers who had developed serious coping problems. At the threshold of adulthood they had developed a sense of coherence in their lives and expressed a continuous desire to improve themselves (see Table 14.4).

Resilient girls differed from high-risk girls with problems in adolescence on a number of additional personality dimensions such as dominance, sociability, achievement via independence, intellectual efficiency and a sense of well-being. For these girls early mother–daughter relationships had been consistently positive, and there were other females present as support for them in the household during childhood and adolescence. Permanent absence of the father and long-term employment by the mother outside of the household seemed to push them into the direction of greater autonomy and competence.

Resilient boys were more often firstborn sons, and grew up in households which were less crowded. There were fewer children, but some adult male models present in their families who provided rules and structure in their lives. Few mothers of resilient males worked for extended periods of time outside of the household and had substitute caretakers for their sons.

Similar characteristics were found to discriminate between the resilient offspring of psychotic parents who were free of learning or behaviour problems in childhood and adolescence, and offspring of psychotic parents who had developed serious problems of their own by late adolescence. The resilient children in this group (13/29) had been perceived by their mothers in infancy 'as good-natured and even-tempered'. Independent observers commented on their advanced self-help skills and autonomy during the 20-month developmental examination. Teachers' classroom observations and test results at 10 years indicated superior problem-solving skills, good impulse control and the ability to focus attention. Self-reports in late adolescence reflected their conviction of being 'in control' of their lives. Like the resilient youngsters who lived in chronic poverty, these youth had *not* been separated from their mothers for extended periods of time during the first year of life and they could draw upon the emotional support of alternate caretakers in the household (for example, older sibs or grandparents).

A TRANSACTIONAL MODEL OF DEVELOPMENT

The results of the Kauai Longitudinal Study appear to lend some empirical support to a transactional model of human development that takes into account the bidirectionality of child–caregiver effects (Sameroff and Chandler, 1975).

In Figure 14.1 we show some of the interrelations between major risk factors at birth, and some of the most common stressful life events in childhood and adolescence that *increased vulnerability* in this birth cohort, and protective factors within the child and his/her caregiving environment that *increased stress resistance*.

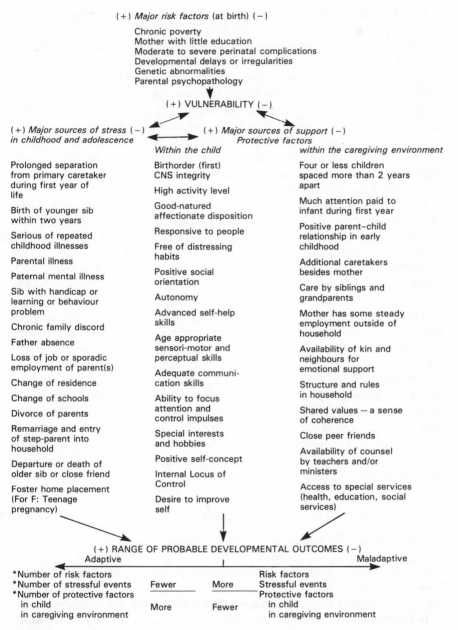

(+) *Major risk factors* (at birth) (−)

Chronic poverty
Mother with little education
Moderate to severe perinatal complications
Developmental delays or irregularities
Genetic abnormalities
Parental psychopathology

(+) VULNERABILITY (−)

(+) *Major sources of stress* (−)
in childhood and adolescence

(+) *Major sources of support* (−)
Protective factors

Within the child

within the caregiving environment

Prolonged separation
from primary caretaker
during first year of
life

Birth of younger sib
within two years

Serious of repeated
childhood illnesses

Parental illness

Paternal mental illness

Sib with handicap or
learning or behaviour
problem

Chronic family discord

Father absence

Loss of job or sporadic
employment of parent(s)

Change of residence

Change of schools

Divorce of parents

Remarriage and entry
of step-parent into
household

Departure or death of
older sib or close friend

Foster home placement
(For F: Teenage
pregnancy)

Birthorder (first)
CNS integrity

High activity level

Good-natured
affectionate disposition

Responsive to people

Free of distressing
habits

Positive social
orientation

Autonomy

Advanced self-help
skills

Age appropriate
sensori-motor and
perceptual skills

Adequate communi-
cation skills

Ability to focus
attention and
control impulses

Special interests
and hobbies

Positive self-concept

Internal Locus of
Control

Desire to improve
self

Four or less children
spaced more than 2 years
apart

Much attention paid to
infant during first year

Positive parent–child
relationship in early
childhood

Additional caretakers
besides mother

Care by siblings and
grandparents

Mother has some steady
employment outside of
household

Availability of kin and
neighbours for
emotional support

Structure and rules
in household

Shared values — a sense
of coherence

Close peer friends

Availability of counsel
by teachers and/or
ministers

Access to special services
(health, education, social
services)

(+) RANGE OF PROBABLE DEVELOPMENTAL OUTCOMES (−)
Adaptive   Maladaptive

*Number of risk factors			Risk factors
*Number of stressful events	Fewer	More	Stressful events
*Number of protective factors			Protective factors
in child			in child
in caregiving environment	More	Fewer	in caregiving environment

*Changes with stage of life cycle, sex of individual, cultural context.

Fig. 14.1 Model of interrelations between risk, stress, sources of support and coping
(based on data from Kauai Longitudinal Study. Reproduced by permission of McGraw-
Hill Book Co.)

It is the balance risk factors, stressful life events, and protective factors in the child and his caregiving environment that appears to account for the range of adaptive or maladaptive outcomes encountered in this birth cohort.

For the children in our study biological factors appeared to pull their greatest weight in infancy and early childhood, ecological factors (household structure and composition) gained in importance in childhood, inter- and intra-personal factors, such as self-esteem and locus of control, in adolescence, judging from the weight assigned to these variables in our discriminant function analyses.

The relative impact of risk factors, stressful life events and protective factors within the child and his/her caregiving environment differs not only with the stage of the life cycle, but also with the sex of the child and the socio-cultural context in which he or she grows up.

As disadvantage and the cumulative number of stressful life events increased, more protective factors in the children and their caregiving environment were needed to counter-balance the negative aspects in their lives and to insure a positive developmental outcome.

To the extent that the men and women were able to *elicit* predominantly positive responses from their environment, at each stage of their life cycle, they were found to be stress-resistant, even if they had experienced perinatal stress, and lived in chronic poverty or in a home with a psychotic parent. To the extent that they elicited negative responses from their environment, they were found to be vulnerable, even in the absence of biological stress or serious financial constraints.

Optimal adaptive development appears to be characterized by a balance between the power of the person and the power of the (social and physical) environment (Wertheim, 1978). Intervention on behalf of children and youth may thus be conceived as an attempt to restore this balance, either by *decreasing* a young person's exposure to risk or stressful life events or by *increasing* the number of protective factors (competencies, sources of support) that *one* can draw upon within oneself or one's caregiving environment.

DISCUSSION

The results of our study, based on a whole population of children in a community over two decades of their lives, provides us with a more hopeful perspective than many short-term studies of problem children found in the clinical literature. As we watched this birth cohort grow from babyhood to adulthood we could not help but respect the self-righting tendencies within them that produced normal development under all but the most persistent adverse circumstances. We were also impressed by the support they received from family, kith and kin.

We were impressed by the pervasive effect of the quality of mother–child interaction in infancy and early childhood that could be documented as early as year 1 by public-health nurses who observed in the home and which were verified independently by observations before, during and after developmental screening examinations at age 2 years. The role of the father appeared more crucial in middle childhood and adolescence, especially for the children with learning disabilities (most of whom were boys) and for the pregnant teenagers. His perceived understanding and support, or lack of it, his consistent enforcement of rules or lack of it, appeared to play a crucial role in the positive or negative resolution of the developmental problems of his children. Parental attitudes (i.e. perceived understanding and support) differentiated significantly between youths with learning and behaviour problems who improved in adolescence and those who did not, while exposure to different types of intervention by community agencies had a lesser impact.

We had not anticipated the considerable influence of alternate caretakers, such as grandparents, older siblings, aunts and uncles, parents of boy- or girlfriends and peers on the children and youth in this cohort. The emotional support of such elders or peer friends was a major ameliorative factor in the midst of poverty, parental psychopathology and serious disruptions of the family unit.

Among the people of Kauai, an informal network of kin and neighbours and the counsel and advice of ministers and teachers were more often sought and more highly valued than the services of the mental-health professionals, whether they were counsellors, psychologists, psychiatrists or social workers.

Equally pervasive appeared to be the effects of competence in reading and writing 'standard English' among the children of Kauai. Competence in these skills was a major ameliorative factor among the resilient youth who coped well in spite of poverty or serious disruptions of their family unit. Lack of these skills led to cumulative problems in coping with cognitive as well as with affective demands in middle childhood and adolescence.

Finally, the degree to which these youth had faith in the effectiveness of their own actions was related not only to the way in which they utilized their self-help skills and intellectual resources but also to positive changes in behaviour. An internal locus of control was a significant correlate of improvement. An external locus of control, i.e. a pronounced lack of faith in the effectiveness of one's own actions, was especially notable among the serious and persistent learning disabilities and childhood mental-health problems. Crucial for these children was not failure *per se*, but loss of control over reinforcement, a lack of synchrony between their actions and feedback from their environment. On the contrary, the experience of the resilient children in *coping with* and *mastering stressful life events* by their actions, appeared to build immunity against such 'learned helplessness', and an attitude of 'hopefulness' instead.

Even among the high-risk children, who were exposed to significant perinatal stress, chronic poverty and parental psychopathology, there were the resilient ones who could draw on a number of protective factors within themselves and their caregiving environment.

The results of our study have made us cognizant of the importance of recognizing and constructively dealing with differences in problem-solving skills and parental socialization styles and values. Emphasis on harmony and co-operation, on spontaneity and expressive role behaviour and preferences for personal relationships among the non-Western subcultures represented in the Hawaiian Islands as well as on the US mainland, can easily come in conflict with demands for competition, individualized achievement and impersonal relationships in the society at large.

The majority of the youth on Kauai successfully coped with the demands of the school system and acquired the cognitive skills needed and valued by the larger society without sacrificing their affective ties with their family and their ethnic identity. For those with serious learning and behaviour disorders, however, intervention programmes may well have to address themselves to their need to acquire two cultural response repertoires. But any attempts at intervention cannot succeed unless all parties concerned, the helping agencies, the parents, and the youth themselves, reach a consensus on their mutual expectations.

IMPLICATIONS

What then are some of the implications of our findings? At present we need to know more about a wide array of what Antonovsky (1979) has called 'generalized resistance resources' that seem to be as important as sources of strength for the survivors of concentration camps (which he studied in Israel) as for the making of resiliency and stress resistance in children and adolescents.

Among them are: *adaptability* on the biological, psychological, and sociocultural levels; *profound* ties to *concrete*, immediate *others*; (formal or informal) *ties* between the *individual* and his/her *community*.

We need to identify more systematically the positive effect of these variables in contributing to 'resiliency' and 'invulnerability', and provide some additional support where they are lacking.

There is an urgent need to re-evaluate present efforts to deal with the load of educational and mental-health problems encountered among the young in most communities of the industrialized world. Available professional skills, time and resources need to be allocated according to the magnitude of the needs and the critical time periods at which intervention appears to be most effective.

Professionals, in turn, need to consider child development within a larger context—they cannot overlook the needs and expectations of the parents and the presence (or lack of it) of informal sources of support, within the family, the neighbourhood and the community at large.

The results of our study (and those of other longitudinal investigations reported in this book) suggest that the critical time for intervention—that time which offers the greatest promise of substantially reducing the number of 'casualties' among the young—should come early in childhood, *before* damage is done, rather than depending upon remedial measures later, as is still the predominant present practice.

Need for closer co-operation between the various professions attending the birth and early care of the child is indicated in order to spot early developmental failures in children suffering from deleterious perinatal conditions, and to provide them and their parents with a supportive and stimulating environment to minimize the effects of early damage.

Hospital, birth and physician's records contain information about the newborn, indicating potential trouble-information that is seldom available to community agencies for utilization in planning with the family for the special needs of high-risk infants.

The results of our two-year examination suggest that every young child in the community should have at least one thorough medical and developmental examination in early childhood. Our analysis of the relationship between the developmental status of the children and the quality of their early family environment leaves little doubt that parental concern and involvement with the young child, language stimulation and parental attitudes toward achievement, have a significant impact on development *before* a child enters school.

Since many of the key predictors of potential problems were already recognizable by the time of the developmental examinations at age 2, it appears reasonable to suggest that the critical time period for intervention for such 'high-risk' children should be in early childhood, preferably between the ages of one and two, the time at which language emerges. Recent reviews of the effectiveness of early intervention programmes (Brown, 1978; Caldwell and Stedman, 1977; Gray and Wandersman, 1980) have shown that such early programmes for high-risk children are strengthened by the involvement of parents.

Some of the most effective interventions have focused on enhancing language development and intellectual skills and on techniques that enhance a mother's sense of control over her own life and that of her child. However, the quality and motivation of the staff and the volunteers who deliver these services to young handicapped and high-risk children appears directly related to the success of early intervention programmes and are therefore primary factors in determining the extent to which a programme is replicable and exportable.

But not all intervention needs to be limited to early childhood. In reviewing the school records of the 10 year olds, we were impressed by the great amount of useful information that had been accumulated about these children through routine group testing. School failures could have been successfully spotted in the first three grades if better use had been made of the information already available on the children. More than half of the school failures detected at age 10 years in our study could have profited substantially from short-term remedial work in the first three grades by teachers' aides and by volunteer tutors at the critical period when the motivation to achieve and future levels of achievement are stabilized.

During middle childhood and especially in adolescence, there is need to explore the support that could be provided by older children tutoring younger ones, by teenagers assisting in running day-care centres and recreational facilities for children of working mothers, by peer counsellors and the growing reservoir of retired persons. Peer counsellors and concerned older volunteers could also relieve pressing manpower needs by helping children cope with temporary emotional distress and would be helpful in meeting the pressing mental-health needs of pregnant teenagers.

Thus, in many situations, it may make better sense to strengthen available informal ties to kin and community than to introduce additional layers of bureaucracy into the delivery of social services, and it might be less costly as well.

A strengthening of already existing informal support systems could focus especially on those children and families in a community that appear most vulnerable because they—temporarily or permanently—lack some of the essential social bonds which appear to buffer stress.

Working mothers of young children, with no dependable alternatives for child care; single, divorced or teenage parents, with no other adult in the household; hospitalized children in need of special care, who are separated from their families for extended periods of time; children of psychotic parents (and the 'well' spouse in such a marriage); immigrant and refugee children.

Future research needs

Future research in the study of vulnerability and stress resistance needs to consider the consequences of *changing demographic trends* (such as later age of marriage and childbirth, smaller families and single parenthood) as well as *changing sex role expectations* that may alter substantially the nature of the caregiving environment and the stress resistance of contemporary children and youth in the 'modern', industrialized world.

We need to know more about the role of *alternate caregivers*, whether they are siblings, grandmothers, kith or kin, as sources of support in times of stress. Outside of the family unit, there is need to explore other *informal sources of support*. Among the most frequently encountered in our study were peer friends, teachers, ministers, and neighbours.

The central component of effective coping with the multiplicity of inevitable life stresses appears to be a *sense of coherence* (Antonovsky, 1979), a feeling of confidence that one's internal and external environment is predictable, that life has meaning and that things will work out as well as can be reasonably expected. The real issue may well be whether the families and the societies in which the children grow up and live their daily lives, facilitate or impede the development and maintenance of such a sense.

A young child maintains a relatively small number of relationships that give him feedback and shape his sense of coherence. We have seen that even under adverse circumstances change is possible when an older child or adolescent develops new competencies and meets people who give him positive reinforcement and a reason for commitment and caring.

REFERENCES

Antonovsky, A. (1979). *Health, Stress and Coping: New Perspectives on Mental and Physical Well-being*, Jossey-Bass, San Francisco.

Brown, B. (1978). *Found: Long-term Gains from Early Intervention*, Westview Press, Boulder.

Caldwell, B. N. and Stedman, D. J. (Eds) (1977). *Infant Education: A Guide for Helping Handicapped Children in the First Three Years of Life*, Walker, New York.

Gray, S. W. and Wandersman, L. P. (1980). The methodology of home-based intervention studies: Problems and promising strategies, *Child Development*, **51**, 993–1009.

Sameroff, A. and Chandler, M. J. (1975). Reproductive risk and the continuation of caretaking casualty, in *Review of Child Development Research*, Vol. IV (Ed. F. D. Horowitz), pp.187–243, University of Chicago Press, Chicago.

Werner, E. E., Bierman, J. M. and French, F. E. (1971). *The Children of Kauai: A Longitudinal Study from the Prenatal Period to Age Ten*, University of Hawaii Press, Honolulu.

Werner, E. E. and Smith, R. S. (1977). *Kauai's Children Come of Age*, University of Hawaii Press, Honolulu.

Werner, E. E. and Smith, R. S. (1982). *Vulnerable, but Invincible: A Longitudinal Study of Resilient Children and Youth*, McGraw Hill, New York.

Wertheim, E. S. (1978). Developmental genesis of human vulnerability: Conceptual re-evaluation, in *The Child in his Family: Vulnerable Children*, Vol. IV (Eds E. J. Anthony, C. Koupernik and C. Chilan), pp.17–36, Wiley, New York.

Longitudinal Studies in Child Psychology and Psychiatry
Edited by A. R. Nicol
© 1985 John Wiley and Sons Ltd.

Chapter 15

Family and School Influences: Meanings, Mechanisms and Implications

M. Rutter

Numerous studies have shown that children with various kinds of behavioural and learning problems in middle childhood tend to come from homes or schools that are disadvantaged or deviant in some respect (see reviews by Birch and Gussow, 1970; Hinde, 1980, Rutter, 1975, 1981a, 1983; Rutter and Madge, 1976; Rutter and Giller, 1983). As a result it has come to be widely accepted that family difficulties—as reflected in such factors as broken homes, child neglect, discord and lack of stimulation—*cause* children to have psychiatric or educational disorders. Similarly, many parents endeavour to choose where they will live or to which schools they will send their children on the basis that certain environments are thought to provide better opportunities than others for optimal psychological development. But what evidence is there that family, school and community environments do truly *influence* children's behaviour and learning? And, in so far as they do, which aspects of the environment matter? Do the effects vary according to the child's age and personal qualities? To what extent do such environmental influences persist and how far are the ill-effects reversible? It is only through answers to questions such as these that the crude statistical associations between family (or school) deviance or disadvantage and child disorder can be translated into useful guidelines for policy or practice. In this overview of some of the main issues and findings in this large topic, therefore, these are the matters that require particular attention.

ALTERNATIVE EXPLANATIONS

The first question of whether the statistical associations between environmental variables and children's disorders represent causal connections requires an examination of three main alternatives—namely, (a) that the associations represent hereditary rather than environmental influences, (b) that the main effect is from the child to the family rather than the other way round, and (c) that both the family (or school) characteristics and the children's disorders

357

are due to some third variable, such as social disadvantage or physical hazards in the environment. Let us consider each of these in turn.

Genetic transmission

The suggestion that the associations reflect genetic rather than experiential factors constitutes a very real possibility. In recent times, passions have tended to run high on this matter because of possible political misuses of genetic findings and because of the unwarranted extrapolation of the findings on individual variation *within* societies to supposed genetic explanations for differences *between* ethnic groups. But, these important sociopolitical implications should not blind us to the hard evidence that hereditary influences do indeed play an important role in the determination of individual differences in most kinds of psychological characteristics (see Rutter and Madge, 1976; Shields, 1977, 1980, for reviews of the findings and concepts). That can no longer be in doubt. But, still we have to ask whether genetic variables account for the associations between family or school variables and child disorder. That question needs to be tackled by means of several rather different research strategies.

Animal studies

First, environmental effects may be examined directly by means of experiments in which the circumstances of rearing are deliberately altered. For obvious ethical reasons, usually this can be done only in animals. Nevertheless, the findings are clear-cut in showing that marked changes in the environment do indeed have important effects on psychological development (see Rutter, 1981a). For example, a period of total social isolation in infancy leads to gross behavioural, social and sexual deficits in rhesus monkeys (Mineka and Suomi, 1978; Ruppenthal *et al.*, 1976); early separation experiences in the same species lead to emotional changes (Hinde and McGinnis, 1977); and severe restrictions in sensory experiences have been found to impair intellectual growth in rats and other animals (Hunt, 1979; Thompson and Grusec, 1970). It is clear then, that gross alterations in the environment can have quite marked and lasting effects on psychological functioning. In these studies we know that the effects were environmental rather than genetic because of the experimental conditions. But, of course, many of the environmental changes were severe and for this reason, as well as because of biological differences between species, the results cannot be directly applied to the human situations. Nevertheless, they provide a sound basis for the environmental effects hypothesis.

Heritability estimates

A second approach is provided by *heritability* estimates. These refer to the proportion of the variation in some attribute among individuals in a population that is genetically determined. These estimates are based on the extent to which resemblances between family members (and especially between monozygotic and dizygotic twins within pairs) are a function of the extent to which they share the same genes. The estimates necessarily apply only to the populations studied and within the circumstances operating at the time the data were collected. That is to say, the heritability measure will be influenced by the extent to which the sample studied varied genetically and environmentally—it is not and cannot be an absolute. Also, it is a parameter that describes *populations*, and not individuals. For these and other reasons, it has been subjected to a good deal of criticism (Madge and Tizard, 1980; Rutter and Madge, 1976). Nevertheless, heritability measures continue to provide useful information.

To begin with, in no case is the heritability of psychological attributes so high that there is no room for environmental effects. For example, it may be calculated that if IQ has an 83 per cent heritability (an estimate that is rather higher than generally accepted) it would still be expected on *environmental grounds alone* that the most-advantaged million people in Britain would have a mean IQ some 24 points above the least-advantaged million (see Burks, 1928)! Heritability estimates are also useful in showing differences between attributes in the extent of the environmental contribution. For example, it is clear that environmental effects are considerably greater for educational achievement than for IQ (see Jensen, 1973). Also, although genetic factors play a part in delinquency (especially delinquency associated with personality disorder that persists into adult life), environmental factors predominate (see Rutter and Giller, 1983). Hence, it is with delinquency and educational difficulties that we may expect to find some of the most marked environmental influences.

But, family resemblances also provide another important datum—namely the extent to which the environmental influences operate *within* or *between* families (Rowe and Plomin, 1981). If children in the same family tend to be rather similar in their characteristics the implication is that they share the most important environmental influences and hence that the crucial factors are likely to be ones that effect the family as a whole. This is very much the situation with respect to juvenile delinquency and conduct disorders where it is common for several children in the family to show similar behaviour. The expectation that follows from this observation is that the families of delinquents are likely to differ markedly from the families of non-delinquents in the overall environments they provide for the children. As we shall see, that is indeed what has been found.

In contrast, if brothers and sisters tend to be *dis*similar in their attributes, the implication is that the environmental influences are likely to be ones that impinge *differently* on each member of the family. That is what seems to be the case with personality features and possibly also emotional disturbance (Loehlin and Nichols, 1976; Scarr *et al.*, 1981). The suggestion, here, is that it will be factors such as ordinal position, or differential treatment by parents, or stresses specific to the individual, or extra-familial influences that will be most important. But, systematic differences *between* families according to the personality characteristics of the children are not to be expected. The findings on educational attainment suggest that they fall into somewhat of an intermediate position with both shared and non-shared environmental influences operative.

Studies of adopted/fostered children

The study of familial influences on adopted or fostered children separated from their parents in infancy constitutes a third research strategy for determining whether effects are likely to be genetic or environmental. If it is deviance in the biological parents (who did not provide the rearing) that is associated with disorder in the child then the association is likely to represent a genetic effect; if it is deviance in the adoptive parents then the effect is likely to be environmental. This comparison has shown very clearly that the link between schizophrenia in the parents and schizophrenia in the children is genetically, rather than environmentally determined (Gottesman and Shields, 1976). The same applies to alcoholism (Cadoret *et al.*, 1980). However, also it has shown that the link between criminality in the parents and criminality in the offspring reflects both genetic and environmental factors (Hutchings and Mednick, 1974). Most strikingly, the *environmental* effect of criminality in the adoptive parent seems to be largely operative when the children are *genetically* vulnerable by virtue of criminality in the biological parent. The implication is that some kinds of genetic factors may operate by making an individual more vulnerable to adverse environmental influences; and similarly, environmental factors may have their greatest impact on those who are genetically susceptible. It is possible that the effect of the biological parent could be environmental if it arose through prejudiced treatment of the child as a result of the adoptive parent's knowledge of the biological parents. Similarly, the association with the adoptive parent could be genetic if there had been selective placement according to the characteristics of the biological parents. Even so, the cross-fostering design provides one of the best ways of differentiating between genetic and environmental influences.

Apart from deviance or disorder in the adoptive parents, there has been surprisingly little study of possible environmental influences on the development of adopted or fostered children—an unfortunate lack as this is a particularly suitable situation for studying non-genetic effects. However, there are some relevant data. Thus, Cadoret and Cain (1980) showed that psychiatric disorder and divorce in the adopting families, as well as rearing during infancy in an institution with changing caretakers, were significantly associated with antisocial disorder in boys who had been separated at birth from their biological parents. Interestingly, this was not so for girls. The findings indicate that these family effects were indeed environmentally mediated but also pointed to the possibility of sex differences in vulnerability to environmental stressors. Similar findings stem from other studies (Crowe, 1974), although Bohman and Sigvardsson (Chapter 7, this volume), found only slight effects attributable to institutional rearing in infancy (in relation to rather 'soft' and general measures of the children's behaviour). A similar comparison may be made by comparing children reared in an institution with those reared in foster-families. Roy (1983) found that the former were more likely to show behavioural disturbance. As both groups had been separated from their biological parents at birth and as 'blind' ratings of the protocols showed no group differences in the characteristics of the biological parents, the strong inference is of an environmental effect.

Several of the early studies of adopted children show that their IQ correlated significantly with various measures of the qualities of the adoptive home (Burks, 1928; Leahy, 1935) — indicating an environmental effect. However, the finding from the same studies that the IQ of adopted children showed a much lower correlation with the characteristics of the homes in which they were reared than did the IQ of children brought up by their own biological parents (0.21–0.23 compared with 0.42–0.53) also shows that part of the association between family variables and children's IQ is due to genetic factors. This is also suggested by a recent study of children reared by their biological parents in which it was found that correlation between home environment measures and children's IQ scores was largely explicable in terms of the mother's IQ (Longstreth et al., 1981). Whereas maternal IQ continued to show a significant correlation (0.33) with child IQ after controlling for the home environment, that for the home environment dropped to a non-significant level (0.18) when maternal IQ was controlled. The strong implication is that genetic factors predominant but this is not certain in that the possibility remains that maternal IQ exerted an environmental effect through mechanisms not reflected in the home environment measures.

The importance of genetic factors is also evident in the finding that within adoptive families that have both biological and adoptive children, the parent–child correlations are substantially stronger for the biological offspring than for the adopted offspring (Scarr, 1981; Willerman, 1979).

Rearing in biological and adoptive homes compared

A further variant of the same strategy consists in the comparison of children from similar biological backgrounds according to whether or not they were reared by their biological parents or were adopted in infancy. The findings are consistent in suggesting that when the biological background is seriously deviant or disadvantaged, children who are adopted have a better outcome than those who remain with their biological parents (see Rutter and Madge, 1976; Rutter and Giller, 1983). Genetic factors still play a part in determining *individual differences* in behaviour and attainment, but the superior environment of the adoptive homes seemed to result in a *general raising* of the outcome for the group as a whole. For example, Skodak and Skeels (1949) showed that children born to parents of low IQ, if adopted and reared in homes somewhat above average, attain normal levels of intelligence. On the basis of their parents' IQ, they could have been expected to have a mean IQ of about 90–95 whereas in fact it was 106. Scarr and Weinberg's (1976, 1978) study showed the same general rise in IQ for children born to disadvantaged parents but reared in average or above-average adoptive homes. Both sets of findings strongly suggest an environmental effect. Similar benefits from adoption have been claimed with respect to protection against delinquency and disturbances of behaviour (see studies cited in Rutter and Giller, 1983). Certainly, several investigations have shown that adopted children have lower rates of problems than children from disadvantaged and deviant backgrounds reared by their biological parents. However, the value of these comparisons is limited by the considerable difficulties entailed in ensuring that the groups are comparable in their genetic background. The evidence is suggestive of an environmental effect but rather better controlled studies are needed to examine the matter more rigorously.

Studies of non-genetic variables

A quite different approach to the disentangling of genetic and environmental effects is afforded by the study of variables that could not be genetically determined. There are several well-established examples of this kind. For example, numerous investigations have shown that, on average, firstborn children have a higher level of scholastic and occupational achievement than do the later born children (see Rutter and Madge, 1976). Taken in conjunction with the evidence that parents tend to treat their first child differently from subsequent children (Rutter, 1981a), the observation clearly indicates an environmental effect on achievement. It should be noted, however, that the ordinal position effect on measured intelligence is both weaker and less consistent.

But, ordinal position affects psychiatric risk as well as cognitive performance. Eldest children have an increased risk of emotional disturbance and of some forms of conduct disorder (Rutter *et al.*, 1970). Again, this is an effect that must be non-genetic. The precise mechanisms remain somewhat uncertain but it seems likely that the stresses associated with adaptation to the birth of a younger sibling play a part. The recent systematic study by Dunn and her colleagues (see Chapter 2 this volume) showed that more than half of 2–3-year-old children become more tearful after the birth of a sibling, a quarter develop sleeping difficulties and nearly half show new toileting problems. It was also found that the development of emotional and behavioural problems in the firstborn was linked with changes in the pattern of mother–child interaction (following the birth of a second child mothers tend to play less with the first child and to become more controlling and negative with him). The causal inference, here, is much strengthened by the combination of three different types of evidence showing, (a) that the association was unlikely to be caused by other non-hypothesized variables, (b) that the link between the hypothesized variable and the predicted outcome showed a close and consistent time relationship, and (c) that the link was associated with changes in variables that constitute a plausible mediating mechanism (see Rutter, 1981b).

Hospital admission constitutes another non-genetic variable. There are many studies showing that preschool children frequently show emotional distress as a consequence of admission to hospital; and, particularly when there are multiple admissions, sometimes this may lead on to more persistent psychosocial problems (Rutter, 1981a). The causal inference, here, is further strengthened by a different type of evidence—namely, that the risks to the child can be reduced by changes in the admission experience (see Rutter, 1981a,c). For example, distress is reduced by daily visiting, the presence of one of the parents during the hospital stay, a supportive relationship with a consistently present nurse, and by measures to better prepare the child and family for the admission.

Bereavement provides another example of a 'non-genetic' variable. The St Louis follow-up study of young widows and widowers together with appropriate controls (van Eerdewegh et al., 1982) provides the best data regarding the effects on children. The great majority (77 per cent) of the bereaved children showed depressed mood during the year following bereavement compared with only a third (34 per cent) of controls, and 14 per cent (compared with 4 per cent) exhibited a depressive syndrome. Over twice as many of the bereaved children wet the bed (19 per cent versus 7 per cent) and far more (18 per cent versus 0 per cent) showed a fall-off in school performance. The findings point to the importance of bereavement as a precipitating factor for at least short-term distress. However, the more limited data on persistent sequelae suggest that long-term disturbance is likely to be related to the changes in the family subsequent to parental death (depression in the surviving parent, break-up of the family, etc.) as much as to the direct stress of the bereavement itself (Rutter, 1966).

Change of environment

Environmental effects may also be studied through the consequences of *changes* in the environment. Three rather different examples of this research strategy may be given. First, the most impressive evidence of the importance of the social group comes from investigations of the effects of a total change in the non-familial environment. For example, West (1982) in his prospective study of London boys found that delinquent activities (whether assessed through self-reports or convictions) tended to diminish following a move to somewhere outside London. Similarly, another study (Buikhuisen and Hoekstra, 1974) found that the reconviction rate of male offenders was significantly less for those who, on discharge from a correctional institution, moved away from their previous neighbourhood (as compared with those who returned to the same address). This benefit from moving was greatest in the case of those who moved away from an unstable family or an asocial environment. Or again, Elliott and Voss (1974) found that although future school drop-outs had an increased rate of delinquency while still at school, there was a reduction in delinquent activities following drop-out. This was particularly likely to occur if the drop-out obtained regular work and, even more so, if he married. All these findings suggest that young people's delinquent activities are influenced by the social group in which they find themselves.

Secondly, it has been found that changes in *family* circumstances are also associated with effects on the children's behaviour. For example, my colleagues and I (Rutter, 1971) investigated children, all of whom had been separated from their parents as a result of family discord or family problems. Within this group who had experienced severe early family stresses, a change for the better, in terms of a return to harmony or at least a cessation of open discord, was associated in a marked reduction in the risk of conduct disturbance. Similarly, it has been shown by Hetherington *et al.* (1982) that whether or not disorders in the children of divorcing parents diminished was a function of whether or not divorce improved family relationships. When the divorce brought harmony, the children's problems tended to improve, but when parental discord and difficulties continued so, too, the children's disorders tended to persist. Most other studies (see Rutter and Giller, 1983) have given rise to similar findings all of which point to environmental effects associated with changes in the quality of family relationships. However, there are circumstances in which children's behaviour disturbance seems to develop a self-perpetuating quality and improvements in patterns of family interaction are not necessarily followed by equivalent improvements in the child's behaviour (Richman *et al.*, 1982; see also Chapter 6 this volume).

The third type of environmental change is that brought about as a result of treatment. It might be thought that this would provide the clearest demonstration of environmental effects but for a variety of reasons the findings are difficult to interpret. In part this is because there is a paucity of well-controlled therapeutic studies (see Robins, 1973; Rutter, 1982b; Rutter and Giller, 1983) but, even when therapeutic benefits have been demonstrated, in most cases there has been a lack of evidence on which *elements* in the treatment brought about the change in the children's behaviour. This issue is also discussed in Chapter 13 of this volume. Obviously, too, the fact that some environmental change improved the child's behaviour does not necessarily mean that some abnormality in that feature of the environment caused the disorder in the first place. The observation that electro-convulsive therapy may relieve depression tells one nothing about the causes of depression and the finding that stimulants aid concentration and improve behaviour in hyperkinetic children does not identify the causal mechanisms (if only because somewhat similar effects are seen in non-hyperkinetic children — see Rapoport, 1983; Taylor, 1983). In the same way, the improvements following behaviour therapy are uninformative regarding causal mechanisms. Nevertheless, therapeutic studies can be informative provided that the *mechanism* involved in the therapeutic change can be identified and provided that this is the same mechanism postulated in the genesis of the disorder. No very clear-cut evidence of that type is available but the findings on the benefits, in terms of a reduction in the children's aggression and disturbed behaviour, of improving family functioning as a result of behavioural interventions begin to provide relevant data for this chain of argument (see Patterson, 1982; Rutter and Giller, 1983).

Perhaps the most dramatic demonstration of the effects of therapeutic environmental change is provided by the results of rescuing children from conditions of extreme deprivation and maltreatment (see Clarke and Clarke, 1976; Rutter, 1981a; Skuse, 1984a,b). There are now a number of well-documented reports of children reared in isolation in cellars, attics and cupboards under the most appalling circumstance of neglect, restriction and punishment. At the time of their discovery, at ages up to 13 years, they were mute, severely retarded and grossly abnormal in their social behaviour. However, within months of their removal to a normal environment there was evidence of remarkable recovery of cognitive and social functions in most (but not all) cases. In these cases, the extent and timing of the recovery in precise relationship to the change of environment provides very convincing documentation of the major effects on development of very major changes in conditions of rearing.

Non-familial environments

The final strategy to be mentioned as a means of disentangling genetic and environmental effects concerns the study of non-familial environments. There is now a substantial literature showing major differences in the behaviour and attainments of children according to the characteristics of the institutional environment in which they find themselves. Thus, studies of institutions for delinquents, such as probation hostels or correctional schools, have shown large differences between them in rates of absconding and reconviction (see Rutter and Giller, 1983). Broadly speaking, the successful institutions were characterized by a combination of firmness, warmth, harmony, high expectations, good discipline and a practical approach to training. Similarly, other studies (see Rutter *et al.*, 1979; Rutter, 1983) have shown that secondary (high) schools vary greatly in a host of different measures of pupil success — behaviour in the classroom, rates of attendance, low level of delinquency, exam success, entry to college, and even employment during the year after leaving school.

Furthermore, these differences in outcome have been shown to be systematically associated with the qualities of the schools as social organizations. In general, the more successful schools have been characterized by a student body with a balanced intake (i.e. they have had an appropriate mix of both able and less-able youngsters), a substantial academic emphasis, effective techniques of classroom management, good discipline (with ample use of praise and encouragement and not too much punishment), good working conditions for the pupils, plenty of opportunities for student participation and responsibility, and a style of staff organization that combines firm leadership at a senior level with a decision-making process in which all teachers feel that their views are represented and seriously considered.

Obviously, in these institutional studies, there can be no question of genetic transmission in the ordinary sense in that the staff and pupils have no biological relationship. The consistent association between the characteristics of the institution and the behaviour and attainments of the pupils strongly suggests a causal connection that represents an environmental effect. The query here is of a different kind — namely, in which direction does the causal arrow run? Did the institution shape the children's behaviour or, rather, did the qualities of the children make the institution what it was? Of course, that question also arises with the family associations, and we need to consider the various ways in which the problem of how to determine the direction of causation may be tackled.

Child effects on the environment

As with genetic transmission, the first question is whether there is any evidence in favour of the alternative explanation — that is, is there any reason to suppose that children can have effects on how adults behave? This question was first raised in a systematic fashion by Thomas *et al.* (1968) with respect to the rôle of child temperament and by Bell through his reanalysis of the direction of effects in studies of socialization (1968, 1974). Since Bell's critique, evidence has accumulated to show that there *are* important child effects (Bell and Harper, 1977; Lerner and Spanier, 1978; Lewis and Rosenblum, 1978; Rutter, 1977a), although it has to be added that our knowledge on these effects remains rather rudimentary. Nevertheless, there is no doubt that they exist and the question is whether or not they account for the observed associations between environmental variables and child disorder.

Input differences to schools

We may begin our consideration of that issue by looking at the research strategies used in studying possible school effects. The first issue, perhaps, is to ask whether the differences in pupil outcome are simply a function of differences in intake.

It could be that the schools with more successful outcomes had better results just because they had a more favoured intake of intelligent, well-behaved pupils from advantageous family backgrounds. If so, the association would not provide any kind of measure of the schools' effectiveness as educational institutions. It is obvious that school outcomes can be compared meaningfully only if the school intakes are made comparable in some way. A variety of different methods have been used for this purpose (see Rutter, 1983). They have shown that schools do indeed vary in their intakes and that, to some extent, the outcome variations reflect that fact. However, also they are agreed in showing that the differences between schools in pupil outcome are *not* merely a function of variations in intake. Of course, the validity of that conclusion depends on whether or not investigators have chosen the most appropriate intake (or predictor) variables to examine. A review of the evidence suggests that they have, but one can never be entirely sure that some unmeasured intake variable was not responsible for the school outcome differences. Accordingly, it is necessary to turn to other research strategies to take the matter further.

Timing and patterning of associations in schools

The main reason for considering intake differences was the possibility that the differences in outcome were artefactual—that is, no change had taken place, it was just that the outcomes reflected a continuation of children's behaviour already well-established before entry to school. As we have seen, the findings indicate that this was not so, but, in any case, the repeated observation of a systematic association between school characteristics and child behaviour makes a purely artefactual variation in pupil outcomes quite implausible. Rather the query concerns which caused which. This question may be tackled by determining the timing and patterning of the associations between school characteristics and pupil behaviour or attainments. If the schools influenced the pupils, the correlations should be weak at the time of school entry but strong at the time of school leaving. Conversely, if the pupil characteristics shaped teacher behaviour the reverse should occur, that is the strongest association should be with the intake measures. In our own study (Maughan *et al.*, 1980) the former proved to be the case. Thus, for example, the school measures correlated 0.44 with academic attainment at intake but 0.76 with those at the end of secondary schooling. For obvious practical reasons the child measures could not be entirely comparable on the two occasions but both in that study and in others (Maughan *et al.*, 1980) the findings on timing and patterning provide strong circumstantial evidence of a causal effect of the school on the child. That is not to say that the reverse does not also occur (almost certainly it does) but it appears that there is a true influence on the child stemming from characteristics of the school environment. Of course, to be sure on this point we would require experimental studies in which school practices are deliberately changed. These have not yet been undertaken but there is supporting evidence from experimental studies in the classroom, as distinct from the school as a whole (see Rutter, 1983).

Timing and patterning of associations in families

Much the same issues arise with respect to the associations with family variables. Did family discord cause the child to develop behavioural problems or did the presence of a difficult child in the family lead to quarrelling and discord? Did harsh and inconsistent punishment cause the boy to be aggressive or was it that the parents were led to take extreme measures just because the boy's disruptive behaviour failed to respond to more ordinary methods of discipline? Again, there are reasons for supposing that both may occur. For example, Patterson (1982) found that aggressive boys were indeed less responsive than other boys to disciplinary measures; Gardner (1977) showed experimentally that autistic children *elicited* different patterns of interaction (as compared with those with normal children) from the adults with whom they were placed; and there is some evidence that the stresses associated with having a mentally retarded child may increase the risk of emotional disturbance in other family members and of parental discord (Howard, 1978; Korn et al., 1978). So how may we determine how far and under what circumstances the family factors influence the child rather than vice-versa?

Of course, the matter is clear-cut in the case of the many family variables that could not have been caused by the child. Thus, it is obvious that such variables as being the oldest child, having a younger sib born, or being bereaved could not conceivably have resulted from the child's behaviour. In other cases, the fact that the family factors *antedated* the child's disturbance makes the direction of causation equally clear. This would be so, for example, with many instances of parental criminality or mental disorder and, equally, it would apply in many cases of marital discord. But, often, it is difficult to be at all sure about the timing. For example, prospective longitudinal studies of high-risk populations—such as the West and Farrington (1973, 1977) study of working-class London boys—have been able to obtain parental measures before the children became delinquent. But, we know that many of the boys showed difficult and troublesome behaviour when they were younger—some years before they appeared in court. It might be thought that a study of the timing of changes in the behaviour of the child and of his parents would help. Potentially it could (Rutter, 1981d) but in practice it has not done so both because of the statistical problems in such analyses and because in so many instances there has been so little change. The families remain discordant and disorganized and the children continue to be aggressive and difficult.

There is no easy way out of this dilemma and often there has to be a reliance on an interpretation of the overall pattern, together with an assessment of which causal process is more likely. Perhaps the situation where this problem arises most obviously concerns the associations between conduct disorders in boys on the one hand and family discord, poor parental supervision and inefficient discipline on the other. A key feature here is that in such families it is usual for *several* sons to show behavioural disturbance. As already noted, genetic factors do not seem to play a major rôle in these disorders and hence there is no ready explanation of why so many of the children should show problems if the association with family discord stemmed from the children's behaviour. Rather, it is more plausible that the association stemmed from a general effect of the family on the children resulting from problems in the parents. But this suggestion demands some explanation of why the parents should show such severe difficulties in parenting and in marital relationships. Is it possible to predict these difficulties in advance of the children's birth? Empirical findings show that to some extent it is.

For example, our own study following London children into early adult life (Rutter *et al.*, 1983) provides relevant data. It was found that those who experienced severe adversities in their own childhoods were the ones most likely to grow up to show difficulties in many aspects of adult functioning — including marked problems in parenting. People's experiences of rearing when they were young were important determinants of their own qualities as parents when they reached adulthood. To complete this causal chain, we need to know whether adverse experiences in one generation are linked with adverse experiences in the next and in turn with the development of disorder in the offspring. No one study has really good data for all links in that causal chain but there are indications that the chain exists. For example, Robins (1966) showed that antisocial children who grew up to be sociopathic adults had children with a much-increased rate of disturbed behaviour. If we can predict the behaviour of a second generation by information on the first generation *before* they had children, as to some extent we can, it is clear that the parenting problems must be causes, and not consequences, of the children's disorders.

Planned therapeutic or preventive interventions

As in other situations, experimental manipulations in which one variable is systematically altered in order to determine if this leads to consequent changes in the other variable constitute the best test of causation. Child effects have been studied in this way by using drugs to alter children's behaviour and then determining if this changes patterns of parent–child interaction (Barkley, 1981). The same can be done for parent effects by focusing the intervention on parental behaviour. One example of this kind is provided by Tizard *et al.*'s (1982) study of children's reading. In a cross-sectional study of inner-London primary-school children, they found that children who read badly were much less likely to have parents who listened to them reading. The question arose as to which was cause and which effect. To answer that question they set up an intervention study in which some school classes were involved in a programme to get parents to listen to their children read regularly; these were then systematically compared over the next few years with classes run in the usual way and with classes given extra teaching input (but no involvement of parents). The striking finding was that the children given daily opportunities to read to their parents, although similar to the other groups at the beginning of the experiment, were reading much better at the end. The implication is that the parents' listening to children read had a causal effect in increasing the children's reading skills.

Association with some third variable

The third main alternative to family effects to be considered is that both the parents' behaviour *and* that of the children are due to some third variable. Thus, one might postulate that the association between parental criminality and delinquency in the sons or that between marital discord and aggressive behaviour in the children are due, not to any causal link between the two, but rather to the fact that both are caused by some other influence such as poverty or poor housing. Of course, this is a possibility that must be borne in mind in any study of hypothesized causal influences, and analyses to investigate the matter were undertaken in all the research considered so far.

In essence, the strategy required is one in which possible changes in the association between the first two variables are looked for in relation to changes in the third. This may be done in several different ways. The easiest and most straightforward is to undertake some appropriate multivariate statistical analysis that determines whether the initial association is still maintained after 'taking account of' or 'controlling' or 'holding constant' the third variable. This is an essential precaution in any study that deals with multiple intercorrelated variables. Nevertheless, inevitably, however fancy the statistics, it is a somewhat artificial procedure that is heavily reliant on the ways in which the variables happen to group in the particular sample studied. Accordingly, whenever possible, it is highly desirable to replicate the findings in different populations deliberately chosen to vary on the hypothesized third variable. Thus, in our own studies we compared the associations between family variables and child disorder in two general population samples—socially disadvantaged inner London and the more affluent small-town communities of the Isle of Wight (Rutter *et al.*, 1975)—and both of these with a sample of families with a mentally ill parent (Rutter, 1971; Rutter and Quinton, 1981). The family associations were strikingly similar in all three studies, making it very unlikely that they were due to either social circumstances or parental mental illness. That has been the general finding with all the main parent–child associations considered (see Rutter and Giller, 1983). The patterns have been found to be remarkably consistent across a wide range of social, cultural and ethnic groups. It is clear that it is most unlikely that the family links are an artefact of some broader sociocultural variable.

However, there are circumstances in which some third variable has been found to account for at least some of the association initially supposed to be causal. For example, to some extent (but only some), the association between multiple hospital admissions and child disorder is explicable in terms of the fact that children from chronically deprived and disadvantaged homes are more likely to be admitted to hospital repeatedly (Quinton and Rutter, 1976). Or again, the link between parental criminality and delinquency in the children could be a consequence of greater police surveillance of criminal families so that the sons are more likely to be caught and convicted. There is some evidence that this does occur (West and Farrington, 1973; West, 1982) but it cannot be the whole story in that there is a strong link with self-reported delinquency even after controlling for convictions (Farrington, 1979).

However, there are two supposedly causal variables that may not be directly causal—namely, social disadvantage and large family size. Although low social status, poverty and poor housing are statistically correlated with delinquency it seems probable that the association is indirect. The point is that social disadvantage is connected with a variety of other features that predispose to delinquency—such as parental criminality or poor supervision of the children. It is known that these other features still predispose to delinquency even after taking into account social conditions but the converse is less clearly the case. Moreover, historical analyses show that there is no connection between changes in economic conditions and changes in crime rates—indeed the big post-Second World War increase in delinquency came at a time of high employment and a rise in the standard of living. The question of whether and how social disadvantage might have a role in the genesis of children's problems remains unanswered. Probably, it operates by making good parenting more difficult and hence only indirectly affects the children—but this remains uncertain.

The effects of large family size on delinquency remain somewhat of an enigma. To begin with this association largely applies to socially disadvantaged sections of the population—so that it may not be large family size as such that matters but rather the multiple adversities that tend to accompany large family size in poorer sections of the community. But also, the link with delinquency may be indirect in a different sense. Large family size is associated with educational backwardness which is in turn linked with delinquency. It could be that that chain provides the association with delinquency. However, once again, the data to resolve the matter are not yet available. Another alternative, suggested by Offord's (1982) finding that delinquency is associated with the number of brothers in the family but not with the number of sisters, is that the mechanism may lie in some form of deviant modelling that potentiates delinquent behaviour.

The suggestion that social disadvantage and large family size may have only indirect causal links with delinquency is also supported by the findings on the *course* of delinquent activities. Whereas many of the other family variables that are associated with whether or not someone becomes delinquent are also predictive of recidivism, this has not been found to be a consistent factor in the case of socioeconomic conditions or family size (see Rutter and Giller, 1983).

Conclusions on environmental effects

Let me draw the threads of the argument together in relation to the issues considered thus far. First, it is apparent that the three main types of alternative explanation do have some validity. There are associations between family or school variables and child disorder that constitute artefactual links—that is connections, which, in reality, are due to a prior association with some third variable. That is always an important possibility to consider but it does not explain most of the associations that are commonly supposed to represent causal mechanisms. Similarly, it is evident that children can and do have an influence on parental behaviour and on family functioning generally. It would be seriously misleading to regard the causal process as uni-directional—it is not. Rather, all human interactions, including parent–child interaction, have to be seen as reciprocal, with two-way effects. But even that constitutes an over-simplified view in that the dyadic interaction will also be influenced by the social context and milieu within which it takes place. As Bronfenbrenner (1979) has made clear an *ecological* perspective is needed. Or, as Hinde (1980) puts it, relationships must be viewed in terms of networks with both self-regulating and interactive properties. Nevertheless, when due account has been taken of child effects on parents (or other adults), it is apparent still that major parent effects remain. But, as the genetic analyses have shown, not all of these represent environmental effects. Rather some reflect biological heredity. This applies, for example, to the links between schizophrenia in parent and child and, probably, at least in part, to those between alcoholism in parent and child. Also, the evidence shows that much of the association between the home environment and children's intellectual development is in truth a function of the genetic links between parent and child intelligence. However, not all of the association is explicable in this fashion; there *are* important environmental influences on intellectual development, even if they are not quite as strong as sometimes supposed.

But, in addition to these outcome variables for which reservations have to be expressed about the power of environmental effects, there are others for which no such serious reservations are needed. These include scholastic achievement, conduct disorders and emotional disturbances. On the face of it, the environmental factors that have most impact are rather different in these three cases. With scholastic achievement, those that stand out include various school variables, aspects of parent–child interaction, and ordinal position. With emotional disturbance, the key factors include various acute stresses that tend to alter patterns of parent–child interaction or involve a loss of an important relationship (such as bereavement, admission to hospital or birth of a sibling), parental mental disorder and, once again, ordinal position. The picture with conduct disorders involves much more gross disturbance of family functioning, with family discord and disharmony, parental criminality, lack of supervision, inefficient and inconsistent discipline, neglect and hostility. But, in addition, peer group influences also seem important. We need to consider now the evidence that might indicate which mechanisms and processes are involved with these three rather different outcomes.

MECHANISMS AND PROCESSES

Scholastic achievement and cognitive performance

Most studies of children's cognitive performance do not make a clear distinction between general intelligence and scholastic achievement; hence, to some extent, we need to consider these together. This is appropriate in so far as many of the environmental variables are the same for both. However, as already noted, environmental influences seem more important with the latter, and where possible the focus will be on scholastic achievement as the outcome variable.

It is convenient to begin with a discussion of the mechanisms and processes that can be *excluded*, as largely inoperative. Studies of children reared in modern institutions have shown that the children attain roughly normal levels of intellectual functioning (Tizard and Rees, 1974; Tizard and Hodges, 1978; Roy, 1983). There is the clear implication that continuities in family relationships do not have the central role in intellectual development that they do in social development (see below). Whether personal relationships are as unimportant for scholastic achievement is less certain. The finding in the same studies that institutional children tend to have poor task involvement in the classroom, together with the reports of poor school progress in the year following bereavement (van Eerdewegh *et al.*, 1982) suggest that there might be effects on achievement. On the other hand, Douglas *et al.* (1968) found that parental death had no apparent effect on educational attainment. The evidence taken as a whole suggests that neither family disruption nor loss of an important relationship have a very direct effect on scholastic achievement, although the long-term family adversities that sometimes follow break-up of the family may have more impact (Rutter and Madge, 1976).

Rather than relationship variables, it seems that perceptual and linguistic experiences are most crucial. The evidence on this point comes from several different sources. First, there are the findings from educational interventions all of which focus on such experiences combined with direct teaching of some kind. Both the preschool compensatory education programmes (Darlington *et al.*, 1980; Lazar and Darlington, 1982; Schweinhart and Weikart, 1980) and the much more intensive and prolonged interventions in the Heber and Garber project (Heber, 1978; Garber and Heber, 1977) have been of this kind and both have had positive effects on school progress, as well as less-lasting effects on IQ. But it should be noted that the children in these projects have seemed to differ in their task involvement and their attitudes to learning and to schooling, as well as in their scholastic achievements. The implication is that the scholastic benefits may stem from behavioural effects as well as from gains in cognitive competence.

Secondly, there are the statistical studies concerned with the associations between the home environment and the children's cognitive functioning. As noted already, these associations are not very strong but the variables found to be important mainly relate to some aspects of play and conversation between caretaker and child, the availability of toys, or learning experiences in or outside the home. Much the same was found in Tizard et al.'s (1972) study of children in residential nurseries. The children's language scores were better in those nurseries with more 'informative' staff talk, more reading and playing with the children, more answering of children's remarks and more play in which the child was actively rather passively involved.

The last point raises an important issue. It is usually said that what is needed for cognitive growth is cognitive 'stimulation'. The impression conveyed is of the need for parents to do things *to* children; to talk at them, to read to them, and to provide them with stimulating experiences. However, the available evidence suggests that this is a quite misleading picture. Animal studies have shown that it is *active* as distinct from passive, experiences that are most important (see Rutter, 1981a). Similarly, it is not doing things *to* children that is beneficial; rather the benefits come from helping them to learn how to do things for themselves. I have already mentioned the Tizard et al. (1982) study of reading which showed the importance of getting parents to encourage children to read aloud to them — note that it was the children who did the reading and not the parents. In humans, it also seems that *talking* with people is as important as (if not more important than) doing things with objects. Also, mere sensory stimulation is not helpful (to be reared in an environment of booming cacophony is not likely to aid cognitive growth); rather the experiences must be *meaningful* and require the child's active participation. Perhaps it is time that the term 'stimulation' ceased to be used in this connection.

A further set of data come from the school studies. Once again active learning experiences stand out as influential. For example in our own study (Rutter *et al.*, 1979) the variables associated with exam success were the regular setting and marking of homework, children's use of the school library, children's work displayed on the walls, full use of lesson teaching time and frequent school outings. But also, the crucial variables included the children's active participation in school life as a whole (as shown by their holding positions of responsibility), good conditions for pupils, and staff–pupil relationships that were such that children felt they could consult ordinary teachers about personal problems.

Taken together with the evidence already considered, we may conclude that what is needed for optimal scholastic achievement is a combination of active learning experiences that promote cognitive competence, and a social context in which the style of interaction and relationships promotes self-confidence and an active interest in seeking to learn independently of formal instruction.

However, before leaving the topic of scholastic achievement there are two other variables that must be considered—ordinal position and family size. How do they fit in with that tentative formulation? Why should firstborn children tend to have superior educational achievement? The answer probably lies in the findings on the differences in the ways parents respond to their first child compared with the ways in which they deal with their later-born children (see Rutter, 1981a). It has been found that parents tend to have a more intensive relationship with their first children, interacting with them more and showing more social, affectionate, and caretaking behaviours. They are more anxious and controlling but also they talk with them more and pay them more attention than they do to later children. It is not necessarily an easy relationship but probably it provides the characteristics of active learning experiences, high expectations and high demands that seem to facilitate achievement.

What about family size? Here, the evidence shows that children reared in large families (four or more children) tend to achieve less well on average. The association is probably less marked in upper social groups but, with the odd exception, it has been remarkably consistent across a wide variety of populations and holds up even after controlling for ordinal position and social class (see Rutter and Madge, 1976). The fact that the association between large family size and low attainment is strongest with verbal and language-related skills and that it is already maximal during the early years of schooling has led to the suggestion that the explanation lies in the child's linguistic environment during the pre-school years (Nisbet, 1953; Douglas et al., 1968). Thus, it has been suggested that, because as family size increases parents have to share their time among a larger number of children, there is probably less intensive interaction and communication between parents and children in large families. The suggestion is certainly plausible but it has to be said that there is a lack of direct evidence to show whether or not this is in fact the case. Until that is available, the mechanisms involved in the family size associations remain speculative. But, so far as one can tell, they are likely to be in keeping with the general formulation that active meaningful experiences are the most important environmental factors concerned with cognitive growth, and that the social context of learning is likely to influence children's task involvement and attitudes to education in ways that may affect scholastic achievement.

Conduct disorders and delinquency

As we have seen, several rather broad aspects of family functioning have been found to be associated with conduct disorders and delinquency, but five may be picked out for more detailed consideration (see Rutter and Giller, 1983). First, there are characteristics of the parents. Of these, criminality (and especially recidivist criminality) is the most striking and consistent but it is not the only one. The association applies also to the persistent social difficulties (as shown by excessive drinking, poor work record and reliance on social welfare) and serious abnormalities of parental personality. Secondly, there is intra-familial discord—as evidenced by frequent and prolonged quarrelling, temporary or permanent family break-up, expressed hostility and negative feelings between family members, rejecting attitudes towards the children, frequent shouting and punishment of the children, and a marked tendency for minor specific disagreements between two family members to escalate into prolonged and unproductive hostile exchanges which come to involve everyone in the vicinity. Thirdly, weak family relationships have been reflected in such items as a lack of joint family leisure activities, lack of intimate family communication, lack of affectional identification with parents, lack of parental warmth and a parental failure to identify with the rôle of parent. Fourthly, there is harsh, inconsistent and ineffective discipline or supervision of the children. Fifthly, there seem to be important peer-group influences. These variables cover a wide range and it is necessary to ask which are the crucial dimensions. This is particularly important because the five features overlap greatly. Criminal parents often have discordant families with weak family relationships and chaotic patterns of discipline; moreover many of the families are large and socially disadvantaged. Which of these elements is most important in the genesis of conduct disturbance or do they all play a crucial rôle? That is not an easy question to answer but several research strategies have proved fruitful. However, the common feature in all of them has been the search for means to 'pull apart' variables that ordinarily tend to go together. The procedures may be illustrated by taking just a few specific examples.

Broken homes and family discord

At one time, much emphasis was placed on the supposed importance of broken homes as a cause of delinquency. The notion was that it was the fact of family break-up that was damaging. The idea seemed plausible in that broken homes were indeed statistically associated with delinquency. But what alternative explanations should be considered? One obvious contender is the presence of family discord and quarrelling (see Rutter, 1971, 1981b). In order to differentiate the two it is necessary first to split broken homes into those where discord was a prominent feature and those where it was not. Divorce and separation constituted causes that meet the first criterion and parental death meets the second. Several large-scale studies have data that differentiate these two causes of a broken home; the findings of all of them are agreed in showing that whereas divorce/separation is strongly associated with delinquency, death is only very weakly so. It seems that perhaps discord is more important than break-up *per se*. But if that were so, it should follow that discord in *un*broken homes should also lead to delinquency. It has been found that it does. It might also be predicted that temporary separations should predispose to conduct disorders if they arose as a result of discord but not if they occurred for other reasons. Again that has been confirmed. Also, if discord is indeed a causal factor it might be expected that a *reduction* in discord should be followed by a diminution in the risk of conduct disturbance. Once more, empirical findings show this to be so. On the basis of this very consistent body of evidence from a range of different studies, in good agreement with one another, we may conclude that the relevant mechanism is likely to involve discordant relationships rather than break-up *per se*. However, the matter cannot be left there.

First, we need to ask, if it is the discord that is crucial, why is divorce still associated with a continuing increased risk of delinquency? Surely, resolution of the marital conflict ought to have removed the risk factor. Recent studies of divorcing families have shown that the answer lies in the error of the assumption (Wallerstein and Kelly, 1980; Hess and Camera, 1979; Hetherington *et al.*, 1982). All too often, divorce does *not* bring marital conflict to an end; disputes continue over housing, finance and access to the children. Moreover, the risk to the children is related to whether or not discord does continue. In the long term (meaning after several years), most families are better off with divorce than with unabating discord and quarrelling but frequently things get worse before they get better. Also, it is clear that although the break-up of the marriage may solve some problems it may create others that also carry risks for the children.

Secondly, it is important to move from broad statistical associations to more molecular analyses of what actually goes on in families. The work of Patterson (1977, 1982) and his colleagues is most informative in this connection. By means of sequential analyses of observations of family interaction in the home, they have shown that a hostile response to an aggressive act serves to perpetuate the aggression. This seems to be so whoever in the family is involved. In other words, if a punitive response is part of a hostile interchange, far from stopping the aggression, it may actually make things worse. It is necessary to go beyond a reward and punishment framework for behaviour. The consequence of this accelerating effect of hostile reactions is a family pattern of coercive negative interchanges that spreads to involve other family members.

This provides the basis for one sort of mechanism but is that the only means by which discord predisposes to conduct disturbance and delinquency? Probably not, in that often discord is also associated with diverse other family problems. Possibly alternative mechanisms are most conveniently considered by focusing on a few of these other problems.

Weak family relationships

As already noted, weak family relationships have also been found to be associated with delinquency. The possible importance of personal relationships is also shown by the finding that a good relationship with one parent has an ameliorating effect (reducing the risk of conduct disorder) even in the presence of general family discord (Rutter, 1971; Rutter et al., 1983). However, discord and weak relationships so often accompany one another that it is difficult to separate their effects. When this is the situation, it is necessary to seek special circumstances where this is not the case. Rearing from infancy in a good quality group home or other institution with multiple changing caretakers provides the nearest approach. Because of the frequent changes in parent-figure and because of the more 'professional' approach to child-rearing, children are less likely to form close bonds and attachments with their caretakers in this setting than if they were brought up in a nuclear family. On the other hand, usually such institutions are not particularly discordant and quarrelsome environments. So the question is what happens to young people reared in that way? Data on that point are somewhat limited but they are all agreed in showing that conduct disorders are much increased in frequency among children reared from infancy in an institutional setting (Rutter et al., 1983; Wolkind, 1974; Yule and Raynes, 1972). Accordingly, it appears that weak family relationships are important in their own right quite apart from their association with discord. The precise mechanisms remain uncertain but two are generally favoured in the literature. First, early bonding is thought to constitute an important part of the basis of social development as a whole so that children who lack secure attachments in infancy are likely to be impaired in their friendships with peers and in their love relationships later (see Rutter, 1981a). Secondly, it is supposed that the development of internal controls (or conscience formation) depends on an affectional identification with parents. Hence, individuals who lack close family ties may lack the internal controls that prevent involvement in delinquent activities (see Hirschi, 1969). There is a certain amount of evidence that provides partial support for both those views but neither constitutes an entirely satisfactory complete explanation.

Supervision and discipline

This is because moral development cannot be viewed entirely in terms of the strength of controls, nor social development solely in terms of social skills and qualities. It is necessary also to consider some of the specific influences that shape particular behaviours—the role of adult supervision and discipline. At one time, attention was focused on the use of specific practices (whether it is better to smack children or deprive them of privileges), on the severity of discipline, and on matters of consistency (see Becker, 1964). But it became clear that these were not the most relevant dimensions and the focus has shifted in recent years. Empirically, it has been found that the parents of problem children differ from other parents in being more punitive, issuing more commands, providing more attention following deviant behaviour, being less likely to perceive deviant behaviour as deviant, in being more involved in extended coercive hostile interchanges, in giving more vague commands, and in being less effective in stopping their children's deviant behaviour (see Patterson, 1982; Rutter and Giller, 1983). It is not yet certain how these (and other) findings are best conceptualized but Patterson (1982) plausibly suggests four dimensions as likely to be most important, (a) the lack of 'house rules' (so that there are no clear expectations of what children may and may not do), (b) lack of parental monitoring of the child's behaviour (so that the parents are not adequately informed about his acts or emotions and hence are not in a good position to respond appropriately, (c) lack of effective contingencies (so that parents nag and shout but do not follow through with any disciplinary plan, and do not respond with an adequate differentiation between praise for prosocial and punishment for antisocial activities), and (d) a lack of techniques for dealing with family crises or problems (so that conflicts lead to tension and dispute but do not result in resolution). The points, then, are that we need to focus on an *awareness* of what children are doing, the *process* of disciplinary management (including problem-solving methods), and the *efficiency* of the techniques used.

Models of behaviour

So far, most of the dimensions considered have been concerned with one or other aspect of control (either internal or external). But it is clear that control concepts, on their own, provide an inadequate explanation for the specific form or content of children's behaviour (see Hirschi, 1969; Elliott *et al.*, 1979). In that connection, we need to turn to the rôle of parental criminality and of peer-group influences. Doubtless, they exert their effects through several different means—including those considered already. But, in addition, we need to add the dimension of modelling. Both delinquent peers and criminal parents provide a model of aggression and of antisocial attitudes. Their behaviour constitutes something to be copied and identified with by the children, as well as a setting in which delinquent solutions to problems are regarded as acceptable, or at least to be tolerated. There is an extensive body of experimental and naturalistic studies to show that imitation and identification do indeed occur (Bandura, 1969); and also of course, many investigations have shown the power of social-group influences (Kelvin, 1969; Sherif and Sherif, 1969). People show a strong tendency to form social groups with their own rules, values and standards of behaviour, and there is a general tendency for people to act in accord with these social group 'norms'. The evidence on the importance of peer-group influences at school (Rutter *et al.*, 1979) and that showing the effects on delinquent behaviour of moving to a less delinquent neighbourhood (see above) both suggest that these social forces operate with respect to delinquency. Experimental studies also suggest the importance of individual models of aggressive behaviour and naturalistic studies seem to confirm their effect. For example, we found (Rutter *et al.*, 1979) that schools in which the teachers unofficially (and indeed illegally) slapped and cuffed the pupils had higher rates of disturbed behaviour—the teacher actions seemed to set models of violence for the students to follow. Similarly, the same study showed that schools where the staff were poor timekeepers had worse rates of pupil non-attendance. Again, modelling seems to constitute a plausible mechanism.

To summarize the findings on conduct disorder, it appears that the operative mechanisms probably include discordant patterns of interaction, weak family relationships, inefficient supervision and discipline, and deviant models of behaviour. It should be noted that these mechanisms probably apply as much to school influences as to family effects.

Emotional disturbance

In turning now to the possible mechanisms involved in the genesis of emotional disorders it is immediately apparent that we are on much weaker ground. To some extent there is an overlap with the factors associated with conduct disturbances, but it is clear that the gross family problems that are characteristic of delinquents and of aggressive children are *not* usually found with emotional disorders. Either the family features that predispose to depression and anxiety states are much more subtle than those that lead to delinquency or else they are of a different kind. There are various reasons for suggesting that to a considerable extent the latter is likely to be the case. First, as already noted, emotional disorders commonly affect just one child in the family whereas conduct disorders usually affect several. This suggests that the mechanisms are likely to involve *within*-family differences that cause one child to be dealt with in a way that differentiates him from his siblings—rather than *between*-family differences that reflect general variables that impinge similarly on all children in the family (Rowe and Plomin, 1981). Secondly, emotional disorders are more likely to be acute conditions with a shorter course and a better prognosis (Rutter, 1975; Rutter and Garmezy, 1983). This suggests that acute and transient stressors (as distinct from chronic adversities) may play a greater rôle in their genesis. What little evidence there is seems to fulfil these expectations.

Ordinal position and sibling rivalry

Emotional disorders are linked with ordinal position, with disorders most frequent in the firstborn. Also, it has been shown that the birth of a younger sib commonly provokes at least short-lived emotional difficulties in many children. The mechanisms underlying these two observations may well be connected. As already noted, the patterns of parent–child interaction tend to be different with the firstborn (see Rutter, 1981a). Usually, the relationship with the firstborn is both closer and more involved, and also tenser and more controlling. With subsequent children, parents tend to be more relaxed, more consistent and less punitive—although also they interact with them less. This is reflected, for example, in family photographs—most families have many more pictures of the first child as an infant than they do of later children. But, also as Dunn and Kendrick (Chapter 2 this volume) showed, the arrival of the second child tends to change the parents' interaction with the first one. Having been very actively involved with the eldest child, they come to interact less with him when the new baby is born. At the same time, they become more negative and controlling—expecting the older child to show responsibilities and good behaviour not expected of the baby, as well as protecting the baby from overly rough overtures from the firstborn. Having enjoyed the parents' unrivalled attention and affection, the eldest child now has to accept a sharing of parental time and interest, and perhaps, take second place to the baby in some respects.

Acute stressors

Various acute stressors have been identified as ones liable to lead to short-term emotional stress reactions. Bereavement, admission to hospital and parental divorce perhaps constitute the best documented of these but, in addition, it has been suggested that a wide variety of other unpleasant or distressing happenings may also provoke emotional disorders (see Rutter, 1981c). Unfortunately, the evidence on these matters is severely limited in three different respects. First, we lack data on which types of events constitute stressors for children. In adults, happenings that reflect some form of loss or disappointment or that involve disturbed interpersonal relationships seem to be most influential. The evidence with respect to children is consistent with this but the question has been too little studied for any firm conclusions to be drawn. We lack knowledge on the importance of acute fear-provoking events (such as being bitten by a dog or being involved in an accident) that do not involve any loss of a loved person or object. Also we do not know the significance of events that involve some long-lasting change or adaptation (e.g. starting school or moving to a new town or a different country) but that are not obviously positive or negative in affective tone. Secondly, although we know that bereavement and admission to hospital make many children unhappy and distressed we know far less on their rôle in the more serious and persistent emotional disorders that lead to psychiatric clinic referral. There are very few good studies of children with clinically significant emotional disorders and none at all that have studied stressors systematically in this group. Thirdly, we have no good data to indicate whether or not some sorts of stressors lead to one sort of disorder whereas other types predispose to different conditions.

However, such limited evidence as is available does suggest that acute stressors are likely to be more important in the genesis of emotional disorders than of conduct disorders, and that the most influential 'stress' events tend to involve a real or imagined loss of a relationship or a change in the pattern of interaction that may be perceived as a rebuff.

Parental mental disorder

Several studies (Rutter, 1966, 1970; Weissman, 1979) have shown that children of mentally ill parents have themselves a substantially increased risk of psychiatric disorder. To some extent, this linkage will reflect genetic transmission but it is clear that this is not the whole story. The disorders in the children are of various types and several different mechanisms seem to be involved. For example, there is an increased risk of conduct disorders in the boys; this seems to be largely explicable in terms of the parental discord and general family disorganization sometimes associated with adult mental disorder (especially when abnormalities of personality are concerned). But, also there is an increase risk of emotional disorder in both boys and girls and this is not associated with family discord. To some extent, the disorders seem to be associated with the extent to which the parental symptoms directly impinge on the family but this, too, does not constitute a sufficient explanation. It seems that parental mental disorders—perhaps especially depression in the mother—are associated with altered patterns of parenting and of family interaction. It may well be that these changes account for some of the psychiatric risk to the children but the data to determine the mode of operation of these mechanisms is not yet available. The issues are discussed further in Chapter 6.

Family patterns of communication and of dominance

The widespread belief that impaired communications and unsatisfactory patterns of dominance within the family play a major rôle in the genesis of psychiatric disorder has been an important motivating force in the increasing use over recent years of conjoint family therapy as the main means of therapeutic intervention in child psychiatry. Unfortunately, the empirical data to substantiate that belief are largely lacking (see Rutter, 1977b; Hinde, 1980). There is some evidence to show that family communication difficulties are associated with child disorder (although it is not known whether this association is with particular types of disorder) but the findings on patterns of dominance are quite inconclusive. But, with very few exceptions, the research designs employed have been concerned to compare 'normal' families with families having a 'problem' child. At least with respect to emotional disorders, this may not constitute the most appropriate strategy if the hypotheses predict *within*-family, rather than *between*-family, effects. In other words, we need to ask, *not* why the families as a whole differ (which they may well not do), but rather why the pattern of interaction within the family with this child (showing emotional disorder) differs from that with the other normal children. Almost no studies of that kind have been undertaken and hence no useful conclusions can be drawn about possible mechanisms involving the parents' differential treatment of the children.

PERSISTENCE OF ENVIRONMENTAL EFFECTS

Up to this point, the effects of family and school influences have been considered without explicit reference to any time frame. Some years ago it was commonly assumed that the effects of serious family adversity or deprivation in early childhood were very long-lasting and very difficult to reverse. However, research findings over the last decade or so have cast increasing doubt on that view (see Clarke and Clarke, 1976; Rutter, 1981a) and we need to consider now the extent to which ill-effects persist and, more especially, the factors that determine persistence or non-persistence.

Perhaps we need to begin by asking why it was thought that the effects of early deprivation were liable to be enduring and irreversible. There were various theoretical reasons that led to this supposition but also it stemmed from observations on deprived children. It is a commonplace to note that disturbed or delinquent children were seriously deprived or neglected as infants and it is well known that therapeutic interventions in later childhood or adolescence are not very effective in the case of chronic antisocial problems. The inference of persistent effects difficult to reverse seems justified, but it is not. In the first place, in the great majority of cases the deprivation and neglect were not confined to the infancy period—rather they were still operative at the time of clinical referral. Far from an effect lasting years, the situation is simply one of a continuing *current* effect that happens to have lasted for most of the child's life time. In the second place, the supposedly ineffective therapeutic interventions have rarely involved any radical alteration in the environment. Instead of a complete *change* of environment, the therapy has usually comprised some form of *talk* about adaptation or response to family adversity. If we are to examine the persistence of effects we must focus attention on that small subgroup of children who experience severe early neglect, deprivation or disadvantage but who then experience a change of environment followed by a normal pattern of upbringing thereafter.

Cognitive effects

Apart from single case studies of children rescued in middle childhood from cruel isolated rearing in cupboards and attics, studies of late adoption are about the only examples we have of this phenomenon (see Rutter, 1981a). The findings are consistent in showing very substantial recovery in most cases. The case studies provide clear demonstration that, even as late as age 6 or 7 years, many children who were severely retarded when rescued, later attain normal levels of general intelligence. The late-adopted children, too, have usually shown average cognitive functioning. Whether or not recovery has been complete is more difficult to determine. The finding that the IQs of late-adopted children tends to be somewhat lower than those of children adopted in infancy suggests that there may be some slight residual impairment, but equally the effect could be a result of biases in who is left in the institution to be adopted only when older.

The converse question on whether *good* experiences restricted to the infancy period can have a lasting beneficial impact even when experiences during middle or later childhood are disadvantageous is equally difficult to answer conclusively. The evidence on preschool compensatory education programmes provides, perhaps, the most appropriate data with respect to effects on cognitive development. As already discussed, it appears that the effects on IQ are largely or entirely 'washed-out' after the first few years of regular schooling. On the other hand, follow-up studies are beginning to provide evidence of *some* enduring effects in terms of better scholastic attainment and a stronger commitment to education (Darlington *et al.*, 1980; Schweinhart and Weikart, 1980). Pedersen *et al.*'s (1978) demonstration of the remarkable persistence of the effects on children of being taught by one particular first-grade teacher is in keeping with these findings. These results, which provide a more optimistic view of the benefits of early good experiences, should be kept in perspective. Like those on the sequelae of early bad experiences, they show only slight enduring effects. *All* studies are agreed in their finding that the most powerful factor determining whether effects persist is whether or not the experiences (good or bad) continue. If there is a complete change of environment, only minimal persistence can be expected. But, of course, the changes are usually far from complete and where there are continuities in experiences, so also there are likely to be continuities in effects. Does this explain the slight persistence of the effects of preschool compensatory education?

A more detailed analysis of the findings shows that the answer is somewhat more complicated. Pedersen *et al.* (1978) conducted a statistical critical paths analysis of the effects on children of the one outstanding first-grade teacher they studied. This showed that the teacher had a major effect on children's academic achievement, work effort and initiative in both the first and second grades, but that her *direct* effects after that were negligible. On the other hand, her *indirect* effects were considerable because the initial effects led on to further developments yielding a cumulative benefit that lasted very much longer. The children had acquired styles of work and behaviour that brought success, which in turn further reinforced their efforts. Similarly, their behaviour in class made them more rewarding students for the teachers of later classes who then responded to them in ways that facilitated their continuing success. Although not analysed in this way, the preschool studies findings suggest a similar process.

Our own studies of the longer-term effects of different experiences in high school tell the same story (Gray et al., 1980; Rutter et al., 1982). The results showed that there *were* schools effects on employment in so far as schooling influenced attendance, school drop-out, examination success and continuation of schooling into the sixth year. But there were no consistent school effects on employment that did not operate through these mechanisms. In other words, school effects continued after pupils left school, not because they permanently changed children's personality or cognitive potential, but rather because the immediate effects (in terms of school drop-out or educational qualifications) either opened up or closed down further opportunities. Schooling had long-lasting consequences, not because of any 'inoculation' effect or enduring change in the child, but rather because its immediate results set in motion a train of events which then, in turn, resulted in persistent sequelae.

Social and behavioural effects

Much the same story applies to the persistence of social and behavioural effects. Again there is good evidence from studies of late-adopted children that environmental improvements in middle or late childhood can do much to reverse the ill-effects of early neglect, discord and deprivation. The effects of early bad experiences are not necessarily enduring, and to a substantial extent the ill-effects *are* reversible provided that the environmental change is sufficiently great and that the later environment is sufficiently positive and beneficial. Conversely, a good home in the early years does not prevent damage from psychosocial stresses in adolescence. The same general conclusions on enduring sequelae are operative, with persistence of effects dependent on continuities of experiences and on chain reactions.

However, other considerations must be added before the picture can be regarded as at all complete. There is the possibility that certain experiences *have* to occur during the early years for social development to precede normally (see Rutter, 1981a). Although the original notion of fixed and absolute 'critical periods' in development has had to be largely abandoned, the concepts of 'sensitive periods' during which environmental influences have a particularly marked effect has some validity (Bateson, 1979, 1983). The generally favoured candidate for this effect concerns the initial formation of selective bonds or attachments. It has been suggested by Bowlby (1969) that these first bonds *must* develop during the first two years or so if normal social relationships are to be possible later. The evidence to test that hypothesis is quite meagre but the few available data from studies of late-adopted children (Tizard and Hodges, 1978) are most interesting and informative. Two main findings require emphasis. First, even children adopted after age 4 years can develop bonds with their adoptive parents. To that extent, either the 'sensitive period' notion is wrong or it extends to a later age than usually supposed. But, secondly, in spite of this development of parent–child bonds at age 4–6 years, the late-adopted children showed the same social and attentional problems in schools as did those who remained in the institution. The implication is that, although attachments can still develop for the first time after infancy, nevertheless fully normal social development may be dependent on bonding having taken place at an early age.

This possibility is both provocative and important in its apparent rejection of the idea that almost all ill-effects are potentially reversible given a good enough environment. However, it would be premature to reject the idea on the evidence so far. The findings are based on small numbers and, as the children were only 8 years when studied, it is still too early to judge the eventual outcome. Moreover, it is not known whether the children had failed to acquire normal social skills or rather whether they had gained patterns of social behaviour that were adaptive in the institution but maladaptive outside it. All we can state is that the hypothesis of a sensitive period for optimal early socialization remains one worth further testing. Even so, it should be noted that the notion of a sensitive period for the *optimal* acquisition of some psychological function carries with it no necessary implication of irreversibility. Indeed, the empirical evidence (see Rutter, 1981a) suggests that there *is* a potential for an important degree of later change in behaviours that showed a sensitive period effect in their acquisition.

The second major consideration that needs adding to the overall story concerns so-called 'sensitization' and 'steeling' effects (see Rutter, 1981c). In the first place, early events may lead to bodily changes which in turn influence later functioning. For example, it has been shown that rat pups subjected to electric shock showed an enhanced resistance to later stress (see Hunt, 1979). The same effect has been shown with other noxious experiences and it appears that the explanation lies in changes in the neuro-endocrine system that provide a more adaptive response to later stress (Hennessy and Levine, 1979). But, also, early events may operate by altering sensitivities to stress (perhaps through their effect on the individual's appraisal or perception of the event), or in modifying styles of coping which then protect from, or predispose towards, disorder in later life only in the presence of later stress events (Rutter, 1981c). The suggestion, then, is not that there is any direct persistence of good or ill-effects but rather that patterns of response are established that influence the way the individual reacts to some later stress or adversity. If the pattern is one that *increases* the harm from later stress it is termed a 'sensitization' effect. Conversely, if it *decreases* the harm it is spoken of as 'steeling'. The literature contains several examples of both these effects. For example, in both monkeys (Spencer-Booth and Hinde, 1971; Mineka and Suomi, 1978) and humans (Quinton and Rutter, 1976) it seems that the experience of one unpleasant separation may render the individual *more* likely to be affected adversely by later stressful separations. On the other hand, the experience of some types of acute stressful event may *reduce* the effects when the same event is encountered again—parachute jumping constitutes a good example (Ursin *et al.*, 1978). Or with respect to a quite different kind of 'stressor', Elder (1979) reported that some young people gained from their experiences in coping successfully with the many problems involved in the 1930s economic depression. There seems little doubt that early events may protect from or predispose towards later disorder through 'sensitization' or 'steeling' effects, but we lack any adequate understanding of *how* these effects come about, or *what* determines whether they are protective or damaging.

The third element that needs to be included in any consideration of persistence is that there is marked variation in the outcomes following even the most serious early adversities. For example, this is apparent in our own follow-up into early adult life of young people who came from gravely discordant and unhappy homes and who, as a result of breakdowns in parenting, spent their childhoods in and out of institutions (Rutter *et al.*, 1983; see also Chapter 8 this volume). Not surprisingly, they had a worse overall outcome than that of a general population comparison group followed over the same time period—the rates of almost all sorts of psychosocial problem (criminality, psychiatric disorder, marital difficulties, and failures in parenting) were all about double. However, in spite of pretty appalling childhood experiences, about a quarter developed into ordinarily well-functioning adults. These results are typical of findings on the results of stress, deprivation and disadvantage. Some children succumb with the development of disorder, but others escape showing resilience in the face of adversity. The issue is neatly expressed in the title of the latest report of the Kauai study—*Vulnerable But Invincible* (Werner and Smith, 1982—see Chapter 14 this volume). In the last section of this paper, possible reasons for this individual variation are considered.

INDIVIDUAL DIFFERENCES IN RESPONSE TO ADVERSITY

Age-dependent susceptibilities

The first question that arises with respect to any developmental function is whether or not there are developmentally determined age-specific susceptibilities (Rutter, 1981a,c). Of course, the issue here is *not* whether adverse effects are generally greater at one age period than other (it would be absurd to assume that all adversities operate in the same way), but rather whether *particular* environmental influences vary in their effects according to children's social, emotional and intellectual maturity. It seems that some do.

Thus, the effects of age have been found to be particularly marked in the case of hospital admission, where the age period of greatest risk has proved to be about 6 months to 4 years (Rutter, 1981a). It seems likely that children below age 6 or 7 months are relatively immune because they have not yet developed selective attachments and therefore are not able to experience separation anxiety. Children above age 4 years or so, on the other hand, probably are less vulnerable because they have the cognitive skills needed to appreciate that separation does not necessarily mean abandonment or loss of a relationship, and to understand better what is involved in hospitalization and why unpleasant medical or surgical procedures may be necessary (Rutter, 1981c).

The effects on bonding also seem to be largely restricted to the first few years of life. The pattern of social disinhibition and indiscriminate friendships that is seen in some institution-reared children applies to those admitted in the first two years of life and not to those admitted in later childhood (Wolkind, 1974). Animal studies, too, show that, whereas social isolation in infancy leads to severe social, sexual and parenting abnormalities in rhesus monkeys (Ruppenthal *et al.*, 1976), isolation does not have the same effects in older monkeys (Davenport *et al.*, 1966). It appears that once socialization has become well established in early life, it is less readily disrupted by isolation experiences or by rearing characterized by multiple rotating caretakers. Moreover, if disrupted later, it tends to be affected in a *different* way.

Bereavement, in contrast, seems more likely to lead to severe grief reactions in adolescence than in earlier childhood (van Eerdewegh *et al.*, 1982; Rutter, 1981c). This may be because depressive disorders of all kinds become much more frequent during the teenage years (that is that the capacity to express depressive effect may be age-dependent), or the reason may lie in the fact that older children are better able to conceptualize the past and to understand the meaning of death.

On the other hand, the example of bereavement highlights another issue; that is that age may influence short-term and long-term effects in different ways. The point is that although *immediate* grief reactions seem to be milder and more short-lived in younger children, there are indicators that the *delayed* consequences in terms of psychiatric disorder may be greater (Rutter, 1966). Almost certainly this is not a function of the stress of bereavement itself but rather because of the host of adversities that may follow the death of a parent — break-up of the home, depression in the surviving parent, poverty etc. (Furman, 1974; Rutter, 1966).

Also, it is possible that age may be important for reasons separate from age-dependent susceptibilities. It has been argued (with a little evidence in support) that the meaning and impact of events may be affected by whether or not they occur at what are usually regarded as 'appropriate' times in the life cycle (Hultsch and Plemons, 1979) — thus the death of a young person may be felt to be more stressful than that of someone in old age. The suggestion is plausible but it remains uncertain whether it is true and, if true, how it applies to events in childhood.

Sex differences

The sex of children has been found to influence their response to various family stressors and adversities. In general, it has been found that boys are more vulnerable than girls (see Rutter, 1970, 1982a). This is most evident with respect to family discord, disharmony and disruption but also it has been observed with other environmental factors. However, the sex difference may not operate in all circumstances; for example, it does not appear to apply to the effects of an institutional upbringing (Wolkind, 1974). The mechanisms remain ill-understood. In part, the greater susceptibility of boys may be biologically determined but in part, too, it may reflect differences in the ways in which family difficulties impinge on boys and girls or in the ways in which parents respond to and deal with children of either sex.

Temperamental factors

Quite apart from sex and age differences, it is evident that children vary greatly in their temperamental *styles*, that is in their characteristic mode of behaviour and in the manner in which they respond to differing situations (see Porter and Collins, 1982). Various studies have shown the importance of these temperamental differences in the determination of whether or not children develop emotional or behavioural problems in relation to the psychosocial hazards they face (see Rutter, 1977a, 1981a,c).

Coping processes

Many such hazards require some reaction or response from the child. Accordingly, it might be thought that the outcome would be influenced by what he does about the stress situation — that is by the coping process (see Rutter, 1981c). Coping mechanisms, in this connection, need to have the dual function of problem-solving and of a regulation of emotional distress. It is obvious that some coping processes could increase the risk of maladaption or disorder whereas others could improve adaptation and reduce the risks of a deviant outcome. The notion of effective and ineffective coping is a very plausible one. Unfortunately, we lack good data on what differentiates effective and ineffective mechanisms.

Patterning and multiplicity of stressors

We have seen already that the persistence of ill-effects following stress or adversity depends to a substantial extent on whether or not the environmental hazards continue to impinge on the child. However, there is evidence that the patterning and multiplicity of stressors at any one time is also important (Rutter, 1979a, 1981a,c). Thus, the presence of *chronic* psychosocial adversity makes it more likely that a child will suffer ill-effects from *acute* stressors. Biological and social factors tend to interact so that, for example, it has been found that the effects of low birth weight on children's intelligence is most marked in those who have the added disadvantage of poor social circumstances (Sameroff and Chandler, 1975). But, in addition, there are some indications that there are interactive effects between psychosocial adversities so that the presence of one potentiates the effect of a second or third (Rutter, 1979a).

Compensatory good experiences

Another sort of interaction has also been proposed—namely the balance between pleasant and unpleasant events (Lazarus et al., 1980). The notion is that the presence of happy experiences, to some extent, can provide a buffer that reduces the impact of unhappy ones. The suggestion fits in with the general experience that when everything is going well it is easier to ride adversities and difficulties without succumbing to their effects. Nevertheless, reasonable and understandable though it is, there is remarkably little evidence on whether or not day-to-day happenings do balance each other out in that way. The evidence on longer-term experiences is also limited but, here, there are some indications of protective effects. The shielding influence of a good relationship in the midst of discord and disharmony has been mentioned already. In addition, good experiences at school can, perhaps, do something to compensate for difficulties at home (Rutter, 1979a). Success and a sense of self-esteem are important elements in growing up and factors that enhance a person's feelings of their own worth may prove protective. Certainly, the possibility warrants further exploration.

Catalytic factors

Finally, we need to mention the possibility of 'catalytic' factors. The concept is one of factors that are largely inert on their own but, when combined with environmental stresses or hazards, either increase their effect (so-called 'vulnerability' factors), or decrease their impact (so-called 'protective' factors). The presence of a supportive social network and of a cohesive social group are thought to operate in that fashion and there is some indication that in adults they do so (see Rutter, 1981c). The hypothesis of 'learned helplessness' introduces another dimension—that of a person's cognitive attribution style, or self-concept of themselves as in control of life situations. Most of the work on this topic has been with adults (Seligman, 1975, 1978) but there are a few studies with children (cf. Dweck and Bush, 1976; Dweck et al., 1978) that suggest that the concept may have some applicability. Werner and Smith (1982) in their analysis of the Kauai study provide some of the very few data directly relevant to the 'catalytic' notion—namely the identification of factors that are important in counterbalancing stress, deprivation or disadvantage, but that are not important or influential in the absence of such circumstances (see Chapter 14 this volume). Such ameliorating factors included good physical health, autonomy and self-help skills, a positive social orientation and self-concept, a positive parent–child relationship in infancy, and emotional support from other family members during early and middle childhood.

IMPLICATIONS FOR POLICY AND PRACTICE

It is clear from this review of the findings from longitudinal studies of the environmental effects of children's experiences at home and at school that a great deal of knowledge is available on the topic, but also that still we lack an adequate understanding of many issues. It remains for me to consider a few of the policy and practice implications that stem from what we do know.

Environmental effects

The demonstration that there *are* substantial environmental effects is itself important. The clear implication is that if we can alter children's circumstances in the right direction there should be worthwhile benefits in terms of changes in their psychosocial functioning and development. However, also it is necessary that we recognize the limitations on what can be accomplished by most of the actions currently at our disposal. Perhaps the most obvious conclusion is that no amount of environmental manipulation will ever eliminate individual differences. The crucial point is that one of the main ways in which individual differences operate is in terms of an ability to take advantage of opportunities. Hence, if environmental circumstances are greatly improved, biological differences between children will ensure that some will profit more than others. On the other hand, it is apparent that a general improvement in conditions of child rearing *will* have the effect of raising overall standards of scholastic attainment and social behaviour and, in so doing, may well reduce some forms of undesirable unequal opportunities (see Rutter and Madge, 1976; Rutter, 1983). The conclusion serves to emphasize that the issues of social inequality and individual differences are far from synonymous.

Two further limitations should be noted. First, it is clear that some crucial variables have their impact through biological heredity rather than through environmental effects. Schizophrenia and alcoholism in the parents are examples of this kind. They have been found to be associated with the same conditions in the offspring even when the children have been removed at birth and brought up in adoptive families. On the other hand, this should *not* be taken to mean that rearing by a schizophrenic or alcoholic parent is without environmental effects on the children. There is other evidence that such rearing does have an impact involving adverse sequelae, although most of the sequelae do not take the form of schizophrenia or alcoholism. Secondly, although environmental influences *do* influence intellectual development, most of the more ordinary variations in families and schools have their greatest impact on scholastic achievement rather than on IQ. This constitutes an important outcome with consequent effects on life chances and it is time that we ceased using IQ as the main (and often the whole) indicator of cognitive effects.

Mechanisms

Much of the research has been most informative in terms of the possible mechanisms involved in environmental effects. We have come to appreciate that there is a crucial difference between risk *indicators* and causal *mechanisms*. Thus, low social class is associated with an increased risk of educational difficulties and (at least in the USA) black children are more likely to become delinquent, but class and skin colour represent indicators and not mechanisms. No-one supposes that the nature of the father's job causes a child to fail at school and equally it would be ridiculous to suggest that skin colour causes crime. We need to ask what mechanisms or processes underlie the risk indicator associations.

Scholastic achievement

In that connection, two implications stand out as particularly important in relation to environmental effects on cognition. First, it is not 'stimulation' or doing things *to* children that matters. Rather it is talking and playing *with* children that has effects. It seems that *active, meaningful experiences* are most important in facilitating cognitive development. Mere bombardment with sensory stimuli is not beneficial. Secondly, in terms of scholastic achievement, task involvement and attitudes to learning, as well as cognitive capacity, determine outcome. The social context of learning, and the personal relationship between 'teacher' (meaning parent just as much as educators at school) and child probably have an effect on these aspects of cognitive performance. Attainments are a consequence of intellectual capacities, taught skills, a commitment to and interest in learning, and an ability to translate capacity into performance.

Conduct disorders

With conduct disorders and delinquency, three shifts of emphasis require mention. First, it has been recognized that physical separations of parents and children and broken homes are not the key aspects of family relationships. Rather it is *continuity* in parenting (especially during the preschool years) and the *quality* of relationships that matter. Quarrelling and discord are damaging whether in broken or unbroken homes. But with young children quality in parenting is not enough; there must also be substantial continuity. Caretaking may be divided among a few key adults but it cannot be successfully provided by a roster of ever-changing caretakers, however good they may be individually (see Smith, 1980).

Secondly, with discipline, it is not the particular technique or its severity that matters most. Rather, parents need to be concerned with their *perception* and recognition of the deviant behaviours that are most important; their ability to *monitor* and supervise their children's activities (in a manner that enables them to pick up warning signals but yet is not so intrusive as to lead to resentment); and with the *efficiency* of the disciplinary techniques they employ (efficiency, that is, in bringing about the desired behaviour, in doing so in a way that resolves conflicts or difficulties and brings harmony). This last consideration emphasizes the importance of both the affective style and context of disciplinary techniques and also the use of social problem-solving strategies.

Thirdly, it is apparent that children's conduct is affected by factors outside, as well as inside, the family. The peer group and the school stand out as the two most important influences that need to be taken into account. Virtually all children go to school and it is now evident that their experiences in that environment can have either beneficial or harmful effects. The challenge before us is that of ensuring that children's school experiences *are* positive and helpful rather than alienating and discouraging.

There are further implications for preventive policies that stems from the evidence on the importance of continuity in parenting (together with the lack of importance of so-called 'blood ties'). In the case of young children whose parents seem unlikely ever to be able to look after them adequately, an *early* decision should be taken with respect to adoption or long-term fostering (Rutter, 1979b). It is not in the child's interests for there to be vacillation and indecision while he shuffles to and from his parents' in and out of institutions, nor is it in his interests to remain for long periods in an institution in the forlorn hope that the parents who abandoned him and who now visit only sporadically will one day take him back. But also it is important to strive to improve the quality of children's group homes as environments that can meet young children's psychosocial needs. It has proved possible to ensure that institutions provide the range of experiences needed for cognitive growth but it has proved much more difficult to ensure any kind of continuity in parenting. An institutional upbringing should never be a first choice, but when that constitutes the best available alternative, it is important that the experience be as positive and beneficial in its effects as we can make it.

As we have seen, although low social status is a risk indicator for conduct disorders, probably poor socio-economic conditions *per se* do not directly cause delinquency or conduct disturbance. Of course, there can be no question but that social disadvantage makes it more difficult to bring up children in an optimal fashion. But, many parents succeed in spite of socioeconomic difficulties. The implication is that we do not necessarily have to wait for a social revolution before anything can be done. Much the same factors that predispose to conduct disorders in middle-class children do so in working-class families as well. All too often, the plea for a revolutionary approach has a deeply conservative and reactionary effect—it is revolution *tomorrow* and inaction today. That is unhelpful on its own because there *are* things that can be done today within the existing social system. Of course, that is not an argument for not working as citizens to reduce the discriminations and inequities in our society. To the contrary, we *should* strive to improve tomorrow's world but in so doing we should not neglect the steps that can be taken to improve the lot of today's children.

Emotional disorders

We have a less substantial empirical basis for decisions on the policy and practice implications in the field of emotional disorders. However, two features warrant notice. First, circumstantial evidence suggests that is likely that most of the crucial environmental influences concern *within*-family, rather than between-family, factors. That is to say, we need to be more concerned with the variations in the ways in which different children in the same family are treated, than with more general influences that effect the family as a whole. This orientation is consonant with therapeutic approaches that regard the social system of individual families as crucial, but it has to be said that, so far, therapeutic enthusiasm for conjoint family methods has rather run ahead of our understanding of how these within-family mechanisms operate. Secondly, although the evidence is limited, it is probable that various acute stressors may play a part in the precipitation of emotional disorders. The few available data suggest that such events are most likely to have an adverse impact when they interfere with parent–child relationships, or involve some form of loss of a relationship, or involve some lasting change in the environment. However, necessarily this suggestion has to be rather tentative and the matter requires further study.

Persistence of effects

In the past there has been vigorous dispute between those who have urged for the critical importance of the infancy period (Bowlby, 1952) and those who have argued that infantile experiences have no significant relevance for later functioning (Kagan and Klein, 1973). The research evidence reviewed here does not support either one of these extreme positions. On the one hand, there can be no doubt that experiences during middle childhood, adolescence and even adult life all serve to influence psychosocial functioning; the infancy period is *not* one of overwhelming, or even preponderant, importance. Moreover, it is also apparent that children's powers of recovery are far greater than once supposed. For both reasons, it is clear that it is never too late to intervene. There is no excuse for giving up on the grounds that the child is too old for anything to make any difference. On the other hand, equally, it is apparent that experiences in infancy *do* have an impact. It would be wrong to disregard the early years as without any importance simply because many of the effects become greatly attenuated (or even disappear) as children grow older. Early intervention continues to be important for three rather separate reasons. First, it is apparent that the longer the adverse experiences last the more likely it is that the ill-effects will be persistent. The sooner that children's suffering can be reduced the better. Secondly, because infantile experiences come first they may have indirect effects on later development because styles of behaviour and response become established that in turn shape later experiences. Thirdly, although less certainly, the early years may constitute something of a 'sensitive period' for certain types of social experiences.

However, other aspects of the findings on persistence of environmental effects also carry implications for policy and practice. All the evidence shows that, to a very considerable extent, the persistence of ill-effects is a function of continuity in family (and other) adversities. All too often, the child in an unhappy, discordant and disorganized home at age 2 years is still experiencing the same conditions at age 12 years. Moreover, it seems that most environmental influences do not have their effects in terms of some once and for all alteration of personality development. Rather, the effects shape *current* functioning in a particular social *context*. That is to say, many of the effects are partially situation-bound. Furthermore, generalization across situations or persistence over time are the result of the acquisition of habitual modes of functioning rather than of any permanent change in the personality. It is probably for these reasons that most forms of treatment (or punishment or rehabilitation) of delinquents have had such limited benefits if the youths return to the same adverse environment, as usually they do (see Rutter and Giller, 1983). The implication is that for interventions to be effective it is likely that either they will have to bring about a lasting change in the environment or they will have to improve the individual's social problem-solving skills and social competence generally so that he is better able to deal with environmental pressures.

Traditionally, 'bad' environments were thought of in terms of whether or not they brought about some form of disorder, or malfunction, or impaired development in the child. Of course, these direct effects do occur and are important. However, it now seems that also there may be *indirect* effects which influence later behaviour only if there is an interactive effect with some subsequent stress or adversity. The notion here is that early (or later) experiences may alter patterns of response to stress in ways that may either increase vulnerability or provide protection. Greater attention to these patterns of response may help us learn how to intervene more effectively when children are suffering adversity.

Individual differences

Finally, there is the need to consider the implications that stem from the findings on the large individual differences in children's responses to stress and adversity. Perhaps, four are worth special mention. First, there is the evidence on the interactive effects by which one environmental hazard potentiates the damage brought about by another. This suggests that there are likely to be benefits from reducing the overall level of adversities faced by children even if it proves impossible to bring about a really satisfactory environment. This is important if only because we are so rarely in the position do all that we would like to do in improving children's circumstances. Secondly, the evidence on temperamental, sex and age differences means that, in any situation of stress or deprivation, we should avoid assuming that damage is inevitable. Rather we need to look at the *specifics* of how each particular child is responding in order to decide on the actions to take. But, of course, in that connection, it is not only 'constitutional' variables that are important. Coping mechanisms and social problem-solving skills are also influential. As yet, we lack understanding of exactly how they operate, or which methods of coping are superior to others, but clearly, further attention to this dimension of children's responses to environmental hazards is required.

Thirdly, there is a need to be aware of the potential value of compensating positive experiences. Again, our knowledge on this area is quite limited but there are at least two respects in which even the knowledge we have provides leads. In the past most preventive and therapeutic strategies have been preoccupied with *reducing* harmful environmental effects of one kind or another. Of course, that is worthwhile but perhaps as much can be achieved by *increasing* positive experiences. Sometimes it may be both easier and more effective to build on strengths than to eliminate weaknesses. The other implication applies to the situations in which difficult decisions have to be taken on whether or not a child should be compulsorily removed from his family because home conditions are so bad that he is at a serious psychological risk. In these circumstances, it may be as important to weigh in the balance the compensatory good experiences in a bad situation (as, for example, a really secure and positive relationship with one parent in spite of gross discord all around) as to add up all the damaging features.

Lastly, it is important to consider the possible ameliorating or buffering effects of various 'catalytic' factors in the environment — factors that have no necessary effect on their own but which, nevertheless, enable an individual or a family to cope better or to be more resilient when facing adversities. So far we lack a detailed understanding of these mechanisms and we lack knowledge on just which factors carry this protective effect. At present, social support systems are arousing most interest but doubtless there are others that have yet to be identified.

Research and policy

In concluding, there is one final point to be made. It is obvious that there can be no simple and straightforward derivation of policy and practice from empirical research findings (Rutter, 1978). Society must decide for itself what social purposes and values it considers most important. Research cannot decide these matters. Nevertheless, research has a crucial rôle to play in deciding on the effects of decisions taken on the basis of these values. In so doing, it may cause a change in the questions being asked and suggest solutions or remedies that had not entered the policy-maker or clinician's original frame of reference. But, this process of moving from value-expressive questions to empirical data and back to the initial social purposes and values can never come to a neat conclusion. In this chapter, I have sought to provide a survey of the state of the art on the family, the child and the school and in so doing I have raised both possibilities for future action and also a host of questions that require further research.

ACKNOWLEDGEMENTS

This chapter is largely based on an article in the *Journal of Child Psychology and Psychiatry*. I am grateful to the Editors and to the publishers for permission to use it here ('Family and school influences on behavioural development', *Journal of Child Psychology and Psychiatry*, in press). A substantially similar version is due to appear in *Middle Childhood: Development and Dysfunction*, edited by M. D. Levine and P. Satz, Baltimore: University Park Press.

REFERENCES

Bandura, A. (1969). Social-learning theory of identificatory processes, in *Handbook of Socialization Theory and Research* (Ed. D. A. Goslin), pp.325–346, Rand McNally, Chicago.

Barkley, R. A. (1981). The use of psychopharmacology to study reciprocal influences in parent–child interaction, *Journal of Abnormal Child Psychology*, **9**, 303–310.

Bateson, P. (1979). How do sensitive periods arise and what are they for? *Animal Behavior*, **27**, 470–486.

Bateson, P. (1983). The interpretation of sensitive periods, in *The Behavior of Human Infants* (Eds A. Oliverio and M. Zappella), pp.57–70. Plenum Press, New York.

Becker, W. C. (1964). Consequences of different kinds of parental discipline, in *Review of Child Development Research*, Vol. 1 (Eds M. L. Hoffman and L. W. Hoffman), Russell Sage Foundation, New York.

Bell, R. W. (1968). A reinterpretation of the direction of effects in studies of socialization, *Psychological Review*, **75**, 81–95.

Bell, R. W. (1974). Contributions of human infants to care-giving and social interaction, in *The Effects of the Infant on its Caregiver* (Eds M. Lewis and L. A. Rosenblum), Wiley, New York.

Bell, R. W. and Harper, L. V. (Eds) (1977). *Child Effects on Adults*, Erlbaum, Hillsdale, N.J.

Birch, H. G. and Gussow, J. D. (1970). *Disadvantaged Children: Health, Nutrition and School Failure*, Grune & Stratton, New York.

Bowlby, J. (1952). *Maternal Care and Mental Health*, World Health Organization Monograph Series 2, Geneva.

Bowlby, J. (1969). *Attachment and Loss:* I. *Attachment*, Hogarth Press, London.

Bronfenbrenner, U. (1979). *The Ecology of Human Development: Experiments by nature and design*, Harvard University Press, Cambridge, Mass.

Buikhuisen, W. and Hoekstra, H. A. (1974). Factors related to recidivism, *British Journal of Criminology*, **14**, 63–69.

Burks, B. S. (1928). The relative influence of nature and nurture upon mental development: A comparative study of foster parent–foster child resemblance and true parent–true child resemblance, *Yearbook of the National Society for the Study of Education*, **27**, 219–316.

Cadoret, R. J. and Cain, C. (1980). Sex differences in predictors of antisocial behavior in adoptees, *Archives of General Psychiatry*, **37**, 1171–1175.

Cadoret, R. J., Cain, C. A. and Grove, W. M. (1980). Development of alcoholism in adoptees raised apart from alcoholic biologic relatives, *Archives of General Psychiatry*, **37**, 561–563.

Clarke, A. M. and Clarke, A. D. B. (1976). *Early Experience: Myth and Evidence*, Open Books, London.

Crowe, R. R. (1974). An adoption study of antisocial personality, *Archives of General Psychiatry*, **31**, 785–791.

Darlington, R. B., Royce, J. M., Snipper, A. S., Murray, H. W. and Lazar, I. (1980). Pre-school programs and later school competence of children from low-income families, *Science*, **208**, 202–204.

Davenport, R. K., Menzel, E. W. and Rogers, C. M. (1966). Effects of severe isolation on 'normal' juvenile chimpanzees: health, weight gain and stereotyped behaviors, *Archives of General Psychiatry*, **14**, 134–138.

Douglas, J. W. B., Ross, J. M. and Simpson, H. R. (1968). *All Our Future: A Longitudinal Study of Secondary Education*, Peter Davies, London.

Dweck, C. S. and Bush, E. S. (1976). Sex differences in learned helplessness: I. Differential debilitation with peer and adult evaluators, *Developmental Psychology*, **12**, 147–156.

Dweck, C. S., Davidson, W., Nelson, S. and Enna, B. (1978). Sex differences in learned helplessness: II. The contingencies of evaluative feedback in the classroom, and III. An experimental analysis. *Developmental Psychology*, **14**, 268–276.

Elder, G. H. (1979). Historical change in life patterns and personality, in *Life Span Development and Behavior* (Eds P. B. Baltes and O. G. Brim), Academic Press, New York & London.

Elliott, D. S., Ageton, S. S. and Canter, R. J. (1979). An integrated theoretical perspective on delinquent behavior, *Journal of Research into Crime & Delinquency*, **16**, 3–27.

Elliott, D. S. and Voss, H. L. (1974). *Delinquency and Dropout*, Lexington Books, Toronto and London.

Farrington, D. P. (1979). Longitudinal research on crime and delinquency, in *Criminal Justice: An annual review of research*, Vol. 1 (Eds N. Morris and M. Tonry), pp.289–348, University of Press, Chicago and London.

Furman, E. (1974). *A Child's Parent Dies: Studies in Childhood Bereavement*, Yale University Press, New Haven and London.

Garber, H. and Heber, F. R. (1977). The Milwaukee project: indications of the effectiveness of early intervention in preventing mental retardation, in *Research to*

Practice in Mental Retardation, I. *Care and Intervention* (Ed. P. Mittler), University Park Press, Baltimore.

Gardner, J. (1977). Three aspects of childhood autism: Mother–child interactions, autonomic responsivity, and cognitive functioning. PhD Thesis, University of Leicester.

Gottesman, I. and Shields, J. (1976). A critical review of recent adoption, twin, and family studies of schizophrenia: behavioral genetics perspectives, *Schizophrenia Bulletin*, **2**, 360–401.

Gray, G., Smith, A. and Rutter, M. (1980). School attendance and the first year of employment, in *Out of School: Modern Perspectives in Truancy and School Refusal* (Eds L. Hersov and I. Berg), pp.343–370, Wiley, Chichester.

Heber, R. (1978). Sociocultural mental retardation—a longitudinal study, in *Primary Prevention of Psychopathology: 2. Environmental Influences* (Ed. D. Forgays), University Press of New England, Hanover, New Hampshire.

Hennessy, J. W. and Levine, S. (1979). Stress, arousal, and the pituitary-adrenal system: a psychoendocrine hypothesis, in *Progress in Psychobiology and Physiological Psychology* (Eds J. M. Sprague and A. N. Epstein), pp.133–178, Academic Press, New York.

Hess, R. D. and Camara, K. A. (1979). Post-divorce family relationships as mediating factors in the consequence of divorce for children, *Journal of Social Issues*, **35**, 79–96.

Hetherington, E. M., Cox, M. and Cox, R. (1982). Effects of divorce on parents and children, *Nontraditional Families* (Ed. M. Lamb), pp.233–288, Erlbaum, Hillsdale, N.J.

Hinde, R. A. (1980). Family influences, in *Scientific Foundations of Developmental Psychiatry* (Ed. M. Rutter), pp.47–66, Heinemann Medical, London.

Hinde, R. A. and McGinnis, L. (1977). Some factors influencing the effect of temporary mother–infant separation: some experiments with rhesis monkeys, *Psychological Medicine*, **7**, 197–212.

Hirschi, T. (1969). *Causes of Delinquency*, University of California Press, Berkeley and Los Angeles.

Howard, J. (1978). The influence of children's developmental dysfunctions on marital quality and family interaction, in *Child Influences on Marital and Family Interaction: A life span perspective* (Eds R. M. Lerner and G. B. Spanier), pp.275–298, Academic Press, New York and London.

Hultsch, D. F. and Plemons, J. K. (1979). Life events and life span development, in *Life-Span Development and Behavior*, Vol. 2 (Eds P. B. Baltes and O. G. Brim), pp.1–36, Academic Press, New York and London.

Hunt, J. McV. (1979). Psychological development: early experience, *Annual Review in Psychology*, **30**, 103–143.

Hutchings, B. and Mednick, S. A. (1974). Registered criminality in the adoptive and biological parents of registered male adoptees, in *Genetics, Environment and Psychopathology* (Eds S. A. Mednick *et al.*), pp.215–227, North-Holland, Amsterdam.

Jensen, A. R. (1973). *Educability and Group Differences*, Methuen, London.

Kagan, J. and Klein, R. E. (1973). Cross-cultural perspectives on early development. *American Psychologist*, **28**, 947–961.

Kelvin, P. (1969). *The Bases of Social Behavior: An approach in terms of order and value*, Holt, Rinehart and Winston, London.

Korn, S. J., Chess, S. and Fernandez, P. (1978). The impact of children's physical handicaps on marital quality and family interaction, in *Child Influence on Marital and Family Interaction: A Life Span Perspective* (Eds R. M. Lerner and G. B. Spanier), pp.299–326, Academic Press, New York and London.

Lazar, I. and Darlington, R. B. (1982). Lasting effects of early education, *Monographs of the Society for Research in Child Development*, **47**, Serial No. 195.

Lazarus, R. S., Cohen, J. B., Folkman, S., Kanner, A. and Schaefer, C. (1980). Psychological stress and adaptation: some unresolved issues, in *Guide to Stress Research* (Ed. H. Selye), Van Nostrand Reinhold, New York.

Leahy, A. M. (1935). Nature-nurture and intelligence, *Genetic Psychology Monographs*, **17**, 241–305.

Lerner, R. M. and Spanier, G. B. (Eds) (1978). *Child Influence on Marital and Family Interaction: A Life Span Perspective*. Academic Press, New York and London.

Lewis, M. and Rosenblum, L. A. (Eds) (1978). *Genesis of Behavior*, Vol. 1, *The Development of Affect*, Plenum, New York.

Loehlin, J. C. and Nichols, R. C. (1976). *Heredity, Environment and Personality: A Study of 850 Sets of Twins*, University of Texas Press, Austin.

Longstreth, L. E., Davis, B., Carter, L., Flint, D., Owen, J., Rickert, M. and Taylor, E. (1981). Separation of home intellectual environment and maternal IQ as determinants of child IQ, *Developmental Psychology*, **17**, 532–541.

Madge, N. and Tizard, J. (1980). Intelligence, in *Scientific Foundations of Developmental Psychiatry* (Ed. M. Rutter), pp.245–265, Heinemann Medical, London.

Maughan, B., Mortimore, P., Ousten, J. and Rutter, M. (1980). Fifteen Thousand Hours: A reply to Heath and Clifford, *Oxford Review of Education*, **6**, 289–303.

Mineka, S. and Suomi, S. J. (1978). Social separation in monkeys, *Psychological Bulletin*, **85**, 1376–1400.

Nisbet, J. D. (1953). *Family Environment: A Direct Effect of Family Size on Intelligence*, Occasional papers on Eugenics, No. 8. The Eugenics Society, London.

Offord, D. R. (1982). Family background of male and female delinquents, in *Abnormal Offenders: Delinquency and the Criminal Justice System* (Eds J. Gunn and D. Farrington), Wiley, Chichester.

Patterson, G. R. (1977). Accelerating stimuli for two classes of coercive behaviors, *Journal of Abnormal Child Psychology*, **5**, 355–360.

Patterson, G. R. (1982). *Coercive Family Processes*, Castalia, Eugene, Oregon.

Pedersen, E., Faucher, T. A. and Eaton, W. W. (1978). A new perspective on the effects of firstgrade teachers on children's subsequent adult status, *Harvard Educational Review*, **48**, 1–31.

Porter, R. and Collins, G. M. (Eds). *Temperamental Differences in Infants and Young Children*. Ciba Foundation Symposium 89. Pitman Books, London.

Quinton, D. and Rutter, M. (1976). Early hospital admissions and later disturbances of behaviour: An attempted replication of Douglas' findings, *Developmental Medicine and Child Neurology*, **18**, 447–459.

Rapoport, J. (1983). The use of drugs: Trends in research, in *Developmental Neuropsychiatry* (Ed. M. Rutter), Guilford Press, New York.

Richman, N., Stevenson, J. and Graham, P. (Eds) (1982). *Preschool to School: a behavioural study*. Academic Press, London.

Robins, L. N. (1966). *Deviant Children Grown Up*, Williams and Wilkins, Baltimore.

Robins, L. N. (1973). Evaluation of psychiatric services for children in the United States, in *Roots of Evaluation: The Epidemiological Basis for Planning Psychiatric Services* (Eds J. K. Wing and H. Häfner), Oxford University Press, London and New York.

Rowe, D. C. and Plomin, R. (1981). The importance of nonshared (E_1) environmental influences in behavioral development, *Developmental Psychology*, **17**, 517–531.

Roy, P. (1983). Is continuity enough?: Substitute care and socialization. Paper presented at Spring Scientific Meeting, Child and Adolescent Psychiatry Section, Royal College of Psychiatry, March 1983.

Ruppenthal, G. C., Arling, G. L., Harlow, H. F., Sackett, G. P. and Suomi, S. J. (1976). A 10-year perspective of motherless-mother monkey behavior, *Journal of Abnormal Psychology*, **85**, 341–349.

Rutter, M. (1966). *Children of Sick Parents: An Environmental and Psychiatric Study*, Institute of Psychiatry Maudsley Monographs No. 16. Oxford University Press, London.

Rutter, M. (1970). Sex differences in children's response to family stress, in *The Child in His Family* (Eds E. J. Anthony and C. Koupernik), pp.165–196, Wiley, New York.

Rutter, M. (1971). Parent-child separation: psychological effects on the children, *Journal of Child Psychology and Psychiatry*, **12**, 233–260.

Rutter, M. (1975). *Helping Troubled Children*, Penguin, Harmondsworth, Middx.

Rutter, M. (1977a). Individual differences, in *Child Psychiatry: Modern Approaches* (Eds M. Rutter and L. Hersov), pp.3–21, Blackwell Scientific, Oxford.

Rutter, M. (1977b). Other family influences, in *Child Psychiatry: Modern Approaches* (Eds M. Rutter and L. Hersov), pp.74–108, Blackwell Scientific, Oxford.

Rutter, M. (1978). Research and prevention of psychosocial disorders in childhood, in *Social Care Research* (Eds J. Barnes and N. Connolly), Bedford Square Press, London.

Rutter, M. (1979a). Protective factors in children's responses to stress and disadvantage, in *Primary Prevention of Psychopathology*, Vol. 3, *Social Competence in Children* (Eds M. W. Kent and J. E. Rolf), University Press of New England, Hanover.

Rutter, M. (1979b). *Changing Youth in a Changing Society*, Nuffield Provincial Hospitals Trust, London.

Rutter, M. (1981a). *Maternal Deprivation Reassessed* (2nd edn), Penguin, Harmondsworth, Middx.

Rutter, M. (1981b). Epidemiological/longitudinal strategies and causal research in child psychiatry, *Journal of the American Academy of Child Psychiatry*, **20**, 513–544.

Rutter, M. (1981c). Stress, coping and development: Some issues and some questions, *Journal of Child Psychology and Psychiatry*, **22**, 323–356.

Rutter, M. (1981d). Longitudinal studies: A psychiatric perspective, in *Prospective Longitudinal Research: An Empirical Basis for the Primary Prevention of Psychosocial Disorders* (Eds S. A. Mednick and A. E. Baert), pp.326–336, Oxford University Press, Oxford.

Rutter, M. (1982a). Epidemiological-longitudinal approaches to the study of development, in *The Concept of Development* Vol. 15 (Ed. W. A. Collins) The Minnesota Symposia on Child Psychology, Lawrence Erlbaum, Hillsdale, N.J.

Rutter, M. (1982b). Psychological therapies: Issues and prospects, *Psychological Medicine*, **12**, 723–740.

Rutter, M. (1983). School effects on pupil progress: Research findings and policy implications, *Child Development* **54**, 1–29.

Rutter, M. and Garmezy, N. (1983). Atypical social and personality development, in *Socialization, Personality, and Social Development*, Vol. 4, *Mussen's Manual of Child Psychology* (Ed. E. M. Hetherington) (4th Edition), Wiley, New York.

Rutter, M. and Giller, H. (1983). *Juvenile Delinquency: Trends and Perspectives*, Penguin, Harmondsworth, Middx.

Rutter, M., Gray, G., Maughan, B. and Smith, A. (1982). *School Experiences and Achievements and the First Year of Employment*, Final Report to the Department of Education and Science, London.

Rutter, M. and Madge, N. (1976). *Cycles of Disadvantage*, Heinemann Educational, London.

Rutter, M., Maughan, B., Mortimore, P., Ouston, J., with Smith, A. (1979). *Fifteen Thousand Hours: Secondary Schools and their effects on Children*, Open Books, London; Harvard University Press, Cambridge, Mass.

Rutter, M. and Quinton, D. (1981). Longitudinal studies of institutional children and children of mentally ill parents (United Kingdom), in *Prospective Longitudinal Research: An Empirical Basis for the Primary Prevention of Psychosocial Disorders* (Eds S. A. Mednick and A. E. Baert), pp.297–305, Oxford University Press, Oxford.

Rutter, M., Quinton, D. and Liddle, C. (1983). Parenting in two generations: Looking backwards and looking forwards, in *Families at Risk* (Ed. N. Madge), Heinemann Educational, London.

Rutter, M., Tizard, J. and Whitmore, K. (Eds) (1970). *Education, Health and Behavior*, Longmans, London. (Reprinted 1981, Krieger, New York.)

Rutter, M., Yule, B., Quinton, D., Rowlands, O., Yule, W. and Berger, M. (1975). Attainment and adjustment in two geographical areas. III. Some factors accounting for area differences, *British Journal of Psychiatry*, **126**, 520–533.

Sameroff, A. J. and Chandler, M. J. (1975). Reproductive risk and the continuum of caretaking casualty, in *Review of Child Development Research, Vol. 4*. (Ed. F. D. Horowitz), University of Chicago Press, Chicago.

Scarr, S. (1981). *IQ: Race, Social Class, and Individual Differences: New Studies of Old Issues*, Lawrence Erlbaum, Hillsdale, N.J.

Scarr, S., Webber, P. L., Weinberg, R. A. and Wittig, M. A. (1981). Personality resemblance among adolescents and their parents in biologically related and adoptive families, *Journal of Personality and Social Psychology*, **40**, 885–898.

Scarr, S. and Weinberg, R. A. (1976). IQ test performance of black children adopted by white families, *American Psychologist*, **31**, 726–739.

Scarr, S. and Weinberg, R. A. (1978). The influence of 'family background' on intellectual attainment, *American Sociological Review*, **43**, 674–692.

Schweinhart, L. J. and Weikart, D. P. (1980). *Young Children Grow Up: The effects of the Perry preschool program on youths through age 15*, Monographs of the High/Scope Educational Research Foundation No. 7. High/Scope ERF, Ypsilanti, Michigan.

Seligman, M. E. P. (1975). *Helplessness: On Depression, Development and Death*, W. H. Freeman, San Francisco.

Seligman, M. E. P. (1978). Comment and integration, *Journal of Abnormal Psychology*, **87**, 165–179.

Sherif, M. and Sherif, C. W. (1969). *Social Psychology*, Harper and Row, London.

Shields, J. (1977). Polygenic influences, in *Child Psychiatry: Modern Approaches* (Eds M. Rutter and L. Hersov), pp.22–46, Blackwell Scientific, Oxford.

Shields, J. (1980). Genetics and mental development, in *Scientific Foundations of Developmental Psychiatry* (Ed. M. Rutter), pp.8–24, Heinemann Medical, London.

Skodak, M. and Skeels, H. M. (1949). A final follow-up study of one hundred adopted children, *Journal of Genetic Psychology*, **75**, 85–125.

Skuse, D. (1984a). Extreme deprivation in early childhood. I. Diverse outcomes for three siblings from an extraordinary family, *Journal of Child Psychology and Psychiatry* (in press).

Skuse, D. (1984b). Extreme deprivation in early childhood. II. Theoretical issues and a comparative review, *Journal of Child Psychology and Psychiatry* (in press).

Smith, P. K. (1980). Shared care of young children: Alternative models to monotropism. *Merrill-Palmer Quarterly*, **26**, 371–389.

Spencer-Booth, Y. and Hinde, R. A. (1971). Effects of brief separations from mothers during infancy on behaviour of rhesus monkeys 6–24 months later, *Journal of Child Psychology and Psychiatry*, **12**, 157–172.

Taylor, E. (1983). Drug response and diagnostic validation, in *Developmental Neuropsychiatry* (Ed. M. Rutter), Guilford Press, New York.

Thomas, A., Chess, S. and Birch, H. G. (1968). *Temperament and Behavior Disorders in Children*, New York University Press, New York.

Thompson, W. R. and Grusec, J. (1970). Studies of early experience, in *Carmichael's Manual of Child Psychology, Vol. 1* (3rd edn), pp.565–654, Wiley, New York.

Tizard, B., Cooperman, O., Joseph, A. and Tizard, J. (1972). Environmental effects on language development: A study of young children in long-stay residential nurseries, *Child Development*, **43**, 337–358.

Tizard, B. and Hodges, J. (1978). The effect of early institutional rearing on the development of eight-year-old children, *Journal of Child Psychology and Psychiatry*, **19**, 99–118.

Tizard, B. and Rees, J. (1974). A comparison of the effects of adoption, restoration to the natural mother, and continued institutionalization on the cognitive development of four-year-old children, *Child Development*, **45**, 92–99.

Tizard, J., Schofield, W. N. and Hewison, J. (1982). Collaboration between teachers and parents in assisting children's reading, *British Journal of Educational Psychology*, **52**, 1–15.

Ursin, H., Baade, E. and Levine, S. (1978). *Psychobiology of Stress: A Study of Coping Men*, Academic Press, New York.

van Eerdewegh, M. M., Bieri, M. D., Parrilla, R. H. and Clayton, P. J. (1982). The bereaved child, *British Journal of Psychiatry*, **140**, 23–29.

Wallerstein, J. S. and Kelly, J. B. (1980). *Surviving the Breakup: How Children and Parents Cope with Divorce*, Basic Books, New York; Grant McIntyre, London.

Weissman, M. M. (1979). Depressed parents and their children: Implications for prevention, in *Basic Handbook of Child Psychiatry: Vol. 4, Prevention and Current Issues* (Eds I. N. Berlin and L. A. Stone), pp.292–299, Basic Books, New York.

Werner, E. E. and Smith, R. S. (1982). *Vulnerable, but Invincible: A Longitudinal Study of Resilient Children and Youth*, McGraw-Hill, New York.

West, D. J. (1982). *Delinquency: Its Roots, Careers and Prospects*, Heinemann Educational, London.

West, D. J. and Farrington, D. P. (1973). *Who Becomes Delinquent?* Heinemann Educational, London.

West, D. J. and Farrington, D. P. (1977). *The Delinquent Way of Life*, Heinemann Educational, London.

Willerman, L. (1979). Effects of families on intellectual development, *American Psychologist*, **34**, 923–929.

Wolkind, S. (1974). The components of 'affectionless psychopathy' in institutionalized children, *Journal of Child Psychology and Psychiatry*, **15**, 215–220.

Yule, W. and Raynes, N. V. (1972). Behavioural characteristics of children in residential care in relation to indices of separation, *Journal of Child Psychology and Psychiatry*, **13**, 249–258.

Index

Adopted children
  11 years, 142
  15 years, 143–144
  18 years, 148–150
  21–22 years, 150–151
Adopting parents, characteristics, 140, 152
Adoption, relinquishment for, 61
Adversity
  acute and chronic, 389–390
  compensatory good experiences, 390
  counterbalancing factors, 390
  coping processes, 389
  susceptibilities with age, 387–388
  susceptibilities with sex; 388–389
  susceptibilities with temperament, 389
Age and sex, children in different schools, 272
Aggression, continuity of, 45–46
Alternate caregivers, of stress resistant children, 347
'At risk' factors, 55, 230

Balance between stress and protective factors, 349
Behaviour disorders, preschool, 75
Behaviour modification, 319, 321, 322, 323, 324, 325, 329–333
Behaviour, specificity, 3
Bereavement, psychological effects of, 363
Bi-directionality of child-caretaker effects, 342
Biological parents, characteristics, 140

Caregiving environment, 335
Causal chains, 369
Causation
  alternative explanations, 357
  broken homes, 357
  chains of events, 4
  child neglect, 357

direct effects, 3
direction of in criminality, 368
genetic factors, 357
interaction effects, 3, 340
large family size as indirect cause of delinquency, 371
of childhood disorder, 357
social disadvantage as indirect cause of delinquency, 371
study by effect of intervention, 369
third variable, 370–371
transactional effects, 4, 335
Changes
  one-parent family and attainment, 252–253
  poor housing and attainment, 252–254
  social class, age and attainment, 254
  vulnerability to, 15
Child effects on environment, 366
Child guidance, 319
Child psychiatry services
  availability, 265
  evaluation, 265
Class size, effects, 257–258
Cohorts, successive, 241
Conduct disorder causation
  divorce, 377
  family interaction, 377
  harsh discipline, 378–379
  institutional rearing, 378
  parental criminality, 376
  parental discord, 376–377
  peer influences, 376, 379
  weak family relations, 376, 378
Congenital defects, 337
Continuities
  ability, 249
  (11 to 15 years) adopted and fostered children, 145–146
  andiometric thresholds, 246

asthma and wheezy bronchitis, 245
behaviour disorder, 75
distant vision, 245
environmental vs. organismic, 197–198
family structure, 247
genetic, 137, 152
housing, 248
mechanisms, 196–197
sibling relationships, 23, 27
social, 137
Continuities and discontinuities, 10
deprivation, 234
different mechanisms, 158
National Child Development Study,
244–249
'Critical' period, 385

Delinquency, 338
effect of move to non-delinquent area,
364
Deprivation
move into
cognitive factors, 232–234, 235–236
risk factors, 230–234
social factors, 230–231, 232, 235
Design of studies
arrival of a sibling, 16
becoming deprived, 229
child to parent, 57
Down's syndrome, 208–209
family pathology and child psychiatric
disorder, 93, 96
Kauai Longitudinal Study, 335
longitudinal study of adoption, 138–139,
141
National Child Development Study, 243
parenting of mothers raised 'in care',
159–161
school treatment project, 321–323
seriously maladjusted children, 267–268,
273
sex differences in pre-school behaviour
problems, 75–76
suspended children, 36
1000 Family Study, 224–225
Diagnosis, preschool behaviour disorders,
65, 76
Difficult pupils, reading, 35, 37
Down's syndrome
adaptive behaviour scales, 209, 212–213
birth weight, 211, 212–213
changing attitudes to, 203

cognitive development, 204, 212–214
community adjustment, 203
congenital heart disease, 210, 211
cross-sectional studies, 204–205
developmental milestones, 208–209
emotional development, 214–215
incidence, 203
leukaemia, 210
mortality, 210, 217
muscle tone, 211, 213, 217
parental marriage, 209, 215, 217
parental reaction to, 203, 214
predictive factors, 211–212, 217
predictors of intelligence, 213–214
previous longitudinal studies, 205–208
psychiatric disorder, 214–215

Early experience
effect of, 54, 68
mother
accidents in child, 65–66
child behaviour disturbance, 65
circumstances of being in care, 67
hospital admissions of child, 65–66
recovery from adverse, 68
Educational level of mothers, 336
Educational therapies, 319
Emotional disorders
causation, 380–383
acute stress, 381–382
family communication and dominance, 382–383
ordinal position, 380–381
parental psychiatric disorder, 382
sibling rivalry, 380–381
Environmental aspects, intelligence, 361
Environmental effects, 357
Environmental factors, persistence, 383–
387
Ethnicity of Kauai population, 335
Extreme deprivation, reversibility of
effects, 365

Families, direction of causation of
disorder, 368
Family, disruption of unit, 335
Family size, effect on parent, child
interaction, 375
Family stability and outcome of perinatal
stress, 341
Family supports, 29, 59
grandmother, 69

grandparents of stress-resistant children, 347
lack of, 342
marriage, 180
of mothers, 67
stress-resistant children, 347
Family therapy, 319
Father
absence, 348
and siblings, 22
loss of and deprivation, 231, 232
First born, parental interaction with, 375
Follow up
siblings at 3 years, 27
suspended pupils, 44
Foster parents, characteristics, 141
Foster-reared children
11 years, 142–143
15 years, 144
18 years, 148–150
21–22 years, 150–151
outcome, 152

Genetic transmission
alcoholism, 153, 360
animal studies, 358
criminality, 137, 153, 361
delinquency, 359, 363–364
differentiation from disrupted parenting, 171–174
vs. early experience, 157
fostering and adoption in study of, 360
heritability estimates, 358–359
intelligence, 359, 361
marriage state of, 183
psychiatric disorder, 92, 127
schizophrenia, 360
Great Depression, 223, 236, 387
Group therapy, 319, 321, 322, 323–324, 325, 329–333

Headstart projects, 53
Health, school years, 227–228
Health visitors, 225
High risk boys, in childhood, 344
High risk girls, in adolescence, 344
Hospital admission, psychological effects of, 363
Hospital services for maladjusted children, 265–266, 267, 271, 279–282, 283, 289, 293, 297–298, 303–304

Housing, amount of adversity and educational progress, 252–253

Improved family circumstances, effects of, 364
Improvement rate, 343
Improving intellectual function, interactive vs. passive instruction, 373
Institutional upbringing
children's home characteristics, 161–162
discharge from care, 176, 177–178, 192
effects of, 58, 72, 158, 190, 387
effects of characteristics on child, 365
experiences in childhood, 161–162, 190–192
mitigating effects, 158
of mothers, 159
ordinal position and parenting, 169–171
parenting, 159
parenting following, 162–166
psychosocial outcome, 166
parenting and psychosocial outcome, 167
teenage behaviour and later parenting, 168–169
Intellectual development, effect of change, 383–385
Intervention, suspended pupils, 48

Key predictors of coping problems, 345

Large families, deprivation, 230, 235
Learning disabilities, prognosis for, 342
Length of schooling, effects, 251–252
Longitudinal studies, definition, 139
Longitudinal study, 335
Longitudinal designs
catch-up studies, 8
follow-back studies, 9
importance of, 154
real-time studies, 8
Low birth weight, 61, 337

Marriage, state of, 65
assortive mating, 180–182
characteristics of spouse, 178–180
children raised 'in care', 159
Down's syndrome, 215
effect of spouse deviance, 186–187
influence on parenting, 194
in mothers raised 'in care', 178
planning, 183
psychiatric parents, 96, 105, 117–119

Mental retardation, 337
Maternal depression, 22, 29, 59, 63–64
  preschool behaviour problems, 78, 86, 87
Methodology
  ability and attainment tests, 321, 329
  anxiety scales, 232
  attrition, 42, 148, 270, 336
  composite scores of adversity, 228, 275
  definitions, 9
  in psychotherapy research, 320–321
  longitudinal analysis, 242
  measurement
    clinic records, 16, 161
    direct observation, 16, 28, 57, 161
    interviewing, 225–226
    interview, 16, 28, 36, 57, 76–77,
      95–96, 142, 161
    limitations, 139
  observation techniques, 16, 57
  parent interviews, 321
  school behaviour scales, 37, 109, 321
  screening, 35, 269
    difficult children, 36–37
    mothers at risk, 55
    preschool behaviour problems, 76
  selection bias, 141, 146–147
  sociometry, 37, 321
  statistical, 313–315
  Swedish army measurements, 147–148
  timing of follow ups, 272, 322
Models of behaviour, 379–380
Mothering problems, specific disability vs.
  general social disability, 157, 167
Mothers background vs. current environment, 157
Multidisciplinary approach, 241

National longitudinal studies, 241
Natural experiments
  control in, 6, 141, 146
  converging techniques, 8
  generalization from, 6, 27
  inconclusiveness of, 6
Need for care at age 10, 337–338
Neurological impairment, 337
Neuroticism scales, 323
Newcastle 1000 Family Study, 223–227

Occupational level of fathers, 335
Ordinal position, 359
  first-born children, 362
  psychiatric effects, 362

Paediatric examination in second year, 337
Parent–teacher consultation, 322, 323, 328
Parental age, stress-resistant children,
  345–346
Parenting, early months, 61–62
Parenting problems
  associations with material adversity, 69
  following institutional upbringing,
    162–166
  intergenerational effects, 72
  mothers raised 'in care', mechanisms,
    188–189
  possibilities of intervention, 72–73
Parent-reared children
  11 years, 142–143
  15 years, 144
  18 years, 148–150
  21–22 years, 150–151
  outcome, 153
Personality attributes of resilient girls, 348
Physical handicaps, 337
Physical illness, effects on offspring, 92
Planning in child care, 153
Policy implications
  conduct disorders, 392–394
  emotional disorders, 394
  individual differences, 396
  of environmental effects, 391
  persistence of effects, 394–395
  scholastic achievement, 392
Poverty, 335
Pregnancy
  antenatal visits, 60
  attitude to, 60–61
  in mothers raised 'in care', 177
Preparation, adoption and fostering, 153
Prevalence
  emotional and behavioural disturbance,
    118
  of disorder, Down's syndrome, 214–215
  of maladjustment, 269–270
  of psychiatric disorder, 53
  preschool behaviour disorder, 77–78
Prevention
  of disorder, 29, 53–54
  preschool behaviour disorders, 86–87
Preschool behaviour disorders
  fearfulness, 84, 85–86
  predictors of outcome, 81–82
  restlessness, 82–85, 87
  sex differences, 75, 78–79, 82
Professional support, 216

Protective factors, 5, 335
  employment, 349
  family relationships, 176
  good self image, 193, 196, 346, 349
  harmonious marriage, 192–193
  positive school experiences, 175–176, 195–196
  support (*see also* Family supports), 349
  schooling, 195
  temperament, 122, 346, 349
Psychiatric disorder
  changes in classification over time, 299–300
  children of psychiatric patients, 110, 111–112
  children
    persistence of disorder, 109, 110, 115, 117
  classification and severity of disorder, 285–288
  conduct disorder, 308
  diagnosis
    conduct and neurotic disorders, 269, 287, 292, 297–298
    family background, 292–293
  in schools years, 168–169, 228
  maternal mental health problems, 341
  mother
    deprivation, 232
  parents and children, 91–92, 111, 125
  parents
    child's temperament and disorder, 121–123
    correlates of diagnosis, 100–102
    course of disorders, 103–104, 123–124
    depression in parent and child, 113, 127
    hostility to child, 114, 126–127
    marriage, 96, 105
    patients, 96–107
    parent–child relationships, 98
    parents and children, mechanisms, 92–93, 125–128
    persistence of disorder, 103–104, 114–116
    personality disorder and child disturbance, 102, 111–112
    sex differences in children's disturbance, 120
    spouses, 98, 106–107, 119–120
    type of disorder and child, 111

  personality disorder, differentiation from poor current functioning, 172
  psychotic parents
    offspring of, 336
  specificity across generations, 91, 125–127
Psychoanalysis, 1
Psychological examination in second year, 337
Psychotherapy
  effectiveness, 319
  theories of, 320

Remedial education, need for long-term, 338
Reproductive risk (*see* Prenatal–perinatal complications), 339
Resilient children, 335
Resilient offspring of psychotic parents, 248
Resistence to stress, 335

School
  attendance
    suspended pupils, 37
  characteristics
    effects, 257–258
  differences, 33, 46, 196
  effects on achievement and behaviour, 365–366
    causation, 366
  effects of input differences, 366
  for maladjusted children, 265, 267, 271, 274, 276, 278–284, 287, 289, 293–299, 303, 305
  for mildly educationally subnormal, 265, 267–268, 274, 275, 276, 278–284, 287, 289, 293–299, 303, 306, 307–308
  grouping policies, effects, 256–257
  input differences, 366
  ordinary, maladjusted children in, 265, 267, 271, 274, 276, 278–284, 287–289, 293–299, 303, 304
Selection bias
  National Child Development Study, 244
Self concept, 35, 37, 193, 196
  stress-resistant children, 349
  locus of control, 343
Self-righting tendencies, 351
Sense of coherence, 348

'Sensitive' periods, 385
'Sensitization' effects, 386
Separations, as sensitizing effect, 386
Seriously maladjusted children
  conduct disorders management, 308
  differing outcomes, 303–305
  educationally subnormal management, 307
  effectiveness of treatment, 301–303
  family factors, 274–278
  follow-up improvement, 294–297
  follow-up outcome, 292–294
  improvement by diagnosis, 297–298
  initial assessment, 284–292
  intellectual and educational, 281, 288–292, 307
  neurotic disorders management, 309
  physical and neurological, 288–289
  social class and employment, 274
  units and treatment received, 278–284
Sex differences, 335
  children of psychiatric patients, 120
  outcome of preschool behaviour disorders, 75, 78–79, 82
  sibling reaction, 20
Siblings
  age gap, 20, 345, 349
  arrival of younger, 362
  changes in mother–child interaction, 19, 28
  home and hospital delivery, 21
  individual differences in reactions to, 20
  managing reactions to, 25–26, 28
  persistence of problems, 23–25
  preparation for, 22
  reactions to birth of, 17
  relationship with father, 22
  sex differences, 20
  stress-resistant children, 347
  temperament, 21, 23–24, 29
Similarities in siblings, significance, 359
Single parents, parenting capacity, 56
'Sleeper' effects, 237
Smoking
  pregnancy, 60
    association with height, 250–251
    association with reading and maths scores, 250–251
    outcome in child, 250–251
Social and behavioural development
  effect of change, 385–386

Social class, changes in attainment with age, 255–256
Social class change
  educational attainment, 259
Social orientation
  of stress-resistant children, 247
Social support, informal, 352
Socioeconomic Status (SES) and outcome
  of perinatal stress, 339–340
'Steeling' effects, 238, 386
Stress
  perinatal, 335
  psychosocial, 335
Stress-resistant children
  mother's employment, 347
Stress-resistant children and youth
  characteristics of, 345
Success in intervention, variables related to, 353–354
Suspended pupils
  aggressive behaviour, 38–40
  disruptive behaviour, 40
  parental viewpoint, 43
  self reports, 35, 37, 43
  setting of misbehaviour, 41
  social relationships, 35, 37
Suspension, effects of, 33–34

Task-centred casework, 328
Teenage mothers, 336
Teenage pregnancy, 55-56
Teacher–pupil ratio, effects, 257
Temperament
  disorder in offspring of psychiatric patients, 121–123
  infancy, 342
  preschool behaviour disorders, 86
  reactions of siblings, 21, 23–24, 29
Theoretical perspectives, 2
Theories
  developmental, 2
  interactional, 3
  multiple causation, 3
  'social mold', 2
Theory
  changes in, 2
Time-periods for intervention, 353
Treatment
  approaches, 319
  effectiveness with different problems, 326

effects of on delinquency, 364–365
evaluation, 319–320
non-specific effects, 329
pre-school behaviour disorders, 87
school base, 332

Unemployment, deprivation, 235
Uses of longitudinal studies, 10

Vulnerability, 335